T0226997

INTERVENTIONAL CARDIOLOGY CLINICS

www.interventional.theclinics.com

Editor-in-Chief

MARVIN H. ENG

Transcatheter Aortic Valve Replacement

October 2021 • Volume 10 • Number 4

Editor

MARVIN H. ENG

ELSEVIER

1600 John F. Kennedy Boulevard ● Suite 1800 ● Philadelphia, Pennsylvania, 19103-2899

http://www.theclinics.com

INTERVENTIONAL CARDIOLOGY CLINICS Volume 10, Number 4
October 2021 ISSN 2211-7458, ISBN-13: 978-0-323-84866-4

Editor: Joanna Collett
Developmental Editor: Arlene B. Campos

© 2021 Elsevier Inc. All rights reserved.

This periodical and the individual contributions contained in it are protected under copyright by Elsevier, and the following terms and conditions apply to their use:

Photocopying
Single photocopies of single articles may be made for personal use as allowed by national copyright laws. Permission of the Publisher and payment of a fee is required for all other photocopying, including multiple or systematic copying, copying for advertising or promotional purposes, resale, and all forms of document delivery. Special rates are available for educational institutions that wish to make photocopies for non-profit educational classroom use. For information on how to seek permission visit www.elsevier.com/permissions or call: (+44) 1865 843830 (UK)/(+1) 215 239 3804 (USA).

Derivative Works
Subscribers may reproduce tables of contents or prepare lists of articles including abstracts for internal circulation within their institutions. Permission of the Publisher is required for resale or distribution outside the institution. Permission of the Publisher is required for all other derivative works, including compilations and translations (please consult www.elsevier.com/permissions).

Electronic Storage or Usage
Permission of the Publisher is required to store or use electronically any material contained in this periodical, including any article or part of an article (please consult www.elsevier.com/permissions). Except as outlined above, no part of this publication may be reproduced, stored in a retrieval system or transmitted in any form or by any means, electronic, mechanical, photocopying, recording or otherwise, without prior written permission of the Publisher.

Notice
No responsibility is assumed by the Publisher for any injury and/or damage to persons or property as a matter of products liability, negligence or otherwise, or from any use or operation of any methods, products, instructions or ideas contained in the material herein. Because of rapid advances in the medical sciences, in particular, independent verification of diagnoses and drug dosages should be made.

Although all advertising material is expected to conform to ethical (medical) standards, inclusion in this publication does not constitute a guarantee or endorsement of the quality or value of such product or of the claims made of it by its manufacturer.

Interventional Cardiology Clinics (ISSN 2211-7458) is published quarterly by Elsevier Inc., 360 Park Avenue South, New York, NY 10010-1710. Months of issue are January, April, July, and October. Subscription prices are USD 209 per year for US individuals, USD 622 for US institutions, USD 100 per year for US students, USD 209 per year for Canadian individuals, USD 638 for Canadian institutions, USD 100 per year for Canadian students, USD 296 per year for international individuals, USD 638 for international institutions, and USD 150 per year for international students. To receive student/resident rate, orders must be accompanied by name of affiliated institution, date of term, and the *signature* of program/residency coordinator on institution letterhead. Orders will be billed at individual rate until proof of status is received. Foreign air speed delivery is included in all *Clinics* subscription prices. All prices are subject to change without notice. **POSTMASTER:** Send address changes to *Interventional Cardiology Clinics*, Elsevier Health Sciences Division, Subscription Customer Service, 3251 Riverport Lane, Maryland Heights, MO 63043. **Customer Service: Telephone: 1-800-654-2452** (U.S. and Canada); **1-314-447-8871** (outside U.S. and Canada). **Fax: 1-314-447-8029. E-mail: journalscustomerservice-usa@elsevier.com (for print support); journalsonlinesupport-usa@elsevier.com (for online support).**

Reprints. For copies of 100 or more of articles in this publication, please contact the Commercial Reprints Department, Elsevier Inc., 360 Park Avenue South, New York, NY 10010-1710. Tel.: 212-633-3874; Fax: 212-633-3820; E-mail: reprints@elsevier.com.

CONTRIBUTORS

EDITOR-IN-CHIEF

MARVIN H. ENG, MD
Structural Heart Program Medical Director,
Structural Heart Disease Fellowship Director,
Director of Cardiovascular Quality, Banner
University Medical Center, Phoenix, Arizona,
USA

AUTHORS

MOHAMMAD ALKHALIL, MD, DPhil
Department of Cardiothoracic Services,
Freeman Hospital, Vascular Biology,
Newcastle University, Newcastle-upon-Tyne,
United Kingdom

DMITRIOS APOSTOLOU, MD
Division of Cardiothoracic Surgery,
Department of Surgery, Henry Ford Health
System, Detroit, Michigan, USA

COLIN M. BARKER, MD, FACC, FSCAI
Vanderbilt University Medical Center,
Vanderbilt Heart and Vascular Institute,
Nashville, Tennessee, USA

RORY S. BRICKER, MD
Department of Medicine, Division of
Cardiology, University of Colorado School of
Medicine, Aurora, Colorado, USA

BRIAN C. CASE, MD
Section of Interventional Cardiology, MedStar
Washington Hospital Center, Washington,
DC, USA

JOSEPH C. CLEVELAND Jr, MD
Department of Surgery, Division of
Cardiothoracic Surgery, University of
Colorado School of Medicine, Aurora,
Colorado, USA

CHERIE DAHM, MD
Vanderbilt University Medical Center,
Vanderbilt Heart and Vascular Institute,
Nashville, Tennessee, USA

**CHANDAN M. DEVIREDDY, MD, MBA,
FACC, FSCAI**
Division of Cardiology, Emory University
School of Medicine, Associate Professor of
Medicine, Emory University Hospital Midtown,
Atlanta, Georgia, USA

MARVIN H. ENG, MD
Structural Heart Program Medical Director,
Structural Heart Disease Fellowship Director,
Director of Cardiovascular Quality, Banner
University Medical Center, Phoenix, Arizona,
USA

JASON R. FOERST, MD
Structural and Interventional Cardiology,
Virginia Tech Carilion School of Medicine,
Carilion Clinic, Roanoke, Virginia, USA

TIBERIO M. FRISOLI, MD
Senior Staff Physician, Interventional Structural
Cardiology, Center for Structural Heart Disease,
Heart and Vascular Institute, Henry Ford
Hospital, Detroit, Michigan, USA; Medical
Director of Structural Heart Disease, Henry Ford
Allegiance Hospital, Jackson, Michigan, USA

**ANDREW M. GOLDSWEIG, MD, MS,
FACC, FSCAI, FSVM, RPVI**
Assistant Professor, Interventional Cardiology,
Associate Cath Lab Director for Structural
Heart Disease, Division of Cardiovascular
Medicine, University of Nebraska Medical
Center, Omaha, Nebraska, USA

PEDRO ENGEL GONZALEZ, MD
Division of Cardiology, Department of Internal
Medicine, The University of Texas Southwestern
Medical Center, Dallas, Texas, USA

PAUL MICHAEL GROSSMAN, MD
Professor, Department of Internal Medicine,
Division of Cardiovascular Medicine,
University of Michigan, Frankel Cardiovascular
Center, Ann Arbor, Michigan, USA

ERINN HUGHES, MD
Fellow, Interventional Cardiology,
Department of Internal Medicine, Division of
Cardiovascular Medicine, University of
Michigan, Frankel Cardiovascular Center, Ann
Arbor, Michigan, USA

ABEL IGNATIUS, MD
Center for Structural Heart Disease, Henry
Ford Hospital, Detroit, Michigan, USA

AHMAD JABRI, MD
Case Western Reserve University/MetroHealth
Medical Center, Cleveland, Ohio, USA

HASAN JILAIHAWI, MD
Heart Valve Center, Associate Professor of
Medicine and Cardiothoracic Surgery, NYU
Langone Health, New York, New York, USA

ANKUR KALRA, MD
Department of Cardiovascular Medicine,
Heart, Vascular, and Thoracic Institute,
Cleveland Clinic, Cleveland, Ohio, USA;
Section of Cardiovascular Research, Heart,
Vascular, and Thoracic Department,
Cleveland Clinic Akron General, Medical
Director of Clinical Research for Regional
Cardiovascular Medicine, Department of
Cardiovascular Medicine, Heart, Vascular,
and Thoracic Institute, Cleveland Clinic,
Akron, Ohio, USA

GUSON KANG, MD
Stanford University Medical Center, Stanford,
California, USA

JAFFAR M. KHAN, BM BCh, PhD
Cardiovascular Branch, Division of Intramural
Research, National Heart, Lung and Blood
Institute, National Institutes of Health,
Bethesda, Maryland, USA

DHARAM J. KUMBHANI, MD, SM
Division of Cardiology, Department of Internal
Medicine, The University of Texas Southwestern
Medical Center, Dallas, Texas, USA

JOHN C. LISKO III, MD, MPH
Division of Cardiology, Emory University
School of Medicine, Atlanta, Georgia, USA

SHAHBAZ ALI MALIK, MD
Assistant Professor, Interventional Cardiology,
Division of Cardiovascular Medicine,

University of Nebraska Medical Center,
Omaha, Nebraska, USA

GIORGIO A. MEDRANDA, MD
Section of Interventional Cardiology, MedStar
Washington Hospital Center, Washington,
DC, USA

JOHN C. MESSENGER, MD
Department of Medicine, Division of
Cardiology, University of Colorado School of
Medicine, Aurora, Colorado, USA

MAKOTO NAKASHIMA, MD
Heart Valve Center, NYU Langone Health,
New York, New York, USA

WILLIAM W. O'NEILL, MD
Division of Cardiology, Center for Structural
Heart Disease, Henry Ford Health System,
Detroit, Michigan, USA

RISHI PURI, MBBS, PhD
Department of Cardiovascular Medicine,
Heart, Vascular, and Thoracic Institute,
Cleveland Clinic, Cleveland, Ohio, USA

MOHAMMED QINTAR, MD, MSc
Division of Cardiology, Sparrow Hospital,
Lansing, Michigan, USA

TOBY ROGERS, MD, PhD
Section of Interventional Cardiology, MedStar
Washington Hospital Center, Washington,
DC, USA; Cardiovascular Branch, Division of
Intramural Research, National Heart, Lung and
Blood Institute, National Institutes of Health,
Bethesda, Maryland, USA

SALEM A. SALEM, MD
Structural and Interventional Cardiology,
Virginia Tech Carilion School of Medicine,
Carilion Clinic, Roanoke, Virginia, USA

PRATIK SANDESARA, MD
Division of Cardiology, Emory University
School of Medicine, Atlanta, Georgia, USA

NIKOLOZ SHEKILADZE, MD
Division of Cardiology, Emory University
School of Medicine, Atlanta, Georgia, USA

ALAN YEUNG, MD
Stanford University Medical Center, Stanford,
California, USA

CONTENTS

The landmark results of the low surgical risk pivotal transcatheter aortic valve replacement (TAVR) trials fueled speculation that the role of surgical aortic valve replacement (SAVR) would be limited in the future. Instead, the field has pivoted away from reductive surgical risk stratification toward understanding the complex interplay of anatomy, timing, and surgical risk to optimize the lifetime management of aortic stenosis. In this review, we systematically explore the subtleties that influence the choice between TAVR and surgery in the low-risk TAVR era.

Most transcatheter aortic valve replacement procedures are currently performed using a percutaneous transfemoral arterial retrograde approach. Complication rates can be minimized with thorough preprocedure planning, pristine technique, and increased team experience. Vascular complications will continue to happen and require early recognition and treatment.

The article serves to outline the beginnings of transcatheter aortic valve replacement and the pivotal trials that have resulted in this technology's being adopted in a widespread manner. Also detailed in the article are the differences between the various iterations of the balloon-expandable transcatheter heart valve platforms, offering insight into scenarios when a balloon-expandable or a self-expanding prosthesis might be considered based on patient characteristics.

 Video content accompanies this article at http://www.interventional.theclinics.com.

The self-expanding transcatheter heart valve (Medtronic Cardiovascular Corevalve and Evolut) is a supra-annular, trileafet porcine pericardial valves on a diamond lattice nickel-titanium alloy frame. The TAVR device has undergone significant improvements in design and procedural techniques to further increase safety, efficacy, and durability since they it was first released. Unique design characteristics, as well as patient and procedural factors, favor self-expanding over balloon-expandable prostheses in certain situations. The self-expanding transcatheter heart valve has proven to be an excellent option for severe aortic stenosis patients with any level of surgical risk and preliminary data suggest a comparable durability to surgical tissue valves.

Conduction disturbances (CDs) after transcatheter artic replacement remain a clinical concern and relatively common complication. A recent meta-analysis showed both new-onset persistent left bundle branch block and new permanent pacemaker implantation were related to all-cause death with risk ratio 1.32 (95% confidence interval [CI] 1.17 to 1.49; P<.001) and 1.17 (95% CI 1.11–1.25; P<.001) at 1 year, respectively. Preprocedural computed tomography imaging can highlight potential risk factors for CDs, such as membranous septum length, device landing zone calcium, and the annulus size/degree of device oversizing.

Mechanical complications after transcatheter aortic valve replacement are fortunately rare with the current generation of devices. Unfortunately, life-threatening complications will occur and it is the responsibility of operators to be familiar with strategies to prevent and manage these challenging scenarios. Because these cases will not occur often, it is important for us to highlight and talk about those that do occur, to learn best practices in how to manage and prevent them going forward. We can learn much from each other's good crash landings.

Acute coronary obstruction is a rare but devastating complication of transcatheter aortic valve replacement. Key factors identifying patients at risk include aortic root anatomy, type of aortic valve (e.g. tricuspid, bicuspid, surgical bioprosthesis), and type of transcatheter heart valve implanted. Techniques to prevent coronary obstruction include pre-emptive intentional leaflet laceration (BASILICA) or snorkel stenting. If acute coronary obstruction does occur, bailout stenting can be challenging and conversion to emergent open heart surgery may be required, both of which are associated with high morbidity and mortality.

Approximately 51,000 to 65,000 surgical aortic valve replacement (SAVR) cases are performed in the United States anually. Bioprosthetic degeneration commonly occurs within 10 to 15 years, and nearly 800 redo SAVR cases occur each year. Valve-in-valve transcatheter aortic valve replacement (ViV TAVR) has emerged as a safe and effective alternative, as the Food and Drug Administration approved ViV TAVR with self-expanding transcatheter heart valve in 2015 and balloon-expandable valve in 2017 for failed surgical valves cases at high risk of reoperation. We review ViV TAVR, with specific attention to procedural planning, technical challenges, associated complications, and long-term follow-up.

Transfemoral is the most widely used access to perform transcatheter aortic valve replacement (TAVR). However, alternative access is needed in up to 21% of patients with TAVR because of a myriad of factors. The authors provide a comprehensive review on alternative access for TAVR, discussing the relevant data and providing the pros and cons of each access route.

Transcatheter aortic valve replacement (TAVR) has become the mainstay of treatment for severe symptomatic aortic stenosis. Although many TAVR complication rates including mortality and aortic regurgitation have decreased, stroke rates have remained stable for years. TAVR-related strokes are devastating to patients and their families, and very costly for health care systems. The predictors of stroke in TAVR are not yet well defined, although older age, female gender, carotid and peripheral arterial disease, bicuspid aortic valve anatomy, and atrial fibrillation are emerging as risk factors across studies.

All bioprosthetic valves, both surgical and transcatheter, have a finite life-span before their leaflets inevitably degenerate, leading to stenosis or regurgitation. As younger, low-risk patients receive a transcatheter aortic valve, it is expected that they will most likely outlive their bioprosthetic valve. The heterogeneity of studies regarding surgical valve durability makes the interpretation of the data challenging. Leaflet thickening is seen in transcatheter heart valves but currently there is no evidence that it leads to premature valve deterioration or clinical events. Standardized definitions of structural valve deterioration should allow for comparisons between future clinical trials to assess the durability of different transcatheter heart valves.

The paucity of data regarding the use of transcatheter aortic valve replacement (TAVR) in bicuspid aortic valve (BAV) anatomy due to exclusion from pivotal studies and lack of studies assessing the long-term outcomes and valve performance continue to present a significant challenge as we expand TAVR to patients with BAV anatomy. This article discusses the important anatomic and clinical considerations in the selection and management of patients with BAV with TAVR and reviews the emerging evidence that increasingly suggests this procedure is safe, device success is excellent, and procedural outcomes are improving.

> Transcatheter aortic valve replacement (TAVR) is a standard treatment option for patients with severe aortic stenosis. Management of concomitant coronary artery disease (CAD) in these patients remains controversial with no randomized clinical trials to guide decision making in this cohort. The role of CAD in TAVR has been difficult to evaluate given the current heterogeneity in defining CAD, and the used methods to assess CAD. Subsequently, the role of coronary revascularization remains individualized and assessed on a case-by-case basis by the heart team. In this article, the authors discuss the rationale and prognostic role of CAD in patients undergoing TAVR.

> Transcatheter aortic valve replacement (TAVR) is now the dominant form of aortic valve replacement in the United States. Continued innovation has allowed the technique to be safe and democratized. New advances will increase the number of patients eligible to receive this therapy while increasing safety and efficiency. Herein, the authors review new TAVR technologies, approaches to valve deployment, and dedicated devices for cerebral embolic protection and vascular closure.

TRANSCATHETER AORTIC VALVE REPLACEMENT

RELATED SERIES

Cardiology Clinics
https://www.cardiology.theclinics.com/
Heart Failure Clinics
https://www.heartfailure.theclinics.com/
Cardiac Electrophysiology Clinics
https://www.cardiacep.theclinics.com/

THE CLINICS ARE NOW AVAILABLE ONLINE!

Access your subscription at:
www.theclinics.com

PREFACE

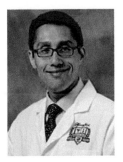

Marvin H. Eng, MD
Editor

We are pleased to introduce this issue of *Interventional Cardiology Clinics*, an in-depth look at contemporary transcatheter aortic valve replacement (TAVR). TAVR has catapulted from a procedure reserved for inoperable/high-risk patients to a standard-of-care procedure extending to low-risk patients. The catalyst to the structural heart revolution, TAVR has eclipsed surgical valve replacement in the United States in terms of volumes and is now a fixture in aortic valve therapy.

This issue reinforces the fundamentals and provides a blueprint for the future of the field. Essentials such as vascular access and alternatives to transfemoral access are necessary for mastery of TAVR. At the time of this publication, two main commercial transcatheter heart valves dominate the US market with some percutaneous valves under clinical development. We provide an in-depth look at the history of their development and detail the analysis of their clinical results. While TAVR for native valve replacement consists of the majority of cases, degenerated surgical bioprosthetic valves require special focus to avoid threats of coronary obstruction and significantly elevated postprocedure gradients. While complications are relatively rare, prevention of mechanical, neurologic, and conduction complications will be essential, especially when extending TAVR to all risk classes. Long-term issues such as durability, leaflet thickening, coronary reaccess and anatomic eligibility for repeat TAVR (ie, TAV-in-TAV) deserve special attention given the widespread implementation of TAVR.

This issue of *Interventional Cardiology Clinics* is a compendium of reviews written by leaders in interventional cardiology. The readership should find this issue to be a comprehensive guide to performing TAVR that provides enhanced learning in all relevant topics.

Marvin H. Eng, MD
Banner University Medical Center
1111 East McDowell Road
Phoenix, AZ 85006, USA

E-mail address:
engm@email.arizona.edu

Intervent Cardiol Clin 10 (2021) xi
https://doi.org/10.1016/j.iccl.2021.07.002
2211-7458/21/© 2021 Published by Elsevier Inc.

Choosing Between Transcatheter Aortic Valve Replacement and Surgery in the Low-Risk Transcatheter Aortic Valve Replacement Era

Guson Kang, MD*, Alan Yeung, MD

KEYWORDS

- TAVR • TAVI • SAVR • Low risk • Lifetime

KEY POINTS

- Transcatheter aortic valve replacement (TAVR) is approved for use across all surgical-risk patients, yet our understanding of which patients benefit most from either modality is incomplete.
- With respect to anatomy, the presence of a heavily calcified bicuspid valve should favor surgery, though emerging data suggest TAVR is a safe alternative in select patients.
- TAVR is associated with lower gradients and less prosthesis-patient mismatch than surgery, suggesting that it should be favored in patients with smaller annular dimensions, though randomized data are lacking.
- Durability remains a key unanswered question, though TAVR prostheses have been shown to be of comparable durability after shorter (5-6 year) follow up.
- Finally, future reoperation or re-intervention strategies should be formulated in younger patients when deciding the index procedure, with close attention given to the feasibility of coronary re-access.

INTRODUCTION

Each pivotal trial since the first-in-man transcatheter aortic valve replacement (TAVR) in 2002 has expanded its use in severe aortic stenosis (AS) by incrementally lower surgical risk, starting with prohibitive/high risk (**Fig. 1**). In 2019, TAVR reached the low-risk milestone with the publication of PARTNER 3 (STS <4%)[1] and Evolut Low Risk (STS <%),[2] which compared conventional open surgery with TAVR in lower surgical risk patients. PARTNER 3 demonstrated TAVR with the Edwards SAPIEN 3 system resulted in a lower rate of death, stroke, or rehospitalization at 1 year compared with surgery; Evolut Low Risk showed TAVR with the Medtronic Evolut system was noninferior to surgery with respect to death and stroke at 2 years. Both platforms were approved just months later in the United States and Europe, opening access to TAVR to the low-risk population.

Outcomes have improved in step. In the 2020 STS-ACC TVT registry update, femoral access has increased to 95.3% and hospital stays have decreased to 2 days.[3] Since 2011, 30-day mortality has decreased from 7.2% to 2.5%, stroke has decreased from 2.75% to 2.3%, and 8 in 10 patients report acceptable outcomes at 1 year. Although overall pacemaker need remains unchanged at 10.8%, refinements in deployment

Stanford University Medical Center, 300 Pasteur Drive, Stanford, CA 94305, USA
* Corresponding author. 3801 Miranda Avenue (111C), Palo Alto, CA 94304.
E-mail address: guson@stanford.edu

Intervent Cardiol Clin 10 (2021) 413–422
https://doi.org/10.1016/j.iccl.2021.05.001
2211-7458/21/Published by Elsevier Inc.

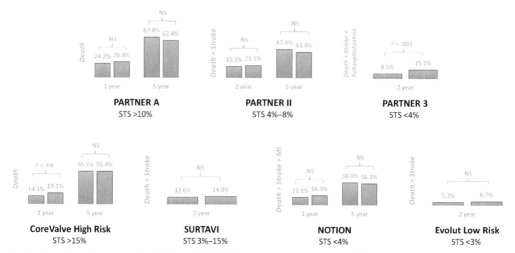

Fig. 1. Pivotal trials comparing TAVR with SAVR. Results from longer-term follow up included where available.

technique with balloon-expandable valves (BEVs; eg, "line of lucency") have decreased pacemaker need to 5% in more recent reports, approximating surgical rates.[4,5]

With TAVR invading the last bastion of surgical AVR (SAVR), how has that affected surgical volumes? Although TAVR has been outpacing SAVR in the United States for isolated AS since 2016 after its approval in intermediate risk,[6,7] total SAVR volumes had held steady at ~65,000/year—until the approval of low-risk TAVR. 2019 was the first year to see (1) a significant decline in total SAVR (n = 57,626) volumes and (2) TAVR outpace total SAVR (n = 72,991).[3]

What then is the role of surgery in the TAVR era? At the end of 2020, the ACC/AHA guidelines were updated to clarify the roles of the respective modalities, moving away from the emphasis on surgical risk, instead focusing on age and the shared decision-making process (Fig. 2). SAVR is now preferred in patients aged less than 65 years, or where the transcatheter evidence base is wanting: asymptomatic very severe with $V_{max} \geq 5$ m/s, abnormal ETT, and so forth.[8,9] The new guidelines otherwise now give a class 1 preference to TAVR in the high/prohibitive risk groups, the elderly (age > 80 years), or patients with a life expectancy <10 years, assuming no anatomic contraindications to TAVR.

But departing from the easily understood framework of surgical risk has anything but clarified the picture, and the bygone times of (ostensibly) simpler decisions have been supplanted with decision-making trees marked by nuances and knowledge gaps. Indeed, deciding between

TAVR and surgery has never been as complex as in the low-risk TAVR era.

ANATOMIC CONSIDERATIONS
Bicuspid Aortic Valves

Despite being the most common congenital heart defect,[10] bicuspid aortic valves (BAVs) were excluded from all pivotal TAVR trials out of concern for potential suboptimal outcomes.[11] With their earlier age at presentation and inherently lower surgical risk, these patients had until recently been largely left to the domain of the surgeon.

The "ellipsoid annulus" in bicuspids was theorized to result in asymmetric expansion and premature valve failure based on a small French series in 2008, where investigators evaluated the deployment of self-expanding nitinol stent frames into bicuspid and tricuspid aortic valve patients intraoperatively, just before aortic valve replacement. Noncircular deployment occurred in 85% of bicuspids, but only 32% of tricuspids, leading to the recommendation that TAVR not be pursued for bicuspids until the long-term results for high-risk tricuspid patients were known.[12]

We understand now that the mechanism of this asymmetric expansion cannot have been related to annular ellipticity. A study of 400 patients (half with BAV) revealed that the bicuspid annulus was *less* ellipsoid than their tricuspid counterparts. Rather, the valves expanded asymmetrically at the level of the leaflets, which are themselves more prone to asymmetric, heavy calcification. The authors also found that bicuspids had larger roots, sinuses, and annuli,

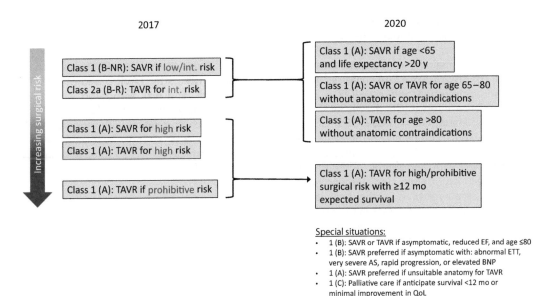

Fig. 2. ACC/AHA treatment of aortic stenosis guidelines before and after low-risk TAVR approval.

although 90% were still eligible for commercially available valves.[13]

The early TAVR-in-BAV cases illustrated that this was not necessarily the case. In a Canadian series of 11 patients, Wijesinghe and colleagues[14] noted symmetric deployments of a BEV in all patients, most of whom had Sievers type 0 valves. Himbert and colleagues[15] found mostly elliptical deployments using self-expanding valves (SEVs) in predominantly Sievers type 1 patients. Hayashida and colleagues reported predominantly ellipsoid deployments after both BEV and SEV in a predominantly Sievers type 1 cohort, although with greater ellipticity after SEV. Although not definitive, these early studies hinted that perhaps SEVs and BAVs with calcified raphes are more prone to asymmetrical expansion.[16]

The larger, modern registries have revealed other risks. The Bicuspid AS TAVR registry reported more frequent aortic root injury (4.5% vs 0%) after early-generation BEVs compared with propensity-matched tricuspid counterparts; early-generation SEVs saw more moderate-to-severe paravalvular leak (19.4% vs 10.5%) in bicuspid anatomy.[17,18] Newer-generation devices have since "closed the gap" with lower rates of aortic injury and significant paravalvular leak, although how much of this can be attributed to the device itself (vs evolving patient selection or valve sizing technique) remains unclear.

TAVR in bicuspid anatomy may also be associated with more stroke. The heavy calcium burden of bicuspid valves requires many operators to routinely predilate the valve to facilitate both crossing and valve expansion; postdilation is also more frequent in this setting. Each additional manipulation of the valve likely poses more risk: degenerated aortic valves demonstrate layered atheroma, thrombus, and calcium, and even minimal instrumentation (such as crossing the valve) has been shown to elevate stroke risk.[19,20] A large, propensity-matched analysis of the STS/TVT registry suggested that while 30-day and 1-year mortality were no different between tricuspid and bicuspid anatomies, the 30-day stroke rate was higher in the bicuspid group, theorizing that either the higher calcium burden or the more frequent use of predilation were responsible.[21,22]

Taken together, the data suggest that TAVR with a newer generation transcatheter valve in select BAV patients may yield short-term results comparable to those of tricuspid patients, with the caveat that (1) periprocedural stroke rates may be slightly higher and (2) no long-term valve durability data exist. Heavily calcified valves should be avoided because of the higher risk of asymmetrical expansion, paravalvular leak, and aortic/annular injury.

Aortopathy

Aortopathy, independent of "bicuspidness," must also be considered. In the largest analysis of its kind to-date, Kassis and colleagues[23] showed that 1% of 171,011 patients undergoing TAVR had concomitant thoracic aortic aneurysms

(TAAs) from the Nationwide Readmissions Database inpatient sample. Although the rate of aortopathy was higher among bicuspids (9.3% vs 0.9%), the vast majority of patients were still tricuspid. The presence of a TAA conferred higher rates of aortic dissection (odds ratio [OR] = 2.117, 95% confidence interval [CI]: 1.304–3.435) and cardiac tamponade (OR = 1.682, 95% CI: 1.1–2.572) after TAVR. Fortunately, the absolute rates of aortic dissection (1%) and tamponade (1.4%) were low even with aortopathy. Although the study lacked key details (eg, ascending vs descending aneurysms), it is the only larger-scale glimpse of TAVR outcomes in the presence of TAA. Although TAVR is feasible and potentially beneficial in aneurysmal patients with higher surgical risk, surgery is favored in their lower risk counterparts.

Porcelain aorta is a well-recognized risk factor for atheroembolism after cardiac surgery.[24–26] Although uncommon in the low surgical risk population, porcelain aorta is not explicitly captured by the most used surgical risk scores (STS, Euroscore II, etc.) outside of being a form of noncoronary arterial disease, despite being an important consideration for the AS population. In some series, up to 7.5% of patients undergoing evaluation for AVR are diagnosed with porcelain aorta,[27] and more than 40% of patients deemed inoperable were turned down because of porcelain aorta, making it the most common reason for technical inoperability.[28] Although TAVR has become the de facto option in this population, for obvious reasons outcomes after TAVR in porcelain aorta will never be compared to surgery in a randomized fashion.

Prosthesis-Patient Mismatch

The concept that a surgical aortic valve prosthesis can be too small for a given patient has been recognized since the 1970s.[29] Although definitions of prosthesis-patient mismatch (PPM) have evolved across the years, the current consensus is that PPM is present with an effective orifice area (EOA) indexed to body surface area (BSA) below 0.85 cm^2/m^2, and is severe below 0.65 cm^2/m^2.[9] Although controversial, PPM has been generally associated with adverse short-term outcomes and reduced LV mass regression.[30–35] Its effect on long-term survival remains unclear.

PPM occurs more frequently in surgical bioprostheses than in mechanical valves,[36] and development has focused on reducing the effect of supporting stents and the sewing ring on EOA. Supra-annular implantations, stentless implantations, leaflets mounted external to the stent, and sutureless valves were all developed with this in mind.[37]

On the transcatheter side, Herrmann and colleagues[38] found that severe PPM was also not infrequent (12%) after TAVR based off STS/TVT registry data, and was associated with higher 1 year mortality and heart failure rates. They found no such correlation with moderate PPM. Severe PPM was strongly associated with a labeled prosthesis sizes ≤23 mm, valve-in-valve procedures, female gender, and larger patient habitus (BSA).

PPM seems to affect TAVR less often than surgery. In the original PARTNER trial, Pibarot and colleagues[39] found that PPM was both more frequent and severe after surgery compared with TAVR, and found worsened survival and less LV mass regression in patients with surgical PPM at 2 years. Similarly, severe PPM was more common after SAVR than TAVR in PARTNER 2.[40] In the low-risk PARTNER 3 population, rates of severe PPM trended higher after SAVR (6.3% vs 4.6%; $P = .30$), although was not statistically significant.[41]

The advantage of TAVR over SAVR with respect to PPM may be even more pronounced with supra-annular designs. The original Core-Valve US High-Risk Pivotal Trial demonstrated significantly less frequent severe PPM after TAVR than SAVR (6.2% vs 25.7%; $P<.0001$). Severe PPM conferred a greater risk of death and acute kidney injury.[42] The intermediate-risk SUR-TAVI trial demonstrated the same.[43] In the Evolut Low-Risk Trial, severe PPM was less frequent in both groups, but still heavily favored TAVR (1.8% vs 8.2%).[2]

Overall, PPM occurs less frequently after TAVR than SAVR, in both BEVs and SEVs. In a meta-analysis of 30 studies, Liao and colleagues[44] reported that TAVR-related severe PPM was associated with an odds ratio of 0.39 (95% CI 0.33–0.48) compared to surgery. Furthermore, they found that self-expanding supra-annular valves were less often associated with PPM than BEVs (32% vs 40%, $P<.0001$). The upcoming SMART ("SMall Annuli Randomized to Evolut or SAPIEN") trial will be the first randomized control trial to address this question by comparing the Evolut and SAPIEN systems head-to-head in patients with small annuli.

Regardless of the approach, care should be taken to recognize and avoid potential PPM.

LONG-TERM MANAGEMENT CONSIDERATIONS

In younger patients, careful consideration must be given to the anticipated lifetime management of their disease. Factors that influence decision-making in this cohort include prosthesis durability, likelihood of failure, feasibility of reintervention after failure or malfunction, future coronary accessibility, and the long-term sequelae of conduction disease.

Durability

Overall, bioprosthetic valve implantations have overtaken mechanical ones across all age groups, constituting the majority (63.6%) of surgical valves implanted in the United States between 2007 and 2011.[45] Although this has in part been driven by the perception of improved durability of newer generation bioprostheses,[46] mechanical valves are still clearly more durable, and present an especially attractive option in younger patients because of the inverse relationship between age at implantation and bioprosthetic durability.[47]

However, their added durability may not translate to better long-term mortality. The existing randomized control trial data were generated in the 1970s and 1980s and are largely obsolete, and the contemporary observational data comparing mechanical and bioprosthetic valves are mixed. A meta-analysis of 32 studies suggested that unadjusted mortality was overall higher with bioprostheses (3.99% vs 6.33% per patient-year), but was equivalent after adjusting for risk.[48] A newer, larger retrospective analysis of 25,445 surgical valve replacements in California found slightly higher mortality in patients younger than 55 years who received bioprostheses compared with mechanical valves at 15 years (30.6% vs 26.4%; $P = .03$), although this did not hold true over age 55 years.[49]

What about TAVR prostheses in the low-risk population? The low-risk pivotal trial data are unfortunately too new to lend insight into their durability in this population. Although 10-year follow-up is planned, the data will not likely be available until 2028. In the only low-risk trial with longer-term follow-up, Søndergaard and colleagues[50] found similar rates of bioprosthetic valve failure between SAVR and TAVR at 6 years in the NOTION trial (n = 274 total).

At the very least, the intermediate and high-risk data seem to suggest that durability is comparable to surgical valves. Blackman and colleagues[51] found very little severe valve degeneration (<1%) at 5 to 10 years in a mix of balloon and self-expanding TAVR prostheses, albeit in an older population, with an average age of 79.3 years. Both the PARTNER and PARTNER 2 echocardiographic data demonstrated similar hemodynamic profiles between SAVR/

TAVR at 5 years, although aortic reintervention was more common after TAVR in PARTNER 2 (3.2% vs 0.8%).[52,53]

The relevance of these durability data may only be limited to younger, low-risk patients. Tam and colleagues published a model examining the PARTNER 3 data and found that TAVR durability would have to be 70% shorter than surgical valves to yield an equivalent life expectancy, suggesting that durability should not be a concern in older low-risk patients. Given the average age in PARTNER 3 was 73 years, this does not necessarily apply to younger low-risk patients.

Overall, the evidence suggests that transcatheter valves are comparably durable to surgical bioprostheses out to at least 5 to 6 years, although longer-term data are needed.

Repeat Intervention

For all their advances, it is still almost certain that any bioprosthetic valve will eventually fail, be it surgical or transcatheter. Whether it occurs within the patient's lifetime is a function of their life expectancy; therefore, the younger the patient, the more critical it is to plan out how the index procedure will influence future reintervention. Which combination of approaches will yield the best outcomes: SAVR after SAVR, SAVR after TAVR, TAV-in-TAV, or TAV-in-SAV?

Data comparing the outcomes of index TAVR versus SAVR in patients who will eventually require reintervention are limited. Although the randomized low-risk pivotal trials lack long-term follow-up, the Redo-TAVR registry reported observational data comparing outcomes of TAVR after index TAVR versus SAVR.[54] After propensity matching, investigators found slightly better procedural success after TAV-in-TAV compared with TAV-in-SAV (72.7% vs 62.4%, $P = .045$), although 1-year mortality was similar (11.9% vs 10.2%, $P = .633$). However, the study should not be interpreted to suggest that TAVR and SAVR were equivalent as index procedures; rather, that TAV-in-TAV was as feasible and safe as the previously established TAV-in-SAV.

Conversely, reoperation after TAVR may be associated with worse outcomes than reoperation after SAVR. In a small study of the STS Adult Cardiac Surgery Database, reoperation after TAVR was associated with higher than expected mortality based on STS-PROM across all risk subgroups.[55] Furthermore, the mean operative time was 321 minutes, nearly double that of the published mean redo SAVR of approximately 200 minutes. The authors propose that surgically explanting a well-incorporated TAVR

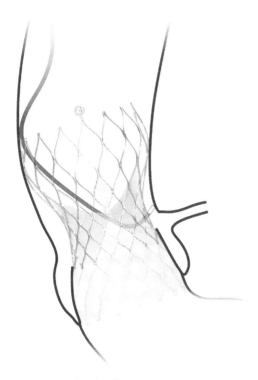

Fig. 3. Example of difficult coronary re-access. Self-expanding prosthesis cells and sealing skirt limit catheter maneuverability in the root, impeding coronary engagement.

valve posed an added technical challenge not seen in typical surgical valves. Although this certainly seems feasible given the abnormally

long operative times, the study is limited by a lack of a comparator arm and its reliance on the accuracy of the STS-PROM model.

Most of the available data compare reintervention strategies after failed surgical bioprostheses, and do not include low-risk patients. In high and intermediate-risk patients, the data support the notion that ViV TAVR is associated with better short-term outcomes, but long-term data are lacking. The largest and most recent study to-date compared ViV-TAVR with redo SAVR in high-risk patients (n = 3443 and n = 3372) and found ViV-TAVR was associated with significantly lower 30-day mortality (OR 0.41, 95% CI 0.23–0.74).[56] Before that, a meta-analysis of 6 observational studies suggested that TAV-in-SAV was essentially equivalent to redo SAVR in high surgical risk patients with respect to mortality at 30 days and 1 year.[57] It should be noted that most of these were with older generation TAVR prostheses, and only 137 of 254 TAVR procedures (54%) were performed transfemoral, with 93 being transapical (37%), an approach known to carry significantly higher morbidity, suggesting outcomes with modern devices and approaches might even favor ViV TAVR.[58] Whether or not the same applies to lower-risk cohorts remains unknown.

Despite its promise, ViV TAVR does not come without a price. Coronary occlusion is a problem unique to TAVR alone, and has been shown to occur at a significantly higher rate after ViV TAVR than native valve TAVR (2.48% vs 0.62%,

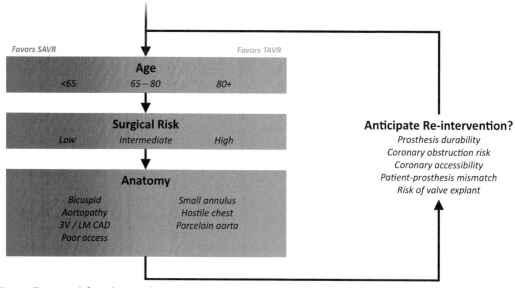

Fig. 4. Framework for selecting the index aortic valve procedure. 3V / LM CAD = three vessel, left main coronary artery disease.

$P = .045$).[59] Although strategies such as chimney stenting or intentional leaflet laceration ("BASILICA") have been demonstrated to mitigate this risk, no single strategy is perfect, and mortality is extremely high when occlusion occurs.[60–62]

Difficulty with coronary reaccess is also unique to post-TAVR patients. The larger profile TAVR prostheses can make future coronary reaccess difficult or even impossible (Fig. 3).[63] Although prosthetic commissures are deliberately oriented away from the coronary ostia during SAVR, the ability to control commissural orientation during TAVR is limited, which may further exacerbate the problem.[64] Techniques to better align the commissures have been developed for specific TAVR systems, but are inconsistent at best.[65] Acute coronary syndromes after TAVR are infrequent but not negligible, and inability to reaccess the coronaries in this setting is associated with poorer outcomes.[66] Although coronary reaccess may be a lower priority to the 95-year-old patient without risk factors, it is highly relevant to the 60-year-old diabetic with potentially decades of exposure to the risk of coronary events, and should be a major consideration in any young patient considering TAVR.

In summary, all 4 "reintervention pathways" are feasible with acceptable outcomes in select patients, but the optimal strategy remains unclear. In the absence of randomized data, the key heart team considerations should be: (1) safety and feasibility of redo sternotomy and valve explantation, (2) potential need for future coronary reaccess, and (3) potential for patient-prosthesis mismatch.

SUMMARY

By now, the reader can appreciate that the low-risk pivotal TAVR trials have not simplified the decision-making process; rather, it has only created new questions about the optimal lifetime management of AS, a concept that had never been as relevant to the high or intermediate-risk populations.

Unfortunately, many of these questions may never be answered with the same rigor. Occurrences such as valve-in-valve-in-valve TAVR are infrequent and would not be feasible to study in a large-scale clinical trial setting. Furthermore, the long-term nature of the problem makes it even more difficult to study given the rapid pace of device advancements: the valves of today may be obsolete by the time we fully understand their optimal use.

We submit that the complexity of these decisions can no longer be captured by simple decision algorithms, and instead require balancing risk within a conceptual framework that accounts for the feasibility of future reinterventions (Fig. 4). Now more than ever is the heart team needed to help navigate patients through these exceedingly complex decision-making pathways.

CLINICS CARE POINTS

- Modern treatment of aortic stenosis must go beyond traditional surgical risk stratification and comorbid conditions.
- When selecting an index modality, consider prosthesis-patient mismatch, durability, and coronary re-access.
- Future re-interventions/reoperations should be planned out with the index procedure.

DISCLOSURE

The authors have nothing to disclose.

REFERENCES

1. Mack MJ, Leon MB, Thourani VH, et al. Transcatheter Aortic-Valve Replacement with a Balloon-Expandable Valve in Low-Risk Patients. N Engl J Med 2019;380(18):1695–705.
2. Popma JJ, Deeb GM, Yakubov SJ, et al. Transcatheter Aortic-Valve Replacement with a Self-Expanding Valve in Low-Risk Patients. N Engl J Med 2019;380(18):1706–15.
3. Carroll JD, Mack MJ, Vemulapalli S, et al. STS-ACC TVT Registry of Transcatheter Aortic Valve Replacement. Ann Thorac Surg 2020. https://doi.org/10.1016/j.athoracsur.2020.09.002.
4. Ramanathan PK, Nazir S, Elzanaty AM, et al. Novel Method for Implantation of Balloon Expandable Transcatheter Aortic Valve Replacement to Reduce Pacemaker Rate—Line of Lucency Method. Struct Heart 2020;4(5):427–32.
5. Sammour Y, Banerjee K, Kumar A, et al. Systematic Approach to High Implantation of SAPIEN-3 Valve Achieves a Lower Rate of Conduction Abnormalities Including Pacemaker Implantation. Circ Cardiovasc Interv 2021;14(1).
6. Leon MB, Smith CR, Mack MJ, et al. Transcatheter or Surgical Aortic-Valve Replacement in Intermediate-Risk Patients. N Engl J Med 2016;374(17):1609–20.
7. Reardon MJ, Van Mieghem NM, Popma JJ, et al. Surgical or Transcatheter Aortic-Valve

Replacement in Intermediate-Risk Patients. N Engl J Med 2017;376(14):1321–31.

8. Nishimura RA, Otto CM, Bonow RO, et al. 2017 AHA/ACC Focused Update of the 2014 AHA/ACC Guideline for the Management of Patients With Valvular Heart Disease. J Am Coll Cardiol 2017;70(2):252–89.

9. Otto CM, Nishimura RA, Bonow RO, et al. 2020 ACC/AHA Guideline for the Management of Patients With Valvular Heart Disease. J Am Coll Cardiol 2020. https://doi.org/10.1016/j.jacc.2020.11.018.

10. Siu SC, Silversides CK. Bicuspid Aortic Valve Disease. J Am Coll Cardiol 2010;55(25):2789–800.

11. Colombo A, Latib A. Bicuspid Aortic Valve. J Am Coll Cardiol 2014;64(22):2340–2.

12. Zegdi R, Ciobotaru V, Noghin M, et al. Is It Reasonable to Treat All Calcified Stenotic Aortic Valves With a Valved Stent? J Am Coll Cardiol 2008;51(5):579–84.

13. Philip F, Faza NN, Schoenhagen P, et al. Aortic annulus and root characteristics in severe aortic stenosis due to bicuspid aortic valve and tricuspid aortic valves: Implications for transcatheter aortic valve therapies. Catheter Cardiovasc Interv 2015; 86(2):E88–98.

14. Wijesinghe N, Ye J, Rodés-Cabau J, et al. Transcatheter Aortic Valve Implantation in Patients With Bicuspid Aortic Valve Stenosis. JACC Cardiovasc Interv 2010;3(11):1122–5.

15. Himbert D, Pontnau F, Messika-Zeitoun D, et al. Feasibility and Outcomes of Transcatheter Aortic Valve Implantation in High-Risk Patients With Stenotic Bicuspid Aortic Valves. Am J Cardiol 2012; 110(6):877–83.

16. Hayashida K, Bouvier E, Lefèvre T, et al. Transcatheter Aortic Valve Implantation for Patients With Severe Bicuspid Aortic Valve Stenosis. Circ Cardiovasc Interv 2013;6(3):284–91.

17. Yoon S-H, Lefèvre T, Ahn J-M, et al. Transcatheter Aortic Valve Replacement With Early- and New-Generation Devices in Bicuspid Aortic Valve Stenosis. J Am Coll Cardiol 2016;68(11):1195–205.

18. Yoon S-H, Bleiziffer S, De Backer O, et al. Outcomes in Transcatheter Aortic Valve Replacement for Bicuspid Versus Tricuspid Aortic Valve Stenosis. J Am Coll Cardiol 2017;69(21):2579–89.

19. Otto CM, Kuusisto J, Reichenbach DD, et al. Characterization of the early lesion of 'degenerative' valvular aortic stenosis. Histological and immunohistochemical studies. Circulation 1994;90(2):844–53.

20. Omran H, Schmidt H, Hackenbroch M, et al. Silent and apparent cerebral embolism after retrograde catheterisation of the aortic valve in valvular stenosis: a prospective, randomised study. Lancet 2003;361(9365): 1241–6.

21. Makkar RR, Yoon S-H, Leon MB, et al. Association Between Transcatheter Aortic Valve Replacement for Bicuspid vs Tricuspid Aortic Stenosis and Mortality or Stroke. JAMA 2019;321(22):2193–202.

22. Halim SA, Edwards FH, Dai D, et al. Outcomes of Transcatheter Aortic Valve Replacement in Patients With Bicuspid Aortic Valve Disease. Circulation 2020;141(13):1071–9.

23. Kassis N, Saad AM, Ahuja KR, et al. Impact of thoracic aortic aneurysm on outcomes of transcatheter aortic valve replacement: A nationwide cohort analysis. Catheter Cardiovasc Interv 2020. https://doi.org/10.1002/ccd.29195.

24. Leyh RG, Bartels C, Nötzold A, et al. Management of porcelain aorta during coronary artery bypass grafting. Ann Thorac Surg 1999;67(4):986–8.

25. Zingone B, Rauber E, Gatti G, et al. Diagnosis and management of severe atherosclerosis of the ascending aorta and aortic arch during cardiac surgery: focus on aortic replacement. Eur J Cardiothorac Surg 2007;31(6):990–7.

26. Osaka S, Tanaka M. Strategy for Porcelain Ascending Aorta in Cardiac Surgery. Ann Thorac Cardiovasc Surg 2018;24(2):57–64.

27. Faggiano P, Frattini S, Zilioli V, et al. Prevalence of comorbidities and associated cardiac diseases in patients with valve aortic stenosis. Potential implications for the decision-making process. Int J Cardiol 2012;159(2):94–9.

28. Makkar RR, Jilaihawi H, Mack M, et al. Stratification of Outcomes After Transcatheter Aortic Valve Replacement According to Surgical Inoperability for Technical Versus Clinical Reasons. J Am Coll Cardiol 2014;63(9):901–11.

29. Rahimtoola SH. The problem of valve prosthesis-patient mismatch. Circulation 1978;58(1):20–4.

30. Pibarot P, Dumesnil JG. Hemodynamic and clinical impact of prosthesis–patient mismatch in the aortic valve position and its prevention. J Am Coll Cardiol 2000;36(4):1131–41.

31. Mohty-Echahidi D, Malouf JF, Girard SE, et al. Impact of Prosthesis-Patient Mismatch on Long-Term Survival in Patients With Small St Jude Medical Mechanical Prostheses in the Aortic Position. Circulation 2006;113(3):420–6.

32. Blackstone EH, Cosgrove DM, Jamieson WRE, et al. Prosthesis size and long-term survival after aortic valve replacement. J Thorac Cardiovasc Surg 2003;126(3):783–93.

33. Tasca G, Mhagna Z, Perotti S, et al. Impact of Prosthesis-Patient Mismatch on Cardiac Events and Midterm Mortality After Aortic Valve Replacement in Patients With Pure Aortic Stenosis. Circulation 2006;113(4):570–6.

34. Jamieson WRE, Ye J, Higgins J, et al. Effect of Prosthesis-Patient Mismatch on Long-Term Survival With Aortic Valve Replacement: Assessment to 15 Years. Ann Thorac Surg 2010;89(1):51–9.

35. Rao V, Jamieson WR, Ivanov J, et al. Prosthesis-patient mismatch affects survival after aortic valve replacement. Circulation 2000;102(19 Suppl 3):Iii5–9.

36. Moon MR, Pasque MK, Munfakh NA, et al. Prosthesis-Patient Mismatch After Aortic Valve Replacement: Impact of Age and Body Size on Late Survival. Ann Thorac Surg 2006;81(2):481–9.

37. Russo M, Taramasso M, Guidotti A, et al. The evolution of surgical valves. Cardiovasc Med 2017;20(12): 285–92. https://doi.org/10.4414/cvm.2017.00532.

38. Herrmann HC, Daneshvar SA, Fonarow GC, et al. Prosthesis–Patient Mismatch in Patients Undergoing Transcatheter Aortic Valve Replacement. J Am Coll Cardiol 2018;72(22):2701–11.

39. Pibarot P, Weissman NJ, Stewart WJ, et al. Incidence and Sequelae of Prosthesis-Patient Mismatch in Transcatheter Versus Surgical Valve Replacement in High-Risk Patients With Severe Aortic Stenosis. J Am Coll Cardiol 2014;64(13): 1323–34.

40. Ternacle J, Pibarot P, Herrmann H, et al. TCT CONNECT-474 Incidence and Impact of Prosthesis–Patient Mismatch after Aortic Valve Replacement in the PARTNER 2 Trial and Registry. J Am Coll Cardiol 2020;76(17):B202–3.

41. Pibarot P, Salaun E, Dahou A, et al. Echocardiographic Results of Transcatheter Versus Surgical Aortic Valve Replacement in Low-Risk Patients. Circulation 2020;141(19):1527–37.

42. Zorn GL, Little SH, Tadros P, et al. Prosthesis–patient mismatch in high-risk patients with severe aortic stenosis: A randomized trial of a self-expanding prosthesis. J Thorac Cardiovasc Surg 2016;151(4):1014–23.e3.

43. Head SJ, Reardon MJ, Deeb GM, et al. Computed Tomography–Based Indexed Aortic Annulus Size to Predict Prosthesis-Patient Mismatch. Circ Cardiovasc Interv 2019;12(4). https://doi.org/10.1161/circinterventions.118.007396.

44. Liao Y-B, Li Y-J, Jun-Li L, et al. Incidence, Predictors and Outcome of Prosthesis-Patient Mismatch after Transcatheter Aortic Valve Replacement: a Systematic Review and Meta-analysis. Sci Rep 2017;7(1). https://doi.org/10.1038/s41598-017-15396-4.

45. Isaacs AJ, Shuhaiber J, Salemi A, et al. National trends in utilization and in-hospital outcomes of mechanical versus bioprosthetic aortic valve replacements. J Thorac Cardiovasc Surg 2015; 149(5):1262–9.e3.

46. Banbury MK, Cosgrove DM, Lytle BW, et al. Long-term results of the Carpentier-Edwards pericardial aortic valve: a 12-year follow-up. Ann Thorac Surg 1998;66(6):S73–6.

47. Stassano P, Di Tommaso L, Monaco M, et al. Aortic Valve Replacement. J Am Coll Cardiol 2009;54(20): 1862–8.

48. Lund O, Bland M. Risk-corrected impact of mechanical versus bioprosthetic valves on long-term mortality after aortic valve replacement. J Thorac Cardiovasc Surg 2006;132(1):20–6.e3.

49. Goldstone AB, Chiu P, Baiocchi M, et al. Mechanical or Biologic Prostheses for Aortic-Valve and Mitral-Valve Replacement. N Engl J Med 2017; 377(19):1847–57.

50. Søndergaard L, Ihlemann N, Capodanno D, et al. Durability of Transcatheter and Surgical Bioprosthetic Aortic Valves in Patients at Lower Surgical Risk. J Am Coll Cardiol 2019;73(5): 546–53.

51. Blackman DJ, Saraf S, Maccarthy PA, et al. Long-Term Durability of Transcatheter Aortic Valve Prostheses. J Am Coll Cardiol 2019;73(5):537–45.

52. Daubert MA, Weissman NJ, Hahn RT, et al. Long-Term Valve Performance of TAVR and SAVR. JACC Cardiovasc Imaging 2017;10(1):15–25.

53. Pibarot P, Ternacle J, Jaber WA, et al. Structural Deterioration of Transcatheter Versus Surgical Aortic Valve Bioprostheses in the PARTNER-2 Trial. J Am Coll Cardiol 2020;76(16):1830–43.

54. Landes U, Sathananthan J, Witberg G, et al. Transcatheter Replacement of Transcatheter Versus Surgically Implanted Aortic Valve Bioprostheses. J Am Coll Cardiol 2021;77(1):1–14.

55. Jawitz OK, Gulack BC, Grau-Sepulveda MV, et al. Reoperation After Transcatheter Aortic Valve Replacement. JACC Cardiovasc Interv 2020;13(13): 1515–25.

56. Hirji SA, Percy ED, Zogg CK, et al. Comparison of in-hospital outcomes and readmissions for valve-in-valve transcatheter aortic valve replacement vs. reoperative surgical aortic valve replacement: a contemporary assessment of real-world outcomes. Eur Heart J 2020;41(29):2747–55.

57. Nalluri N, Atti V, Munir AB, et al. Valve in valve transcatheter aortic valve implantation (ViV-TAVI) versus redo-Surgical aortic valve replacement (redo-SAVR): A systematic review and meta-analysis. J Interv Cardiol 2018;31(5):661–71.

58. Allen KB, Chhatriwalla AK, Cohen D, et al. Transcarotid Versus Transapical and Transaortic Access for Transcatheter Aortic Valve Replacement. Ann Thorac Surg 2019;108(3):715–22.

59. Ribeiro HB, Webb JG, Makkar RR, et al. Predictive Factors, Management, and Clinical Outcomes of Coronary Obstruction Following Transcatheter Aortic Valve Implantation. J Am Coll Cardiol 2013; 62(17):1552–62.

60. Palmerini T, Chakravarty T, Saia F, et al. Coronary Protection to Prevent Coronary Obstruction During TAVR. JACC Cardiovasc Interv 2020;13(6): 739–47.

61. Mercanti F, Rosseel L, Neylon A, et al. Chimney Stenting for Coronary Occlusion During TAVR. JACC Cardiovasc Interv 2020;13(6):751–61.

62. Khan JM, Greenbaum AB, Babaliaros VC, et al. The BASILICA Trial. JACC Cardiovasc Interv 2019; 12(13):1240–52.

63. Ochiai T, Chakravarty T, Yoon S-H, et al. Coronary access after TAVR. JACC Cardiovasc Interv 2020; 13(6):693–705.

64. Fuchs A, Kofoed KF, Yoon S-H, et al. Commissural alignment of bioprosthetic aortic valve and native aortic valve following surgical and transcatheter aortic valve replacement and its impact on valvular function and coronary filling. JACC Cardiovasc Interv 2018;11(17):1733–43.

65. Tang GHL, Zaid S, Fuchs A, et al. Alignment of Transcatheter Aortic-Valve Neo-Commissures (ALIGN TAVR). JACC Cardiovasc Interv 2020;13(9): 1030–42.

66. Faroux L, Munoz-Garcia E, Serra V, et al. Acute coronary syndrome following transcatheter aortic valve replacement. Circ Cardiovasc Interv 2020;13(2). https://doi.org/10.1161/circinterventions.119. 008620.

Femoral Access, Hemostasis, and Complications for Transcatheter Aortic Valve Replacement

Colin M. Barker, MD, FSCAI*, Cherie Dahm, MD

KEYWORDS

• Vascular access • TAVR • VARC • Percutaneous closure • Bleeding • Endovascular repair

KEY POINTS

- Transcatheter aortic valve replacement vascular complications have declined significantly but are still inevitable.
- Preprocedural planning is necessary for predicting and preventing vascular complications.
- Compulsive access and closure techniques are essential.
- Early recognition and treatment of vascular complications can reduce morbidity and mortality.
- Major complications resulting in hemodynamic collapse and hemorrhagic shock require a multidisciplinary approach with vascular surgery and mechanical circulatory support.

BACKGROUND

Percutaneous transfemoral (TF) arterial access has become the most common approach for procedures that require large-bore access. Years ago, as endovascular techniques evolved that required access sheaths that were greater than or equal to 20 Fr, surgical cutdowns with primary arterial repair, as well as temporary conduits, were required and considered part of the procedure. Transcatheter aortic valve replacement (TAVR) has become not just an alternative to surgical aortic valve replacement but often a preferred strategy.[1] Since the first TAVR performed through transseptal access in 2002,[2] the technology has evolved, in that the procedure is now safely performed retrograde transarterial with percutaneous access and closure in 95% of contemporary cases.[3]

Complications from arterial access were frequent and a dominant limitation of adoption and spread of TAVR into intermediate-risk and lower-risk patient populations. The initial series in high-risk and extreme-risk patient populations reported vascular complications of 12% to 16%.[4,5] Since then, as the evidence to treat lower-risk patients has evolved, the vascular complication rate has significantly decreased to 1% to 3%.[3,6,7] Overall, the safety of the procedure is now either noninferior or superior to surgical aortic valve replacement.[6,7] The improvement in reduction of vascular complications is multifactorial: treating lower-risk and healthier patient populations with less vascular disease; the improvement in technology with smaller size catheters with lower profiles; more experience and technical expertise in interventional cardiology with large-bore access.

Over the past 20 years, several alternatives to transfemoral access were explored.[8] Initially, these depended on the TAVR platform. The balloon expandable valves allowed the valve to be mounted and delivered in either a retrograde or antegrade fashion, and therefore a transapical

The authors have no conflicts of interest related to this work.
Vanderbilt University Medical Center, Vanderbilt Heart and Vascular Institute, 1215 21st Avenue South, Medical Center East, 5th Floor, Nashville, TN 37232-8802, USA
* Corresponding author.
E-mail address: Colin.m.barker@vumc.org

Intervent Cardiol Clin 10 (2021) 423–430
https://doi.org/10.1016/j.iccl.2021.07.001
2211-7458/21/© 2021 Elsevier Inc. All rights reserved.

approach with antegrade transaortic delivery was the initial alternative when transfemoral access was prohibitive. The self-expanding platform can only be loaded in a retrograde delivery system, and therefore direct aortic access though a minithoracotomy or sternotomy was the alternative to transfemoral access. Both these techniques came with limitations and increase risk compared with transfemoral access with regard to morbidity, because these required a thoracotomy or sternotomy and had increased risk of stroke. Given these limitations, alternative vascular access approaches that gained popularity included transaxillary artery and transcarotid artery access.[9] These approaches came with less morbidity compared with a strategy that required a thoracotomy, but still had limitations with stroke risk and vascular complications. Subsequently, a transvenous transcaval technique was developed.[10] This technique allowed for transfemoral procedures despite significant peripheral arterial disease that would otherwise be prohibitive. The safety and efficacy of this procedure have been described and are likely more favorable to the transthoracic either direct aortic or transapical approach, but it does have some limitations. Specifically, prohibitive aortic disease, intra-abdominal bleeding, and limited expertise.

Paradoxically, many of the vascular complications that occur during a TAVR procedure can involve the non–delivery system access site, frequently the contralateral femoral artery. For the purposes of this article, the focus is on the issue of delivery system and large-bore access, including a brief review of the anatomy, large-bore access, closure, and complications.

ANATOMY

Familiarity with vascular anatomy, including common variants, is an essential foundation before getting arterial access in any catheter-based procedure. This familiarity is especially important when large-bore catheters and sheaths are required. As part of the work-up for any TAVR procedure, a comprehensive cardiac computed tomography (CT) scan as well as CT angiogram is essential[11] (**Fig. 1**). This imaging allows an assessment of the aortic and cardiac anatomy, and an assessment of the vascular access allowing prediction of any potential challenges. Given the requirement for contrast, alternatives to CT angiography include MRI/magnetic resonance angiography, noncontrast CT, and invasive intravascular ultrasonography.[12] All these modalities have

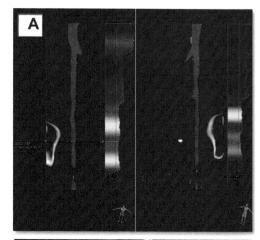

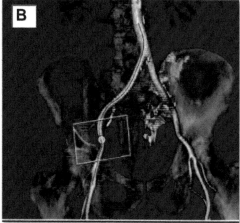

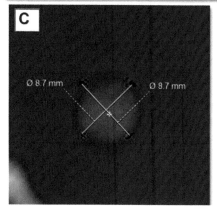

Fig. 1. Example of pre-TAVR computed tomography angiography. Stretched vessel view shows the minimum diameter throughout (*A*); three-dimensional reconstruction shows location of bifurcations, tortuosity, and calcium (*B*); magnified axial view facilitates accurate vessel size measurements (*C*).

limitations. Most patients in contemporary practice can undergo CT angiography with minimal contrast and minimal risk of contrast-induced nephropathy.

When evaluating a patient's preprocedural vascular access, several variables need to be considered: size of the access arteries (diameter), presence of vascular disease, presence and degree of vascular calcification, tortuosity, and location of the bifurcation distal to the common femoral artery between the profunda artery and superficial femoral artery. While assessing the access arteries (common femoral and iliac), attention should be paid to their caliber (mean diameter at least 5.0 mm, ideally 6.5 mm for a 18-Fr delivery system). Smaller-caliber arteries can be used in the absence of significant vascular calcification, but the team should be prepared for a bailout strategy with endovascular repair if needed. In general, a sheath to femoral artery ratio (SFAR) of less than or equal to 1 is ideal; however, in a healthy artery with retained compliance, SFAR greater than >1 can be safely performed. The presence and extension of atherosclerotic plaques and calcifications does not preclude TF access. Expertise in peripheral vascular interventions and equipment, including angioplasty balloons and stents, can help facilitate TF access in the presence of significant occlusive disease. With the availability of intravascular lithotripsy, these procedures can be done safely.[13]

The degree and extension of tortuosity does not exclude TF access but helps with procedural planning. In the presence of severe tortuosity, the procedural team should be aware and may use a longer catheter over a soft wire and then exchange for a stiff wire in the thoracic aorta to straighten the iliofemoral system and safely deliver the large-bore sheath. A good estimation of the caliber of the iliac artery is of paramount importance in balloon size selection when transient occlusion is needed in bailout situations.

LARGE-BORE ACCESS

When deemed suitable for percutaneous TF access, an optimal puncture site is identified in the segment of the common femoral artery extending between the inferior epigastric artery superiorly and the distal portion of the common femoral artery proximal to the bifurcation.[14] The right common femoral artery is used most frequently, but, in the case of potential barriers or higher-risk features, the left femoral artery is good alternative. After the evaluation outlined earlier, the procedural planning execution can now be done with minimal risk. The arteriotomy should be at least 1 cm above the femoral bifurcation and a segment of the artery with minimal

or no calcification. This location can be identified on the preprocedural CT, fluoroscopy, and ultrasonography. All 3 modalities should be used. In case of vascular complications, having enough distance from the femoral bifurcation allows the placement of a covered stent or, if needed, a safe surgical isolation and repair. Additional venous and arterial access to be used during the procedure, other than the delivery system access site, should be done first (pacemaker and pigtail catheter). Historically, many surgeons would place a safety wire up and over the distal aortic bifurcation from the contralateral arterial access site with the wire tip in the ipsilateral superficial femoral artery. This procedure is not necessary anymore because of improved equipment and techniques and is consistent with a minimalist approach to TAVR.

At the time of the procedure, there are several steps that can be taken to enhance success and minimize vascular complications.[15] After careful review of the CT with three-dimensional reconstruction, the ideal puncture spot for arterial puncture is identified: mid–common femoral artery below the inferior epigastric, at least 1 cm above the distal bifurcation, and with the least amount of calcification. CT-fluoroscopy fusion with coregistration of the preprocedural CT and live fluoroscopy can facilitate indirect but accurate visualization of the common femoral artery without additional contrast. Ultrasonography-guided access is imperative and can confirm optimal localization for arterial puncture, including a front-wall arteriotomy. The initial puncture is performed with a small-gauge needle and a microintroducer system with a small sheath and low-profile soft wire (eg, 21-G needle, 4–5-Fr access sheath, and 0.18-mm wire). Angiography can be performed through the small access sheet to confirm optimal localization of the puncture. If the location of the arteriotomy is not ideal, the dilator can be removed and a few minutes of manual pressure can be applied before another attempt.

The next step depends on the strategy for closure.[16] If a percutaneous suture-based closure device is to be used, this would be the time to preclose after dilating the track with a small sheath (6-Fr catheter). In the presence of anterior calcification of the femoral artery, attention should be paid when percutaneous suture-based vascular closure devices are used, because the delivery needles may not adequately penetrate the arterial wall and may fail to deploy. If a percutaneous collagen-based plug device is to be used, this would be the time to measure and note the depth of the puncture.

When it is time to place the large-bore sheath, it is good practice to do this over a stiff wire. This wire can be the same as the one that will be used during valve deployment. To safely position the stiff wire in the thoracic aorta, best practice is to place a small-caliber 4-Fr to 6-Fr catheter over a soft wire into the thoracic aorta and then, using this catheter, exchange for the stiff wire. When advancing the large-bore sheath, it is important to do this under fluoroscopy and confirm that the tip of the wire is ahead of the sheath. More importantly, when resistance is encountered, the surgeon must stop and evaluate. Occasionally provisional angioplasty may be needed to facilitate delivery of the large-bore sheath.[13,17] In addition to traditional angioplasty techniques, peripheral vascular lithotripsy has recently become a valuable tool for facilitating large-bore access in the setting of calcified obstructive peripheral vascular disease.[13] Pushing against significant resistance can result in harm, which in this case could be potentially fatal, as described later. Once the sheath is in place, it should be sutured to the skin, and full-dose anticoagulation should be given.

HEMOSTASIS TECHNIQUES

Proficiency in access management with successful hemostasis at the conclusion of the procedure is essential for many reasons. From a practical standpoint, the only mark that patients see on their bodies after undergoing TAVR is the small incision at the access site (usually the right groin). A successful TAVR deployment followed by a vascular complication or unsuccessful hemostasis can lead to significant morbidity, mortality, and patient dissatisfaction. As discussed earlier, vascular complications were common and a significant limitation as the field evolved in high-risk and extreme-risk patient cohorts. Initially, a significant portion of vascular access and hemostasis was performed via open cutdown and arteriotomy with subsequent open repair. However, in contemporary practice, most procedures are performed with percutaneous closure techniques. In parallel, vascular complications have significantly decreased, as seen by the most recent data from the Society of Thoracic Surgeons (STS)/American College of Cardiology (ACC) Transcatheter Valve Therapy Registry.[3]

Given the frequency of failure during percutaneous closure and hemostasis early in the TAVR experience, several provisional techniques were developed to be prepared. Aside from having all the necessarily vascular complication bailout equipment in the room and readily available, including peripheral angioplasty balloons and covered stents, many clinicians would place a safety wire up and over from the contralateral arterial access site to maintain access after the large-bore sheath is removed and allow for delivery of balloons and stents. Furthermore, many routinely use this wire and a balloon inflation for dry closure.[16] If all else failed, the safety wire and an occlusion balloon allowed for temporary hemostasis to convert to an open repair. At present, a safety wire is rarely used.

Percutaneous suture-based techniques for hemostasis have been the preferred method of closure for TAVR. Initially, this was done with either the Prostar XL percutaneous vascular surgical system or multiple Perclose Prostar or Prostyle devices (Abbott Vascular, United States).[18] The Prostar XL system is cumbersome and requires manual knot tying and has a steep learning curve. Given the ease and reproducibility of the Perclose system, this became the device of choice.[19] After access is obtained with a smaller-caliber sheath (ie, 6 Fr or less), 1 to 2 Perclose sutures are deployed and the sutures put aside until the end of the procedure. At the end of the procedure, when the sheath is removed, the sutures are used to close the arteriotomy. When removing the sheath, it is good practice to reintroduce the inner sheath dilater because this can be reinserted rapidly if bleeding is not controlled. Frequently, additional Perclose devices may be necessary in addition to potentially using a provisional collagen-based vascular plug (Angio-Seal, Terumo, United States). At the conclusion of the procedure, an angiogram of the access site can be helpful to avoid delayed recognition in potential vascular complications.

Recently, a collagen-based closure device specifically designed for large-bore access has become available (Fig. 2). The MANTA vascular closure device (Teleflex, Wayne, PA) is a novel collagen-based technology designed to close large-bore arteriotomies created by devices with an outer diameter ranging from 12 F to 25 F. The SAFE-MANTA (Pivotal Clinical Study to EvaluAte the SaFety and Effectiveness of MANTA Vascular Closure Device) trial evaluated the safety and effectiveness of the MANTA vascular closure device.[20] The results were encouraging with technical success in 257 (97.7%) patients, and a single device was deployed in 262 (99.6%) of procedures. Valve Academic Research Consortium-2 major vascular

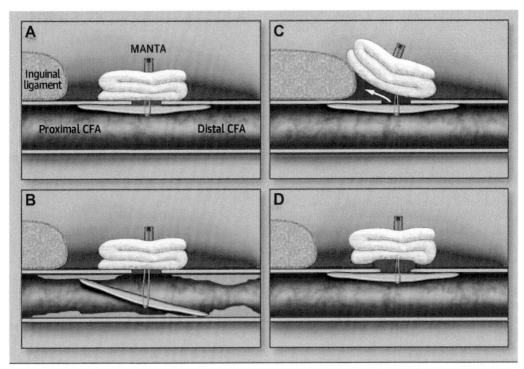

Fig. 2. MANTA closure device (Teleflex, Wayne, PA) with correct final position (*A*), Toggle interaction with intravascular calcium and plaque causing arterial occlusion (*B*), incomplete apposition potentially leading to bleeding (*C*), incomplete apposition potential leading to pseudoaneurysm and delayed rupture (*D*). (*From* Moccetti F, Brinkert M, Seelos R, et al. Insights From a Multidisciplinary Introduction of the MANTA Vascular Closure Device. JACC: Cardiovascular Interventions 2019;12:1730-6.)

complications occurred in 11 (4.2%) patients: 4 received a covered stent (1.5%), 3 had access site bleeding (1.1%), 2 underwent surgical repair (0.8%), and 2 underwent balloon inflation (0.8%). Subsequent evaluation of the MANTA device using the Manufacturer and User Facility Device Experience (MAUDE) database identified 250 reports.[21] The most common failure complication of MANTA is persistent bleeding (48.8%) and vessel occlusion or stenosis (29.6%). Most complications were managed successfully with an endovascular approach (48.4%), but some required surgical intervention (40.4%).

COMPLICATIONS AND MANAGEMENT

As with everything in interventional cardiology, the best way to manage complications is to avoid them. However, any invasive procedure or surgery comes with inherent risks and potential for harm and complications are expected. Therefore, having a sense of an individual patient's risk for potential vascular complication, as well as early recognition and management, is essential. Most access site complications involve bleeding. As soon as possible, usually just before the large-

bore sheath is removed, anticoagulation should be reversed to facilitate hemostasis. Large-bore sheath dwell times during procedures are short, and patients are fully anticoagulated during the procedure. The authors rarely encounter obstructive and ischemic complications. Dissections or injury to the intima during the procedure can be encountered, which are generally retrograde, non–flow limiting, and can be managed conservatively. If the dissection is flow limiting, then it can be treated with balloon angioplasty with provisional self-expanding stent. When these complications occur, they can be managed with standard peripheral endovascular interventional techniques, including a completion angiogram with run-off.[22]

To standardize the definition of a vascular complication during TAVR, not only for clinical research but also to measure quality metrics in practice, the Valve Academic Research Consortium (VARC-2) developed criteria for both major and minor vascular complications during TAVR.[23] In general, major vascular complications involving femoral access include vascular injuries that lead to death, life-threatening or major bleeding, visceral ischemia, or permanent impairment. In contrast, minor vascular complications are those injuries not leading to death, life-threatening or major bleeding, visceral ischemia, or permanent neurologic impairment. In addition, VARC-2 includes percutaneous closure device failure as an event when hemostasis at the arteriotomy site is not achieved as intended and alternative or additional treatments and interventions are required.

Manual external compression and/or endovascular balloon tamponade are the initial maneuvers to control minor access site bleeding. Endovascular balloon tamponade requires maintained arterial access with a wire or a new puncture on the contralateral femoral arterial system to deliver a balloon. If the bleeding persists and the anatomy is favorable, then the arteriotomy can be treated percutaneously with an appropriately sized self-expanding covered stent. A large cohort of patients treated with TAVR who developed an access site vascular complication showed the routine use of a self-expanding nitinol stent graft to be feasible, safe, and associated with favorable short-term and midterm clinical outcome.[24] In the registry, 96 (87.3%) patients were managed by the implantation of a self-expanding nitinol stent graft. In most patients, minor vascular complications triggered the implantation of a stent graft (86.5%), mainly because of bleeding (90.6%) and dissection (5.2%) of the common femoral artery with high rates of primary treatment success (97.9%). Compared with a propensity score–matched cohort of patients without vascular complications, stented patients had comparable long-term mortality, despite the occurrence of a vascular complication (1-year mortality: 17.7% vs 26.6%, stent vs matched cohort, respectively; $P = .1$). If bleeding persists despite these interventions, vascular surgery should be consulted for potential hybrid or open surgical repair.

Major access site complications can be successfully treated when recognized quickly and treated with a multidisciplinary team approach. These complications frequently result in hemodynamic instability requiring active cardiovascular anesthesia support as well as potentially initiating cardiopulmonary resuscitation and mechanical circulatory support. Temporary endovascular hemostasis can be achieved with large-caliber occlusion balloons (Fig. 3). Familiarity with these devices, as well as careful inflation when used, is needed to avoid subsequent complications and potential aortic rupture from the occlusion balloon. Once the patient is somewhat stabilized, angiography can be performed to define the extent of the complication and

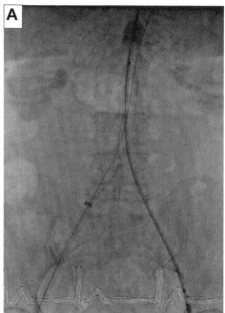

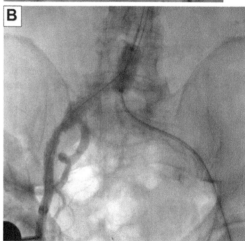

Fig. 3. Coda Balloon Catheter (Cook Medical, Bloomington, IN) deployed for hemostasis in the suprarenal aorta (A), and in the distal abdominal aorta (B) for hemostasis of a right common iliac rupture.

the best treatment approach. In truly hostile and prohibitive surgical anatomy, a percutaneous approach or hybrid approach could be attempted. However, in a major complication resulting in hemodynamics instability from an arterial rupture or evulsion, this frequently requires surgical intervention to successfully resuscitate the patient.

Major vascular complications during TAVR result in increased morbidity and mortality. Consequences of these events include longer procedure times, higher contrast use, longer length of stays, and increase in health care resource use. A recent study examined the incidence, predictors, treatment strategies, and outcomes of vascular complications in a multi-center cohort of patients undergoing transfemoral TAVR.[25] This retrospective review showed patients with vascular complications had a greater need for blood transfusion, longer postoperative length of stay, higher rates of cardiac events, increased vascular-related 30-day readmission, and higher 30-day mortality. Female sex (odds ratio [OR], 3.00; 95% confidence interval [CI], 1.91 to 4.72) and prior percutaneous coronary intervention (OR, 2.14; 95% CI, 1.38–3.31) were the strongest predictors of major vascular complication. Patients with major vascular complication had worse 1-year survival (OR, 79%; 95% CI, 69%–86%) compared with patients with minor vascular complication (OR, 92%; 95% CI, 82%–96%) or no vascular complication (OR, 88%; 95% CI, 87%–90%; $P = .002$).

SUMMARY

Given the improvement in technology with smaller-caliber access catheters for TAVR, as well as a decrease in the patient risk profile and increase in operator experience, the rate of vascular access complications with TAVR has decreased dramatically. However, this is not a reason to become complacent. Although becoming increasingly less frequent, vascular access complications will continue to occur and will have an expected event rate. Given this, TAVR operators must maintain the skill set to evaluate access options preprocedure, use best practices during the procedure, and maintain the knowledge and skills to manage complications. These skills will continue to be valuable as the structural heart landscape continues to grow and evolve.

REFERENCES

1. Otto CM, Nishimura RA, Bonow RO, et al. 2020 ACC/AHA Guideline for the Management of Patients With Valvular Heart Disease. J Am Coll Cardiol 2021;77:e25–197.

2. Cribier A, Eltchaninoff H, Bash A, et al. Percutaneous Transcatheter Implantation of an Aortic Valve Prosthesis for Calcific Aortic Stenosis. Circulation 2002;106:3006–8.

3. Carroll JD, Mack MJ, Vemulapalli S, et al. STS-ACC TVT Registry of Transcatheter Aortic Valve Replacement. J Am Coll Cardiol 2020;76:2492–516.

4. Popma JJ, Adams DH, Reardon MJ, et al. Transcatheter aortic valve replacement using a self-expanding bioprosthesis in patients with severe aortic stenosis at extreme risk for surgery. J Am Coll Cardiol 2014;63:1972–81.

5. Leon MB, Smith CR, Mack M, et al. Transcatheter Aortic-Valve Implantation for Aortic Stenosis in Patients Who Cannot Undergo Surgery. N Engl J Med 2010;363:1597–607.

6. Mack MJ, Leon MB, Thourani VH, et al. Transcatheter Aortic-Valve Replacement with a Balloon-Expandable Valve in Low-Risk Patients. N Engl J Med 2019;380:1695–705.

7. Popma JJ, Deeb GM, Yakubov SJ, et al. Transcatheter Aortic-Valve Replacement with a Self-Expanding Valve in Low-Risk Patients. N Engl J Med 2019;380:1706–15.

8. Abu Saleh WK, Goswami R, Chinnadurai P, et al. Direct Aortic Access Transcatheter Aortic Valve Replacement: Three-Dimensional Computed Tomography Planning and Real-Time Fluoroscopic Image Guidance. J Heart Valve Dis 2015;24:420–5.

9. Reardon MJ, Barker CM. Is Transcarotid an "Alternative" Access? JACC Cardiovasc Interv 2019;12:420–1.

10. Greenbaum AB, Babaliaros VC, Chen MY, et al. Transcaval Access and Closure for Transcatheter Aortic Valve Replacement: A Prospective Investigation. J Am Coll Cardiol 2017;69:511–21.

11. Okuyama K, Jilaihawi H, Kashif M, et al. Transfemoral Access Assessment for Transcatheter Aortic Valve Replacement. Circ Cardiovasc Imaging 2015;8:e001995.

12. Rogers T, Waksman R. Role of CMR in TAVR. JACC: Cardiovasc Imaging 2016;9:593–602.

13. Sardella G, Salvi N, Bruno E, et al. Lithotripsy-Assisted Aortic Valvuloplasty During TAVR. JACC Cardiovasc Interv 2019;12:e131–2.

14. Biasco L, Ferrari E, Pedrazzini G, et al. Access Sites for TAVI: Patient Selection Criteria, Technical Aspects, and Outcomes. Front Cardiovasc Med 2018;5:88.

15. Otto CM, Kumbhani DJ, Alexander KP, et al. 2017 ACC Expert Consensus Decision Pathway for Transcatheter Aortic Valve Replacement in the Management of Adults With Aortic Stenosis: A Report of the American College of Cardiology Task Force on Clinical Expert Consensus Documents. J Am Coll Cardiol 2017;69:1313–46.

16. Kaki A, Blank N, Alraies MC, et al. Access and closure management of large bore femoral arterial access. J Interv Cardiol 2018;31:969–77.

17. Asciutto G, Aronici M, Resch T, et al. Endoconduits with "Pave and Crack" Technique Avoid Open Ilio-femoral Conduits with Sustainable Mid-term Results. Eur J Vasc Endovasc Surg 2017;54:472–9.

18. Haas PC, Krajcer Z, Diethrich EB. Closure of large percutaneous access sites using the Prostar XL Percutaneous Vascular Surgery device. J Endovasc Surg 1999;6:168–70.

19. Toggweiler S, Gurvitch R, Leipsic J, et al. Percutaneous Aortic Valve Replacement: Vascular Outcomes With a Fully Percutaneous Procedure. J Am Coll Cardiol 2012;59:113–8.

20. Wood DA, Krajcer Z, Sathananthan J, et al. Pivotal Clinical Study to Evaluate the Safety and Effectiveness of the MANTA Percutaneous Vascular Closure Device. Circ Cardiovasc Interv 2019;12:e007258.

21. Megaly M, Sedhom R, Abdelmaseeh P, et al. Complications of the MANTA closure device. Insights from MAUDE database. Cardiovasc Revascularization Med 2021. https://doi.org/10.1016/j.carrev.2021.02.013.

22. Samal AK, White CJ. Percutaneous management of access site complications. Catheter Cardiovasc Interv 2002;57:12–23.

23. Kappetein AP, Head SJ, Généreux P, et al. Updated standardized endpoint definitions for transcatheter aortic valve implantation: the Valve Academic Research Consortium-2 consensus document (VARC-2). Eur J Cardiothorac Surg 2012;42: S45–60.

24. Sedaghat A, Neumann N, Schahab N, et al. Routine Endovascular Treatment With a Stent Graft for Access-Site and Access-Related Vascular Injury in Transfemoral Transcatheter Aortic Valve Implantation. Circ Cardiovasc Interv 2016;9:e003834.

25. Ullery BW, Jin R, Kirker EB, et al. Trends in vascular complications and associated treatment strategies following transfemoral transcatheter aortic valve replacement. J Vasc Surg 2020;72:1313–24.e5.

Blowing it up
A Review of Balloon-Expandable Transcatheter Aortic Valve Replacement

Shahbaz Ali Malik, MD[a],
Andrew M. Goldsweig, MD, MS, FSCAI, FSVM, RPVI[b],*

KEYWORDS

- Transcatheter aortic valve replacement • Balloon expandable • Transcatheter heart valves

---

KEY POINTS

- Balloon-expandable transcatheter aortic valve replacement (TAVR) has grown from an experimental therapy in 2002 to become the mainstream therapy for severe aortic stenosis in 2020 for patients at high, intermediate, and low levels of surgical risk.
- The 4 PARTNER trials have shown TAVR has similar outcomes to surgical AVR in terms of mortality and stroke risk.
- Following the original balloon-expandable SAPIEN valve (Edwards Lifesciences, Irvine, CA, USA), subsequent generations of devices have improved upon the design by reducing its access profile from 22F to 24F to 14F to 16F, with a mechanically flexible catheter to facilitate deployment, inner and outer polyethylene terephthalate fabric sealing skirts to reduce paravalvular leak, and open cell stent design to facilitate coronary access.
- Balloon-expandable TAVR is particularly favorable in cases of extremely large aortic annuli, horizontal aorta, baseline conduction system disease, and coronary artery disease due to the flexibility of a low-profile, balloon-expandable valve with a versatile delivery system.

INTRODUCTION

Who indeed will set bounds to human ingenuity?

—Galileo Galilei.[1]

In interventional cardiology, a revolution transpired in 2002 when Professor Alain Cribier performed the world's first transcatheter aortic valve replacement (TAVR). On April 16, 2002, he successfully deployed a Percutaneous Valve Technology (PVT; Fort Lee, NJ, USA) percutaneous heart valve in a 57-year-old man with severe aortic stenosis (AS) who presented with cardiogenic shock, severe left ventricular dysfunction (ejection fraction 12%), and multiple comorbidities contraindicating surgical aortic valve replacement (SAVR).[2] This maiden TAVR was performed via the transeptal route due to the patient's extensive peripheral artery disease. The first device, which was compatible with a 24F introducer sheath, consisted of a stainless steel stent and contained a trileaflet valve made of bovine pericardium, which had been proved for more than 25 years to function well in surgical bioprostheses.[3]

The development of a transcatheter heart valve was prescient; the prevalence of aortic valve stenosis and proportion of patients treated were discordant with up to 48% patients

---

Conflicts of interest: No commercial or financial conflicts of interest for Drs S.A. Malik and A.M. Goldsweig.
[a] Interventional Cardiology, Division of Cardiovascular Medicine, University of Nebraska Medical Center, 982265 Nebraska Medical Center, Omaha, NE 68198, USA; [b] Interventional Cardiology, Structural Heart Disease, Division of Cardiovascular Medicine, University of Nebraska Medical Center, 982265 Nebraska Medical Center, Omaha, NE 68198, USA
* Corresponding author.
E-mail address: andrew.goldsweig@unmc.edu

2211-7458/21/© 2021 Elsevier Inc. All rights reserved.

foregoing aortic valve therapy before TAVR.[4,5] The prevalence of AS increases with age as demonstrated by a prospective population-based study of 3273 participants including 164 subjects with AS: the prevalence of AS increased from 0.2% at ages 50 to 59 years, to 1.3% at ages 60 to 69 years, 3.9% at ages 70 to 79 years, and 9.8% at ages 80 to 89 years.[6] A meta-analysis of studies conducted in Europe, the United States, and Taiwan found a population prevalence of 3.4% for severe AS in those aged 75 years and older.[7] Up to 1.5 million people in the United States have AS, whereas approximately 500,000 within this group of patients have severe AS. An estimated 250,000 patients with severe AS are symptomatic.[8–10] Thus, given the high prevalence of severe AS, Professor Cribier's percutaneous delivery of a stented valve ushered in a new era for interventional cardiology and for patients with AS, with TAVR as a viable alternative to SAVR, traditionally the only approach to treat the disease.

PARTNER TRIAL—COHORT B AND COHORT A

Edwards Lifesciences Corporation (Irvine, CA, USA) acquired PVT in 2004 and launched the PARTNER trials in 2007 to demonstrate the safety and efficacy of TAVR in a randomized controlled manner. The initial PARTNER trial consisted of 2 cohorts—Cohort B and Cohort A. Cohort B was composed of 358 patients with severe, symptomatic AS with a 30-day Society of Thoracic Surgeons predicted risk of mortality (STS-PROM) score of greater than 15% and deemed inoperable by 2 cardiac surgeons. These patients were randomized in a 1:1 ratio to TAVR or standard medical therapy. TAVR was performed under general anesthesia via the transfemoral (TF) approach with transesophageal echocardiographic guidance. A standard balloon aortic valvuloplasty was initially performed, followed by TF sheath insertion used for valve delivery. The bioprosthesis itself was part of the Edwards SAPIEN (Edwards Lifesciences, Irvine, CA, USA) transcatheter heart valve (THV) system, which consisted of a trileaflet bovine pericardial valve mounted on a balloon-expandable (BE), stainless steel support frame. At 1 year, TAVR was associated with lower rates of all-cause mortality (30.7% vs 49.7%, P < .001), as well as the composite end point of all-cause mortality or repeat hospitalization for valve- or procedure-related deterioration at 1 year (42.5% vs 70.4%, P < .001). Major strokes at 30 days (5.0% vs 1.1%, P = .06) and at 1 year

(7.8% vs 3.9%, P = .18) were numerically higher in the TAVR arm.[11]

Published a year later, in 2011, Cohort A consisted of 699 patients with severe, symptomatic AS and a 30-day STS-PROM score of 8% to 15%. These patients were randomized in a 1:1 manner to TAVR or SAVR. TAVR was preferentially performed via TF access, but if a patient had inadequate femoral/iliac vessel diameter, then transapical (TA) access was used. All-cause mortality was not significantly different between TAVR and SAVR at 1 year (24.2% vs 26.8%, P for noninferiority = 0.001). Vascular complications at 1 year were higher with TAVR (18.0% vs 4.8%, P < .001), but major bleeding at 1 year was lower in the TAVR arm (14.7% vs 25.7%, P < .001). The need for new permanent pacemaker was similar at 1 year (5.7% vs 5.0%, P = .68). All strokes were higher with TAVR at 1 year (8.3% vs 4.3%, P = .04), but disabling strokes did not differ significant significantly at the 1-year mark (P > .05).[12]

Based on the PARTNER B results, the Edwards SAPIEN THV delivered via the TF route was approved in November 2011 by the United States Food and Drug Administration (FDA) as a therapy for inoperable patients with symptomatic severe AS. In October 2012, based on the PARTNER A data, the FDA approved an expanded indication to enable the treatment of high-risk patients and also approved TA delivery for patients lacking suitable TF access.

Five-year outcomes of both PARTNER Cohort B and Cohort A trials have been published. For Cohort B, intent-to-treat analysis showed that the primary end point of all-cause mortality was significantly lower in the TAVR arm when compared with the standard medical therapy arm (71.8% vs 93.6%, P < .0001). Mortality between 3 and 5 years was lower in the TAVR arm (38.9% vs 66.7%, P = .028). Cardiovascular mortality (57.5% vs 85.9%, P < .0001) and repeat hospitalizations (47.6% vs 87.3%, P < .0001) were significantly lower in the TAVR arm at 5 years as well. The median survival was 29.7 months in the TAVR arm and 11.1 months in the standard medical therapy arm. Echocardiography after TAVR showed durable hemodynamic benefit with mean aortic valve area 1.52 cm^2 and mean aortic valve mean gradient 10.6 mm Hg at 5 years along with no evidence of structural valve deterioration reported.[13] For Cohort A, all-cause mortality (67.8% vs 62.4%, P = .76), repeat hospitalizations (42.3% vs 34.2%, P = .17), and all strokes (15.9% vs 14.7%, P = .35) were similar between the TAVR and SAVR arms. Echocardiography demonstrated that mean valve area and mean aortic valve gradients were similar between the 2 arms at 5 years, with no structural valve deterioration requiring surgical valve replacement in either group recorded. Patients undergoing TF TAVR had lower mortality and readmission rates compared with those undergoing TA TAVR.[14]

PARTNER 2A TRIAL

The PARTNER 2A trial enrolled 2032 patients with severe, symptomatic AS who had a 30-day STS-PROM score of 4% to 8% and were thus considered intermediate risk for SAVR. These patients were randomized to SAVR or TAVR, which was performed via either TF, transaortic (TAo), or TA access based on the patient's peripheral arterial anatomy. TAVR was performed using the second-generation BE SAPIEN XT THV system. The TF arm of the trial enrolled 1550 patients, randomized to either TF TAVR (775 patients) or SAVR (775 patients). Patients who did not have suitable peripheral anatomy for TF TAVR were included in a parallel arm of the trial. Patients in this arm were randomized to SAVR (246 patients) or TAVR (236 patients) through the TAo or TA approach.

The primary end point of all-cause mortality or disabling stroke was lower with TAVR versus SAVR at 2 years (19.3% vs 21.1%, P = .001 for noninferiority). Disabling stroke was the same for both TAVR and SAVR groups (6.2% vs 6.4%, P = .83). New atrial fibrillation at 30 days was lower in the TAVR arm (9.1% vs 26.4%, P<.001) but moderate to severe paravalvular aortic regurgitation (leak, paravalvular leak [PVL]) at 2 years was increased with TAVR (8.0% vs 0.6%, P<.001). Thus the PARTNER 2A trial showed that, at 2 years, TAVR was noninferior to SAVR with regard to its primary end point. Importantly, in the TF access cohort alone, the primary end point at 2 years was lower for TAVR compared with SAVR (16.8% vs 20.4%, P = .05).[15] In August 2016, based on data from PARTNER 2A, the FDA approved TAVR for patients with severe, symptomatic AS at intermediate risk for death or complications associated with SAVR.

Five-year outcomes from the PARTNER 2A trial showed that there was no significant difference in the incidence of death from any cause or disabling stroke between the TAVR and SAVR groups (47.9% vs 43.4%, P = .21). Results were similar when comparing the TF TAVR and SAVR cohorts (44.5% vs 42.0%, P = .80), but the incidence of death or disabling stroke was higher after transthoracic access TAVR than after surgery (59.3% vs 48.3%, P = .03). Aortic valve reinterventions were also more frequent after TAVR than after surgery (3.2% vs 0.8%, P = .006). By echocardiography, mean aortic valve mean gradients were similar between TAVR and SAVR (11.4 vs 10.8 mm Hg, P = non-significant); however, more patients in the TAVR group than in the surgery group had at least mild paravalvular aortic regurgitation (33.3% vs 6.3%).[16]

Long-term follow-up regarding structural valve deterioration (SVD) showed that with an echocardiographic follow-up of ~ 4 years, SAPIEN-XT was observed to have higher rates of SVD when compared with surgical valves. The 5-year Kaplan-Meier rate of SVD was 9.5% versus 3.5% for SAPIEN XT and SAVR, respectively.[17] The rates of bioprosthetic valve failure (BVF) were 3-fold higher for SAPIEN XT (4.7%) compared with SAVR.[17] BVF was related to SVD in 64% of cases, PVL in 20%, followed by a combination of valve migration and thrombosis for the remainder of the cases. Overall, SAVR was found to have less SVD and BVF than SAPIEN XT.

PARTNER 3 TRIAL

Nearly 80% of patients with severe AS are at low surgical risk.[18] In keeping with its predecessors, the PARTNER 3 trial was a randomized controlled trial that compared TAVR with SAVR in patients with severe, symptomatic AS. The patients included in this trial, however, were at low risk for SAVR based on 30-day STS-PROM scores of less than 4%. The trial enrolled 1000 patients: 503 randomized to TF TAVR with the third -generation BE SAPIEN 3 THV system and 497 patients randomized to SAVR. The duration of follow-up was 1 year, at which point the primary outcome of all-cause mortality, stroke, or rehospitalization (related to the procedure, valve, or heart failure) was lower in the TAVR group compared with the SAVR group (8.5% vs 15.1%, P<.001 for noninferiority, P = .001 for superiority). Fewer patients who underwent TAVR experienced a stroke by 30 days compared with SAVR (0.6% vs 2.4%, P = .02). Similarly, new-onset atrial fibrillation at 30 days was lower with TAVR compared with SAVR (5.0% vs 39.5%, P<.001). Although patients undergoing TAVR were more likely to have mild PVL compared with those undergoing SAVR at 1 year (29.4% vs 2.1%, P<.05), moderate to severe PVL at 1 year was comparable for both TAVR and SAVR (0.6% vs 0.5%, P = not significant).[19]

On the basis of evidence from the PARTNER 3 trial, in August 2019, the FDA approved TAVR for patients at low risk for SAVR.

Two-year outcomes data from the PARTNER 3 trial were presented at the American College of Cardiology 2020 Virtual Scientific Sessions. The primary outcome of all-cause mortality, stroke, or rehospitalization was lower in the TAVR group compared with the SAVR group (11.5% vs 17.4%, P = .007). As well, death or disabling stroke was lower with TAVR when compared with SAVR (3.0% vs 3.8%, P = .47), as well as rehospitalization (8.5% vs 12.5%, P = .046). Valve thrombosis using the Valve Academic Research Consortium-2 (VARC-2) definition was higher with TAVR compared with SAVR (2.6% vs 0.7%, P = .02).[20] Mean aortic valve mean gradients by echocardiography were 13.6 mm Hg with TAVR versus 11.8 mm Hg with SAVR (P<.001), and mild paravalvular aortic insufficiency was 26.0% with TAVR versus 2.3% with SAVR (P<.001).[21]

Information regarding durability of SAPIEN 3 prosthesis comes from the PARTNER II intermediate-risk single-arm registry. A mean of 4-year echocardiographic follow-up demonstrated that the SAPIEN 3 had an SVD rate of 3.9%, equivalent to SAVR.[17] The rate of all-cause BVF was 2.6%, 2-fold higher than SAVR and bordering on statistical significance (P = .083). BVF was related to PVL in 58% of cases and SVD in 32% at 5 years.[17] All in all, SAPIEN 3 rates of SVD and BVF were equivalent to SAVR at 5 year.

Major findings of the landmark PARTNER trials comparing BE THVs to SAVR are detailed in Table 1.

Table 1
Landmark trials, listed in chronologic order, comparing balloon-expandable transcatheter heart valves with surgical aortic valve replacement

Study	Principal Findings	References
PARTNER Cohort B	All-cause mortality for TAVR vs SAVR at 1 y: 30.7% vs 49.7%, P<.001.	Leon et al,[11] 2010
	Composite end point of all-cause mortality or repeat hospitalization for valve- or procedure-related deterioration at 1 y: 42.5% vs 70.4%, P<.001.	
	Major strokes at 30 d: 5.0% vs 1.1%, P = .06	
	Major strokes at 1 y: 7.8% vs 3.9%, P = .18.	
PARTNER Cohort A	All-cause mortality for TAVR vs SAVR at 1 y: 24.2% vs 26.8%, P for noninferiority = 0.001).	Smith et al,[12] 2011
	Vascular complications: 18.0% vs 4.8%, P<.001.	
	Major bleeding: 14.7% vs 25.7%, P<.001.	
	New permanent pacemaker: 5.7% vs 5.0%, P = .68.	
	All strokes: 8.3% vs 4.3%, P = .04	
	Major strokes: 5.1% vs 2.4%, P = .07	
PARTNER 2A	All-cause mortality or disabling stroke for TAVR vs SAVR at 2 y: 19.3% vs 21.1%, P = .001 for noninferiority.	Leon et al.[15] 2016
	Disabling stroke: 6.2% vs 6.4%, P = .83.	
	Moderate to severe PVL: 8.0% vs 0.6%, P<.001.	
	New atrial fibrillation at 30 d: 9.1% vs 26.4%, P<.001.	
PARTNER 3	All-cause mortality, stroke, or rehospitalization (related to the procedure, valve, or heart failure) for TAVR vs SAVR at 1 y: 8.5% vs 15.1%, P<.001 for noninferiority, P = .001 for superiority).	Mack et al,[19] 2019
	Stroke at 30 d: 0.6% vs 2.4%, P = .02.	
	New-onset atrial fibrillation at 30 d: 5.0% vs 39.5%, P<.001.	
	Mild PVL at 1 y: 29.4% vs 2.1%, P<.05	
	Moderate to severe PVL at 1 y: 0.6% vs 0.5%, P = not significant	

DEVICE EVOLUTION

With each trial, and accumulating experience, the BE Edwards SAPIEN THV system underwent design modifications. The first-generation SAPIEN valve was a trileaflet bioprosthesis made of bovine pericardium, mounted on a BE stainless steel stent with an inner skirt made of polyethylene terephthalate (PET) fabric covering the ventricular side. This first-generation valve was available in 2 sizes, 23 and 26 mm. The valves were compatible with a 22F or 24F sheath, respectively, and TF delivery occurred via the RetroFlex catheter (Edwards Lifesciences, Irvine, CA).

The second-generation SAPIEN XT valve consisted of a BE cobalt chromium stent supporting a trileaflet bovine pericardial valve and an inner PET fabric skirt on the ventricular side. In addition to 23 and 26 mm valve sizes, SAPIEN XT included a 29 mm size as well. With design refinements, and the procedural modification to mount the valve on the deployment balloon in the thoracoabdominal aorta, the delivery system sheath was reduced in size, ranging from 16F to 20F depending on the valve size. Delivery occurred using the NovaFlex catheter (Edwards Lifesciences, Irvine, CA).

The third-generation SAPEIN 3 valve consists of a BE cobalt chromium stent with a trileaflet bovine pericardial valve. The valve comes with both an inner skirt and an outer sealing skirt made of PET to help minimize PVL. SAPIEN 3 is available in 4 sizes: 20, 23, 26, and 29 mm. The SAPIEN 3 delivery system consists of an expandable sheath (eSheath) with a hydrophilic coating; the 20-, 23-, and 26-mm valves are compatible with a 14F eSheath, and the 29-mm valve is compatible with a 16F eSheath. Furthermore, TF valve delivery occurs through the eSheath (Edwards Lifesciences, Irvine, CA) using the Commander delivery system, which has a distal flex point to allow safe passage across the aortic arch and coaxial alignment of the bioprosthesis. For TA or TAo valve delivery, the Certitude system is used, with an 18F sheath for the 20-, 23-, and 26-mm valves and a 21F sheath for the 29-mm valve.

The latest iteration of the SAPIEN valve is the SAPIEN 3 Ultra THV; this remains a BE cobalt chromium stent with a trileaflet bovine pericardial valve. The PET inner skirt remains unchanged, but the outer sealing skirt is now 40% taller compared with the SAPIEN 3 valve. The frame design has an open cell geometry to facilitate coronary access post-TAVR should the need arise. The valve is available in 20, 23, and 26 mm sizes, all of which are delivered through a 14F eSheath.

The generations of SAPIEN THVs, current Commander delivery system, SAPEIN 3/Ultra THV sizing chart, and expandable eSheath specifications are depicted in **Figs. 1–3**.

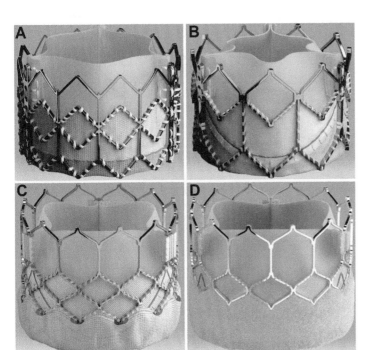

Fig. 1. Balloon-expandable Edwards SAPIEN transcatheter heart valves. SAPIEN valve (*A*); SAPIEN XT valve (*B*); SAPIEN 3 valve (*C*); SAPIEN 3 Ultra valve (*D*). (All images reproduced with permission from Edwards Lifesciences for both electronic and print format.)

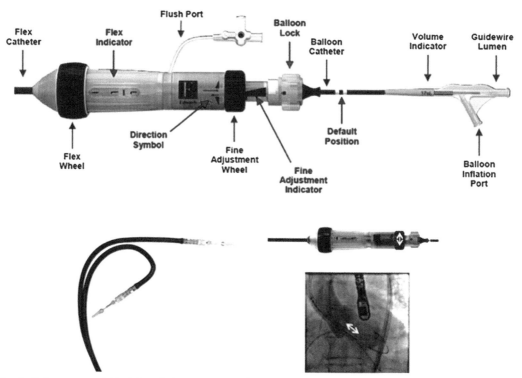

Fig. 2. Balloon-expandable Edwards SAPIEN transcatheter heart valve Commander delivery system. (All images reproduced with permission from Edwards Lifesciences for both electronic and print format.)

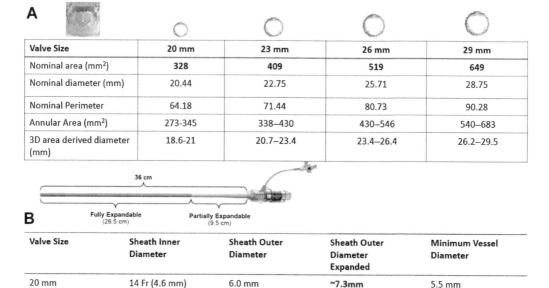

A

Valve Size	20 mm	23 mm	26 mm	29 mm
Nominal area (mm²)	**328**	**409**	**519**	**649**
Nominal diameter (mm)	20.44	22.75	25.71	28.75
Nominal Perimeter	64.18	71.44	80.73	90.28
Annular Area (mm²)	273-345	338–430	430–546	540–683
3D area derived diameter (mm)	18.6-21	20.7–23.4	23.4–26.4	26.2–29.5

B

Valve Size	Sheath Inner Diameter	Sheath Outer Diameter	Sheath Outer Diameter Expanded	Minimum Vessel Diameter
20 mm	14 Fr (4.6 mm)	6.0 mm	~7.3mm	5.5 mm
23 mm	14 Fr (4.6 mm)	6.0 mm	7.6 mm	5.5 mm
26 mm	14 Fr (4.6 mm)	6.0 mm	8.0 mm	5.5 mm
29 mm	16 Fr (5.3 mm)	6.7 mm	8.6 mm	6.0 mm

Fig. 3. Balloon-expandable Edwards SAPIEN 3 and Ultra transcatheter heart valve sizing chart (A) and eSheath specifications (B). (All images reproduced with permission from Edwards Lifesciences for both electronic and print format.)

WHEN TO USE A BALLOON-EXPANDABLE TRANSCATHETER HEART VALVE

Concomitant to the PARTNER series of trials comparing the SAPIEN family of THVs to SAVR, a series of trials comparing a self-expanding (SE) transcatheter aortic valve bioprosthesis (CoreValve, Evolut R, Evolut PRO, Medtronic, Dublin, Ireland) were conducted. Based on their results, the SE THVs received FDA approval for use in all risk strata of patients with severe, symptomatic AS as well.

In the contemporary era, the BE SAPIEN and the SE CoreValve family of THVs are the most commonly used platforms for TAVR. Given the dearth of large-scale, head-to-head comparisons of various TAVR devices and the rapid evolution of new device iterations, there is insufficient evidence to claim superiority of one device type over another. Nonetheless, as each TAVR platform has unique design characteristics, certain patient anatomic factors may slightly favor one platform over the other.[22]

A BE THV may be favored in cases of an extremely large annulus beyond the manufacturer recommendations because BE THVs may be postdilated larger without the recoil observed with SE THVs. A study including 74 patients with a mean aortic valve annular area of 721 ± 38 mm^2 showed that TAVR with the 29-mm SAPIEN 3 valve overexpanded beyond the recommended range was safe, with acceptable PVL and pacemaker rates. Postdilatation occurred in 32% of patients in the study, with final balloon overfilling (1–5 mL extra) in 70% of patients.[23] A horizontal aorta (>70°) favors a BE THV, which has a distal flex point present in the delivery system to allow coaxial implantation.[22] As BE THVs have exhibited lower rates of post-TAVR permanent pacemaker implantation than SE THVs, a BE platform may be favored for patients with baseline conduction disease.[22]

The prevalence of coronary artery disease (CAD) ranges from 41% to 75% in patients with severe AS undergoing TAVR.[24] A study of 411 patients sought evaluated the geometric interaction between THVs (the SE Evolut R and Evolut PRO [n = 66] and the BE SAPIEN 3 [n = 345]) and the coronary ostia to assess the incidence of unfavorable coronary access after TAVR by analyzing post-TAVR computed tomography (CT) in a large cohort. Coronary access was defined as unfavorable if the coronary ostium was below the sealing skirt or in front of the THV commissural posts above the skirt in each coronary artery. CT-identified features of unfavorable coronary access were observed in 34.8% (n = 23) for the left coronary artery and 25.8% (n = 17) for the right coronary artery in the Evolut R/Evolut PRO group, whereas those percentages were 15.7% (n = 54) for the left coronary artery and 8.1% (n = 28) for the right coronary artery in the SAPIEN 3 group. In an engagement-level analysis, the success rates of selective coronary engagement were significantly lower in patients with CT-identified features of unfavorable coronary access compared with those with favorable coronary access in both the Evolut R/Evolut PRO (0.0% vs 77.8%, $P = .003$) and SAPIEN 3 (33.3% vs 91.4%, $P = .003$) groups.[24] A BE THV may thus be favored in patients with significant CAD because BE THVs permit easier catheter access for subsequent percutaneous coronary intervention.[22]

Table 2 Summary of various factors to consider when deciding whether to use or avoid a balloon-expandable transcatheter heart valve system	
Factors Favoring BE THV Use	**Factors not in Favor of BE THV Use**
In case of an extremely large aortic annulus	In case of a small aortic annulus
Patients with a horizontal aorta (>70°)	Presence of dense annular or subannular calcium
Patients with baseline conduction disease	Patients with diminutive or tortuous illeofemoral arteries
Patients with significant coronary artery disease or in whom coronary access need is anticipated post-TAVR for percutaneous coronary intervention or interventions	Patients with low ventricular ejection fraction or those anticipated to tolerate rapid ventricular pacing poorly
Only BE THVs may be deployed inside degenerated surgical valves, rings, and calcium present in the mitral, tricuspid, and pulmonic valve positions	

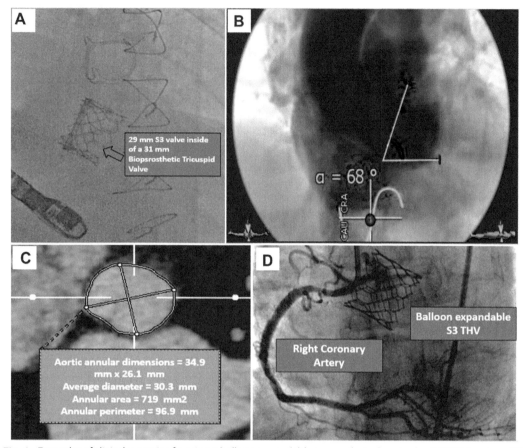

Fig. 4. Examples of clinical scenarios favoring a balloon-expandable transcatheter heart valve (BE THV) system. SA-PIEN 3 (S3) valve implanted percutaneously via the transjugular venous approach inside a degenerated bio-prosthetic surgical tricuspid valve (A); computed tomographic image of a horizontal aorta (B); computed tomographic image of an extremely large aortic annulus (C) fluoroscopic image of invasive coronary angiography following BE THV implantation (D).

A BE THV may be less desirable in the presence of dense annular or subannular calcium because of an increased risk of incomplete valve expansion or annular rupture. In smaller annuli and valve-in-valve TAVR, BE valves with intra-annular leaflets may yield higher post-TAVR gradients than SE valves with supra-annular leaflets.[25,26] As rapid ventricular pacing is required for BE valve deployment, patients with low left ventricular ejection fractions may tolerate BE deployment poorly. BE platforms may also navigate diminutive or tortuous illeo-femoral arteries less easily than their SE counterparts because the former platforms include both an inflexible THV and a balloon, whereas the latter only include a more flexible THV.[22] Only BE valves may be deployed inside degenerated surgical valves, rings, and calcium present in the mitral, tricuspid, and pulmonic valve positions.[22]

A summary of the aforementioned factors is provided in Table 2, and clinical case examples are provided in Fig. 4.

SUMMARY

It used to be that TAVR was really a therapy that was appropriate for patients who were not good candidates for surgery. We think that's turned around, and that probably TAVR should be the therapy considered, and surgery should be used in patients that are not good candidates for TAVR.
—*Martin B. Leon*

The past 2 decades have seen a paradigm shift in therapy for aortic valve disease. The advent of TAVR has not only revolutionized interventional cardiology but also, more importantly, has given patients recourse for a disease that previously had limited therapeutic options. The coming years may bring even smaller BE valve delivery systems, THVs for aortic insufficiency and moderate AS, and improved transcatheter therapies for dysfunction of other heart valves. Answers regarding the durability of THVs, BE and self-expanding, should be available. What is certain is that BE THVs will continue to evolve rapidly and to play an important and ever-expanding role in interventional cardiology.

CLINICS CARE POINTS

- An aortic valve is considered severely stenotic when the maximum aortic transvalvular velocity is ≥ 4 m/sec, typically with an aortic valve area ≤ 1 cm2, accompanied by a mean gradient across the aortic valve of ≥ 40 mm Hg.

- Balloon-expandable transcatheter aortic valve replacement (TAVR) is an approved modality for aortic valve replacement across all surgical risk strata, i.e. prohibitive, high, intermediate, and low risk surgical patients.

- Balloon expandable TAVR should be avoided in case of a small aortic annulus, presence of dense annular or subannular calcium, in patients with diminutive or tortuous illeofemoral arteries and in patients with low ventricular ejection fraction or those anticipated to tolerate rapid ventricular pacing poorly.

- Balloon expandable TAVR may be favorable in case of an extremely large aortic annulus, in patients with a horizontal aorta ($>70°$), patients with baseline conduction disease, patients with significant coronary artery disease or in whom coronary access need is anticipated post TAVR for percutaneous coronary intervention(s). Only balloon expandable transcatheter heart valves may be deployed inside degenerated surgical valves, rings, and calcium present in the mitral, tricuspid, and pulmonic valve positions.

DISCLOSURE

Dr. Goldsweig is supported by a grant from the National Institute of General Medical Sciences, 1U54GM115458, and the UNMC Center for Heart and Vascular Research. Dr. Malik reports no funding to disclose. The content is solely the responsibility of the authors and does not necessarily represent the official views of the NIH.

REFERENCES

1. Galilei G. Letter to the grand duchess Christina of Tuscany 1615.
2. Cribier A, Eltchaninoff H, Bash A, et al. Percutaneous transcatheter implantation of an aortic valve prosthesis for calcific aortic stenosis: first human case description. Circulation 2002;106:3006–8.
3. Cribier A. The development of transcatheter aortic valve replacement (TAVR). Glob Cardiol Sci Pract 2016;2016(4):e201632.
4. Nkomo VT, Gardin JM, Skelton TN, et al. Burden of valvular heart diseases: a population-based study. Lancet 2006;368:1005–11.
5. Bach DS, Cimino N, Deeb GM. Unoperated patients with severe aortic stenosis. J Am Coll Cardiol 2007;50:2018–9.
6. Eveborn GW, Schirmer H, Heggelund G, et al. The evolving epidemiology of valvular aortic stenosis. the Tromsø study. Heart 2013;99(6):396.
7. Osnabrugge RL, Mylotte D, Head SJ, et al. Aortic stenosis in the elderly: disease prevalence and number of candidates for transcatheter aortic valve replacement: a meta-analysis and modeling study. J Am Coll Cardiol 2013;62:1002–12.
8. Bach D, Radeva J, Birnbaum H, et al. Prevalence, referral patterns, testing, and surgery in aortic valve disease: leaving women and elderly patients behind. J Heart Valve Dis 2007;16(4):362–9.
9. Iivanainen A, Lindroos M, Tilvis R, et al. Natural history of aortic valve stenosis of varying severity in the elderly. Am J Cardiol 1996;78(1):97–101.
10. Aronow W, Ahn C, Kronzon I. Comparison of echocardiographic abnormalities in african-american, hispanic, and white men and women aged >60 years. Am J Cardiol 2001;87(9):1131–3.
11. Leon B, Smith C, Mack M, et al. Transcatheter aortic-valve implantation for aortic stenosis in patients who cannot undergo surgery. N Engl J Med 2010;363:1597–607.
12. Smith C, Leon B, Mack M, et al. Transcatheter versus surgical aortic-valve replacement in high-risk patients. N Engl J Med 2011;364:2187–98.
13. Kapadia SR, Leon MB, Makkar RR, et al. 5-year outcomes of transcatheter aortic valve replacement compared with standard treatment for patients with inoperable aortic stenosis (PARTNER 1): a randomised controlled trial. Lancet 2015;385(9986):2485–91.
14. Mack MJ, Leon MB, Smith CR, et al. 5-year outcomes of transcatheter aortic valve replacement or surgical aortic valve replacement for high surgical risk patients with aortic stenosis (PARTNER 1): a randomized controlled trial. Lancet 2015; 385(9986):2477–84.
15. Leon B, Smith C, Mack M, et al. Transcatheter or surgical aortic-valve replacement in intermediate-risk patients. N Engl J Med 2016;374:1609–20.

16. Makkar RR, Thourani VH, Mack MJ, et al. Five-year outcomes of transcatheter or surgical aortic-valve replacement. N Engl J Med 2020;382:799–809.

17. Pibarot P, Ternacle J, Jaber WA, et al. Structural deterioration of transcatheter versus surgical aortic valve bioprostheses in the PARTNER-2 Trial. J Am Coll Cardiol 2020;76:1830–43.

18. Thourani VH, Suri RM, Gunter RL, et al. Contemporary real-world outcomes of surgical aortic valve replacement in 141,905 low-risk, intermediate-risk, and high-risk patients. Ann Thorac Surg 2015;99(1):55–61.

19. Mack M, Leon B, Thourani V, et al. Transcatheter aortic-valve replacement with a balloon-expandable valve in low-risk patients. N Engl J Med 2019;380:1695–705.

20. Presented by Dr. Michael J. Mack at the American College of Cardiology Virtual Annual Scientific Session Together With World Congress of Cardiology (ACC 2020/WCC), March 29, 2020.

21. Pibarot P, Salaun E, Dahou A, et al. Echocardiographic results of transcatheter versus surgical aortic valve replacement in low-risk patients: The PARTNER 3 Trial. Circulation 2020;141:1527–37.

22. Claessen B, Tang G, Kini A, et al. Considerations for optimal device selection in transcatheter aortic valve replacement: a review. JAMA Cardiol 2021;6(1):102–12.

23. Tang GHL, Zaid S, George I, et al. Impact of aortic root anatomy and geometry on paravalvular leak in transcatheter aortic valve replacement with extremely large annuli using the Edwards SAPIEN 3 valve. JACC Cardiovasc Interv 2018;11:1377–87.

24. Ochiai T, Chakravarty T, Yoon SH, et al. Coronary access after TAVR. JACC Cardiovasc Interv 2020; 13:693–705.

25. Hahn RT, Leipsic J, Douglas PS, et al. Comprehensive echocardiographic assessment of normal transcatheter valve function. JACC Cardiovasc Imaging 2019;12:25–34.

26. Abdelghani M, Mankerious N, Allali A, et al. Bioprosthetic valve performance after transcatheter aortic valve replacement with self-expanding versus balloon-expandable valves in large versus small aortic valve annuli: insights from the CHOICE Trial and the CHOICE-Extend Registry. JACC Cardiovasc Interv 2018;11:2507–18.

Transcatheter Aortic Valve Replacement with a Self-Expanding Prosthesis

Erinn Hughes, MD, Paul Michael Grossman, MD*

KEYWORDS

- Aortic stenosis • Transcatheter aortic valve replacement • Self-expanding valve • CoreValve
- Evolut

KEY POINTS

- Self-expanding transcatheter heart valves, first approved in 2014, have proven to be an excellent option for patients with severe aortic stenosis and any level of surgical risk.
- The supra-annular location of the valve optimizes EOA and valve gradients and allows for maximal leaflet coaptation and minimal leaflet stress, which translates to better valve durability.
- Many patient anatomic and procedural factors favor the use of self-expanding valves over balloon-expandable valves (ie, bicuspid valve, small annulus, high degree of calcium, challenging vascular access, etc).
- Newer generations of devices and improved implantation techniques have been successful at increasing safety, efficacy, and durability. In particular, reducing the need for pacemaker implantation and increasing the rate of successful coronary reengagement post-TAVR.

 Video content accompanies this article at http://www.interventional.theclinics.com.

INTRODUCTION

Globally, aortic stenosis (AS) is the most prevalent acquired valvular heart disease requiring intervention in developing countries.[1] There is an exponential increase in the prevalence of AS with age, with 0.2% in those aged 50 to 59 years, 1.3% in those aged 60 to 69 years, 3.9% in those aged 70 to 79 years, and 9.8% in those aged 80 to 89 years. It is a progressive disease and as the valve obstruction worsens, it can cause decreased cardiac output, heart failure, and even premature death. Once the AS has progressed to severe, there is a 50% 2-year mortality if left untreated.[2]

From the 1960s until the 2000s, the treatment for severe, symptomatic AS was almost exclusively surgical. However, owing to the nature of the procedure and its risks, many patients with advanced age or significant comorbidities were deemed inoperable and had limited treatment options.

Aortic balloon valvuloplasty (BV) was introduced in 1985 as a catheter-based alternative for these high-risk patients, but most patients experienced restenosis within 1-year post-intervention. BV was associated with increased stroke rates and did not improve mortality so was used only for palliation and as a bridge to definitive therapy.[3] In 2002, the field was revolutionized when Alain Cribier performed the first-in-man transcatheter aortic valve replacement (TAVR), finally introducing a reasonable alternative to aortic valve surgery.[4]

Department of Internal Medicine, Division of Cardiovascular Medicine, University of Michigan, Frankel Cardiovascular Center, 1500 East Medical Center Drive, SPC 5869, Ann Arbor, MI 48109-5869, USA
* Corresponding author. University of Michigan, Frankel Cardiovascular Center, 2A, 1500 East Medical Center Drive, SPC 5869, Ann Arbor, MI 48109-5869.
E-mail address: pagross@med.umich.edu

Intervent Cardiol Clin 10 (2021) 441–453
https://doi.org/10.1016/j.iccl.2021.06.004
2211-7458/21/© 2021 Elsevier Inc. All rights reserved.

Since then, data have proven TAVR to be a less-invasive, lower-risk alternative to surgical aortic valve replacement (SAVR). Two broad categories of devices were officially FDA-approved in late 2011 and early 2014, balloon-expandable valves (BEVs) and self-expanding valves (SEVs), respectively. Over the past two decades, significant improvements in the design, delivery, and durability of transcatheter heart valves (THVs) have occurred, improving patient outcomes and increasing the treatment options for severe AS.

This review of the journey of self-expanding TAVR devices will highlight the special features of each generation and briefly discuss the most recent outcome data and best practices of self-expanding transcatheter aortic valves.

SELF-EXPANDING TRANSCATHETER AORTIC VALVE REPLACEMENT FOR HIGH-RISK PATIENTS

The first trials to compare TAVR to SAVR were the PARTNER studies, which showed that balloon-expandable TAVR was superior to medical management in the treatment of inoperable patients (Cohort B),[5] and noninferior to SAVR for the treatment of patients with a high surgical risk (Cohort A)[6] based on Society of Thoracic Surgeons [STS] score $\geq$ 8%.[7] In 2014, the CoreValve US Pivotal Trial became the first of many trials investigating the safety and efficacy of SEVs in aortic valve replacement (Table 1). In the extreme risk cohort, TAVR with SEV was compared to medical therapy in inoperable patients and showed a marked survival benefit in patients treated with TAVR.[8]

Subsequently, TAVR with SEV was compared to SAVR in high-risk patients. In this cohort, similar outcomes were seen with TAVR as with SAVR up to 5 years of follow-up. Permanent pacemaker implantation (PPI) and reintervention rates were higher with TAVR, whereas moderate structural valve deterioration (SVD) was higher with SAVR, likely attributed to patient-prosthesis size mismatch (PPM). Valve hemodynamics (effective orifice area [EOA] and aortic valve area) tended to favor SEV over SAVR.[9]

SELF-EXPANDING TRANSCATHETER AORTIC VALVE REPLACEMENT FOR INTERMEDIATE-RISK PATIENTS

After demonstrating desirable safety and efficacy profiles of TAVR in extreme and high-risk surgical patients, researchers compared TAVR to SAVR in intermediate-risk surgical patients (STS score 3%–8%).[7] Analogous to the PARTNER 2 trial comparing BEV to SAVR,[10] the Surgical Replacement and Transcatheter Aortic Valve Implantation (SURTAVI) randomized trial showed that TAVR with self-expanding CoreValve was noninferior to SAVR when comparing all-cause mortality or disabling stroke at 24 months in intermediate surgical risk patients (median STS 4.5%) with severe AS.[11,12]

Patients reported an earlier symptomatic benefit, better quality of life at 30 days, and showed significant improvement in 6-min walk test at 2 years in the TAVR arm. There were significantly more cases of new-onset atrial fibrillation, acute kidney injury, and severe bleeding requiring transfusions in the SAVR arm. Valve hemodynamics and performance at 2 years was equivalent between the 2 arms. Echocardiographically, patients achieved lower aortic-valve gradients and larger aortic-valve areas after TAVR, presumably due to the supra-annular location of the TAVR bioprosthesis.[11]

Notably, there were more vascular complications in the TAVR arm at 30 days and the need for a permanent pacemaker at 30 days was nearly 4 times higher in the TAVR arm.[11,12] These findings were attributed to the fact that 84% of patients in the TAVR arm were enrolled before 2015 and received the first-generation CoreValve. The second-generation Evolut R underwent significant modifications[13] to further improve the safety and efficacy of self-expanding TAVR devices, which translated to a decreased pacemaker requirement.[14]

Along with the results from PARTNER 2,[10] these findings led to a broader indication and wider patient population for TAVR devices, offering transcatheter therapy to intermediate surgical risk patients who would not have had that option only a few years prior.

SELF-EXPANDING TRANSCATHETER AORTIC VALVE REPLACEMENT FOR LOW-RISK PATIENTS

In 2019, the Evolut Surgical Replacement and Transcatheter Aortic Valve Implantation in Low-Risk Patients Trial sought to further explore the use of self-expanding TAVR to patients at low surgical risk (STS <3%).[7] Results confirmed Evolut (R or Pro) was noninferior to SAVR when comparing all-cause mortality or disabling stroke at 24 months in low surgical risk patients (median STS 1.9%) with severe AS.[15]

Much like in the SURTAVI trial, the Evolut Low-Risk results showed higher rates of disabling strokes, new-onset atrial fibrillation, acute kidney injury, and severe bleeding in the

Table 1
Evolut platform clinical trials results

Study	N	Age	STS	30-Day Mortality	1-Year Mortality	30-Day All Stroke	1-Year All Stroke
CoreValve US Pivotal Extreme-Risk Trial	483	83.2 ± 8.7	10.3 ± 5.5	8.4%	24.3%	4.0%	7.0%
CoreValve US Pivotal High-Risk Trial	390	83.1 ± 7.1	7.3 ± 3.0	3.3%	14.2%	4.9%	8.8%
Evolut R US Pivotal Trial	241	83.3 ± 7.2	7.4 ± 3.4	2.5%	8.6%	5.0%	7.7%
Evolut Forward Study	1040	81.8 ± 6.2	5.5 ± 4.5	1.9%	8.9%	2.8%	3.4%
SURTAVI Clinical Trial SURTAVI	864	79.9 ± 6.2	4.4 ± 1.5	2.0%	7.0%	2.6%	5.5%
Continued Access Study	274	79.0 + 6.1	4.1 + 4.5	0.0%	3.5%	1.8%	4.5%
Evolut PRO Trial	60	83.3 ± 7.2	6.4 + 3.9	1.7%	11.8%	1.7%	NA
TVT-Registry- Evolut PRO	2065	81.3 ± 7.7	6.7 ± 4.4	1.4%	NA	2.6%	NA
Evolut Low Risk Trial	725	74.1 ± 5.8	1.9 ± 0.7	0.5%	2.4%	3.4%	4.1%

SAVR arm. Valve hemodynamics and performance at 2 years was, again, equivalent between the 2 arms; however, patients who received TAVR were able to achieve lower mean gradients and higher EOAs than patients in the SAVR arm.[15]

These results, paired with PARTNER 3 trial results,[16] suggested that low surgical risk patients could do as well or better than SAVE with TAVR, essentially ensuring that patients could be safely considered for TAVR over SAVR regardless of their surgical risk.

SELF-EXPANDING TRANSCATHETER AORTIC VALVE REPLACEMENT DEVICES: CoreValve TO EVOLUT R/PRO/+

Medtronic's CoreValve was the first self-expanding heart valve, but it is no longer available for clinical use. Currently, there exist three commercially available self-expanding heart valves, all built on the original CoreValve foundation: the Evolut R, Evolut PRO, and Evolut Pro+ models, as illustrated in Fig. 1.

Unlike the bovine pericardium used in the surgical and balloon-expandable devices, the commercially available CoreValves and all subsequent generations have been made of a porcine pericardial trileaflet valve on a nitinol frame. Compared with bovine, porcine pericardial tissue has a smaller tissue thickness (0.4 vs 0.25 mm), which allows for a smaller introducer size. It has a high tensile strength, exceeding suture and mechanical stress, and a low tissue elongation capacity, providing consistent coaptation of the leaflets. It also has a high tolerance to bending, which helps to accommodate deployment in nonround annuli.[17,18] Nitinol, a nickel-titanium alloy with the unique property of being malleable when cool, but expanding and becoming rigid when heated to body temperatures, is used as the frame to improve the device's ability to conform and seal to the native annulus. The valve becomes functional at only 2/

3 deployment, providing time to assess valve position and performance and allow for recapture if needed, leading to more accurate, controlled deployment (Video 1).[13]

By design, the supra-annular leaflets of the self-expanding devices remain above and unconstrained by the native annulus, maximizing leaflet coaptation and minimizing leaflet stress. This leaflet location leads to increased EOA and lower gradients than achieved with the intra-annular balloon-expandable devices.[13,17]

Over time, each generation of SEVs has been modified and improved upon to address the limitations of the previous generation, as described in Table 2. The first-generation CoreValve devices were bulky, requiring an 18F sheath for deployment.[19] This reliance on large diameter catheters raised the incidence of procedural complications and relied heavily on the expertise of the operators.

The second-generation Evolut R device reduced the overall height of the prosthesis but extended the length of the pericardial skirt to provide a more secure seal and reduce the incidence of perivalvular leak (PVL). This generation was the first to implement the EnVeo R delivery system, which transmits 1:1 torque, allowing for better control during valve position and deployment. It also allows for valve recapture and redeployment if necessary. These devices deliver through either a 14 or 16F in-line sheath, depending on the size of the valve.[13,19]

The third-generation Evolut Pro device introduced an external porcine pericardial wrap around the first 1.5 cells of the skirt to ensure better annular sealing and further prevent paravalvular leak. This advancement came with the trade-off of increased bulk, requiring a larger sheath size (16F) and an inability to accommodate a 34 mm valve. With these changes, the Enveo delivery system was also modernized; however, remained limited in its steerability.[13]

The most recent generation, the Evolut Pro+, retains all features of the prior generations,

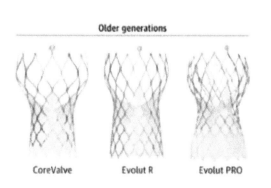
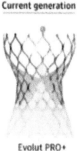

Older generations   Current generation

CoreValve   Evolut R   Evolut PRO   Evolut PRO+

Fig. 1. Four generations of self-expanding valves. (*Modified from* Ref.[20])

Table 2
Overview of self-expanding transcatheter aortic valve replacement (TAVR) prostheses

| Prosthesis | Material | | Valve Sizes, mm | Sheath Sizes | Supra-annular or Intra-annular | Repositionable | Approval Status | Comments |
	Frame	Valve						
CoreValve	Nitinol	Porcine pericardial	26, 29, 31	18F	Supra-annular	Yes	FDA approved	Currently no longer available
CoreValve Evolut R	Nitinol	Porcine pericardial	23, 26, 29, 34	14F equivalent (23, 26, and 29 mm); 16F equivalent (34 mm)	Supra-annular	Yes	FDA approved	NA
CoreValve Evolut Pro	Nitinol	Porcine pericardial	23, 26, 29	16F equivalent	Supra-annular	Yes	FDA approved	Compared with Evolut R, an outer pericardial skirt was added to reduce paravalvular leak
CoreValve Evolut Pro*	Nitinol	Porcine pericardial	23, 26, 29, 34	14F equivalent (23, 26, and 29 mm); 16F equivalent (34 mm)	Supra-annular	Yes	FDA approved	CoreValve Evolut Pro+ is compatible with smaller sheaths and offers a 34-mm valve with an outer pericardial sheath

Modified from Ref.[20]

including recapturability and the external peri-cardial wrap, but conforms to smaller sheaths and thus can accommodate the larger 34 mm valve.

Future modifications of these self-expanding TAVR devices will likely relate to enhanced steering of the delivery system, a shorter stent frame, and larger stent openings to facilitate coronary access.

COMPARISON OF BALLOON-EXPANDABLE TO SELF-EXPANDING TRANSCATHETER AORTIC VALVE REPLACEMENT

Once TAVR proved itself to be a reasonable alternative to SAVR, attention turned to comparing the two different types of TAVR on safety, efficacy, durability, and patient selection. Given the lack of large-scale, head-to-head comparisons of various TAVR devices, the rapid development of new device iterations, and the significant differences in the baseline risk profile between patient populations, there is insufficient evidence to claim the superiority of one device type over another. Even so, as each TAVR device has unique design characteristics, certain patient and procedural factors may favor self-expanding over balloon-expandable prostheses.

Small annular size, a high degree of left ventricular outflow tract (LVOT) and annular calcification, advanced age, intolerance to rapid pacing, and small or challenging iliofemoral arterial access favor self-expanding TAVR devices. In contrast, a horizontal aorta, high preprocedural risk of pacemaker, young age, extensive coronary artery disease, low coronary ostia, and effaced sinuses may deter the use of self-expanding TAVR devices.[20]

Small-sized annuli (perimeter <73 mm) favor SEV because the supra-annular design results in superior hemodynamics. Lower gradients, larger EOA, lower peak velocity, and higher dimensionless index as well as a decreased rate of severe PPM translates into better valve durability.[21–24]

Although a certain degree of calcification is required to adequately anchor, seal and support the TAVR within the aortic root, a heavily calcified LVOT portends a higher risk of PVL and annular rupture, a rare but often fatal complication. Annular rupture occurs most frequently during the deployment of a BEV, particularly when oversized (>20% area) valves are used, or with postdilation for PVL.[25] SEV may be preferable in these patients because they do not require a balloon inflation for deployment; however, they have been associated with a higher

incidence of PVL.[26] The risk of annular rupture should be weighed against the risk and degree of PVL before consideration of postdilation in a heavily calcified patient.

For patients with small or challenging iliofemoral arterial access, SEVs are preferred because of the low-profile delivery system (14–16F) used during deployment.[27] Historically, BEVs have required larger sheath sizes (up to 24F), although newer generations of BEV have been successful at reducing delivery sheath diameter and now have a comparable profile to SEVs.[20,28]

Historically, early generations of SEV were difficult to appropriately position in patients with a high degree of aortic angulation (AA), greater than 48°, referred to as a horizontal aorta. This anatomic complexity led to increased incidence of PVL in these patients, subsequent exclusion of these patients from TAVR clinical trials, and avoidance of clinical use of SEVs in this patient population.[29,30] Recently, data using newer generations of SEV suggest that the degree of AA does not affect procedural success or clinical outcomes.[31]

Owing to increased radial force postdeployment and increased depth of deployment in the LVOT, early trials showed a significantly higher rate of PPI with CoreValve.[14] Given this association of conduction abnormalities and subsequent need for PPI in patients receiving SEV, patients with a high preprocedural risk of pacemaker (ie, pre-existing right bundle branch block, short membranous septum) were deterred from receiving self-expanding TAVR.[32] Data with newer generations of SEV and using improved implantation techniques, including the cusp-overlap model, have shown decreasing rates of conduction abnormalities requiring pacemaker.[14,33] Current trials continue to investigate techniques designed to further reduce the need for a pacemaker post-TAVR.

The longer frame and diamond lattice structure of the SEV also make coronary access more challenging post-SEV TAVR than with BEV. These challenges are even more pronounced in patients with low coronaries (<12 mm) and effaced sinuses (<30 mm). Low coronary arteries and effaced sinuses are associated with an increased risk of coronary obstruction, a rare but devastating complication of TAVR implantation.[26] Preprocedural knowledge of extensive coronary artery disease and a high likelihood of future percutaneous coronary intervention (PCI) may support avoidance of SEV, particularly in patients with unfavorable annuli and coronary ostial locations.[27,34] However, as training, comfort, and success with diagnostic angiography and PCI in patients with prior SEVs improve over time, post-TAVR coronary access may not need to be as much of a concern in the future.[35]

As TAVR use expands, it can be anticipated that younger patients with longer life expectancies will become more frequent TAVR recipients. Specifics on valve durability, feasibility of repeat TAVR in TAVR and future coronary access should be carefully considered. Repeat TAVR within an SEV will carry a higher potential risk of coronary obstruction in patients with a small aortic root and low sinutubular junction. These patients may benefit from initial TAVR with a BEV, which has a shorter frame and intraannular leaflets. Similarly, reducing PVL and conduction abnormalities may be of high importance in younger patients to reduce the need for prolonged pacemaker implantation, and the subsequent long-term complications it may cause.

TECHNICAL CONSIDERATIONS
Valve-In-Valve

As mortality decreases and life expectancy increases in patients who receive SAVRs, more surgically implanted bioprostheses will require reintervention for SVD. Valve-in-valve transcatheter aortic valve replacement (ViV TAVR) has become an alternative to reoperative surgery, currently approved for high-risk and inoperable patients, and is proving to be superior to reoperative SAVR in certain patient populations.[36] Challenges to the technique include higher rates of prosthesis-patient mismatch and coronary obstruction compared with native valve TAVR.[37] Self-expanding TAVR devices may be favorable in patients with small surgical valves (21 mm or less). The supra-annular design helps increase the EOA and leads to a lower rate of PPM with SEV compared to BEV.[38,39] Balloon fracture of the bioprosthetic valve is possible in some surgical valves (eg, Medtronic Mosaic, Edwards Lifesciences Perimount, Magna, Sorin Mitroflow) using a high-pressure balloon to further increase the EOA and facilitate valve-in-valve TAVR.[20] Careful pre-procedure planning, valve selection, and deployment can help to avoid potentially fatal complications. Commissural alignment, pre-emptive coronary protection or Bioprosthetic or Native Aortic Scallop Intentional Laceration to Prevent Iatrogenic Coronary Artery Obstruction during TAVR (BASILICA) are all techniques to consider to maximize procedural success and patient safety.[40,41]

Bicuspid Aortic Valves

Bicuspid aortic valves (BAV) are the most common congenital heart defect, occurring in approximately 0.5% to 2.0% of the general population.[2,20] BAVs are often associated with large, asymmetric annuli, dilated and asymmetric aortic roots, and high degrees of calcification,[27] all of which make any intervention more challenging and lead to poor outcomes. BAV patients have an increased risk of PVL, malposition and embolization due to distorted root anatomy, and an increased risk of annular rupture.[27] In this population, an SEV prosthesis might be preferable to a BEV because of its ability to be retrieved and repositioned, which can reduce the risk of migration or embolization. SEVs are also better able to conform to asymmetric valve orifices, which will decrease the risk and degree of PVL. They are also less likely to cause annular rupture than BEV.[25,26]

Post-Transcatheter Aortic Valve Replacement Coronary Access

The prevalence of coronary artery disease in patients with severe AS enrolled in TAVR trials ranges from 40% to 75%. In previous studies, between 1.9% and 5.7% of aortic valve replacement (TAVR or SAVR) patients required PCI post-TAVR.[42] Patient (aortic root dimensions, leaflet length and thickness, and coronary ostial height) procedural factors (orientation of commissural tab, height of sealing skirt, and depth of valve implantation) make post-TAVR coronary reaccess more difficult.[43] SEVs, with a taller frame that extends over the coronary ostia, make for more challenging coronary engagement after implantation of THV. Notably, the smallest cell on SEVs can accommodate a 10 Fr catheter, which is much larger than standard coronary diagnostic and guide catheters. See **Fig. 2**: Evolut TAVR Frame Cell for Coronary Access. Even so, per the literature, the need to reaccess the coronaries occurs infrequently, and is usually due to a prosthetic commissural after overlapping the native coronary ostium.[35,44] During implantation, attempting to orientation the valve with the native commissural alignment may help to facilitate future coronary engagement.[45–47] Thus, for most TAVR patients, the risk of a future failed PCI attempt is low and may not be as important as other, more acute procedural concerns.[35]

COMPLICATIONS

As more and more TAVR are implanted, and their outcomes compared to SAVR, some

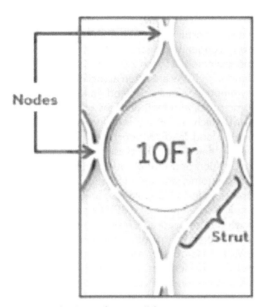

Fig. 2. Evolut TAVR frame cell for coronary access.

similarities and differences in the frequency and type of complications have emerged. The five most-feared complications that have been shown to have the most significant impact on subsequent quality of life are cerebrovascular accidents (CVA), conduction disturbances leading to a need for a permanent pacemaker, valve regurgitation, vascular complications including bleeding, acute kidney injury, and valve regurgitation or leak.[48] Other, more rare complications include annular rupture, coronary obstruction, myocardial infarction, valve malpositioning or migration, left ventricular perforation, cardiac tamponade, need for surgery, infection, hypotension, and death.

Cerebrovascular Events

CVA after TAVR procedures can be serious complications with devastating long-lasting effects. The mechanism is suspected to be multifactorial: due to a combination of intraprocedural hemodynamic instability, thrombosis, bleeding complications, and/or embolic debris showered from the native aortic valve during deployment. Although TAVR procedures have a lower rate of stroke than SAVR, this was not found to be statistically significant. Overall stroke rates for TAVR hover around 2%, without a significant difference between BEVs and SEVs.[49] Initial rates of transient ischemic attack or stroke with the first-generation CoreValve were estimated to be 3.82%. With the newer generation of SEV, this rate has marginally but statistically significantly decreased to 2.36%.[14] Current studies into

additional methods to more dramatically reduce this complication are underway, including ones investigating the efficacy of cerebral protection devices and improved antiplatelet and anticoagulation strategies both periprocedure and postprocedure.[48]

Conduction Abnormalities

Conduction abnormalities like left bundle branch block (LBBB) and/or high-grade atrioventricular block are the most common complication of TAVR. These develop post-TAVR due to trauma by catheters and/or guidewires, mechanical compression of the atrioventricular conduction system or extension of the valve frame into the LVOT.[50,51] A subsequent need for PPI has been shown to prolong hospital length of stay, increase procedural cost, cause LV dysfunction, and portend a poor outcome.[52] Initial rates of PPI in early studies were around 10%; however, most TAVRs were BEV at that time.[51] Conduction abnormalities and need for PPI are more common in SEV than BEV because of the continued radial force exhibited in nitinol self-expanding frames postdeployment and longer stent frame, which leads to the increased depth of deployment.[53] When comparing all studies using the first-generation CoreValve, data suggest an early PPI rate as high as 25%. With the introduction of the newer generation of SEV and improved operator techniques, that number has reverted to ~10% to 14%.[14,51] In an effort to minimize the risk of conduction abnormalities, low valve implantation should be avoided, as it has been directly correlated with PPI.[32,54] Similarly, valve oversizing has been shown to have a direct correlation with increased risk of LBBB and increased mortality.[53,55] Future modifications in SEV design and procedural mechanics will continue to focus on reducing the incidence of conduction abnormalities after SEV TAVR.

Aortic Regurgitation and Paravalvular Leak

Postprocedural aortic regurgitation, due to the residual gap between the annulus, native valve leaflets, and TAVR stent frame, is an important complication that is associated with increased mortality.[56] It is more common in TAVR than SAVR,[5,6,10,15,16,57] and more specifically in SEVs over BEVs, presumably due to their supra-annular location and method of deployment.[14,49] Moderate and severe aortic regurgitation (including PVL) assessed 30 days after self-expanding TAVR occurred in 8.0% of patients in the early, high-risk studies with CoreValve, but has decreased to 1.9% to 3.5% in the moderate-lower risk patient with the newer generation of SEV (Evolut R and Evolut Pro).[11,12,57,58] Mild PVL after TAVR is generally considered clinically benign, and rates have not significantly changed between studies comparing the different generation of SEVs.[56,58] Trials of the most recent generations of SEV, with the outer pericardial wrap, are ongoing to evaluate its efficacy at reducing the incidence of clinically significant PVL.

Bleeding/Vascular Complications

Although TAVR has been shown to have significantly higher rates of vascular injury than SAVR, it has lower rates of major bleeding. In early trials with first-generation valves, life-threatening bleeding rates were 16% and major vascular complications 12%.[59] The smaller delivery sheath profile of early generations of SEV allowed for smaller arteriotomies and translated to fewer bleeding and vascular complications than BEV.[28] As the sheath sizes became more comparable, so did the vascular and bleeding complication rates.[14] Interestingly, recent data have shown that the routine, successful use of closure devices has significantly decreased the rate of vascular complications, bleeding, and AKI.[60]

Annular Rupture

Annular rupture is a rare complication, occurring in 0.5% to 1% of all TAVR procedures.[26] It accounts for 7% of cases that require conversion to open surgical procedure. It carries a high mortality rate ranging from 45% to 78% of cases depending on the nature of the rupture and timing of identification.[25] Unless postdeployment balloon dilation is performed, SEVs have extremely low association with annular rupture. Thus, SEVs are preferable in cases with a high-risk LVOT calcification pattern, bicuspid anatomy, and shallow sinuses of Valsalva, as those cases carry a higher risk of annular rupture if BEVs are used.[20,26,49]

Coronary Obstruction

Coronary artery obstruction, caused by displacement of the bulky native aortic valve leaflets toward the sinotubular junction, sealing off the coronary sinuses and obstructing one or both coronary ostia, complicates TAVR less than 1% of the time but carries a 40% to 50% 30-day mortality rate if it occurs acutely.[14,61,62] This complication is more likely during valve-in-valve procedures or in patients with low coronary height (<8 mm), short sinuses of Valsalva (<15 mm), effaced sinuses of Valsalva, or excessive calcification.[26] In patients at high risk, due to low coronaries or prior TAVR, use of an SEV can further complicate future coronary access and therefore may be avoided.[20] Certain techniques like pre-emptive wiring, ostial stenting, stenting with large protrusion, and BASILICA leaflet laceration can be used before valve deployment in patients at high risk of coronary obstruction to protect the coronary ostia.[40,41]

DURABILITY—STRUCTURAL VALVE DETERIORATION AND BIOPROSTHETIC VALVE FAILURE

Compared to surgical valves, which have been around for decades, THVs have only been widely available since 2007, so robust long-term durability data on THV is still forthcoming. As younger, more low-risk patients receive TAVR, long-term durability of these valves becomes more important. The physical and physiologic differences between surgical and transcatheter valves could correlate to significant differences in the need for repeat valve intervention.

Structurally, TAVR leaflets are thinner (~0.25 mm in THVs vs ~ 0.4 mm in surgical BHVs) and are exposed to higher stress and strains than surgical BHVs, particularly in the presence of native aortic annular calcification or nonround and asymmetric annuli.[63] The valve and leaflets also undergo a crimping and folding process to allow for delivery, which may have an effect on the overall durability and function of the valve.[64] Owing to these differences, it was initially feared that up to half of all TAVR patients who survive for 5 years would have SVD by 10 years after implantation.

Previously, comparing durability between studies of SAVR and TAVR had been difficult because of the speed and frequency of release of new generations of THV with significant design modifications. Durability data on older models were still being collected, even as new and improved models were being released.[20] Furthermore, heterogeneity of criteria for SVD between professional societies made comparison and analysis between studies nearly impossible.

In 2017, EAPCI/ESC/EACTS proposed a uniform consensus definition of SVD and bioprosthetic valve failure (BVF) to allow more cross-study comparisons. Hemodynamic SVD, changes in valve function, assessed by echocardiography, was stratified into two severities: Severe SVD was defined as a mean gradient $\geq$40 mm Hg or a change in gradient $\geq$20 mm Hg or new severe AR. Moderate SVD was defined as an AV gradient $\geq$20 mm Hg but less than 40 mm Hg, a change in mean gradient from discharge or 1 month of $\geq$10 mm Hg but less than 20 mm Hg or moderate new central AR. BVF was defined as the composite of the following[1]: development of severe SVD[2]; need for repeat intervention for bioprosthetic valve dysfunction; and/or[3] valve-related death.[65]

Several recent studies have accepted these definitions to compare the durability of TAVR to SAVR, and then further compare SEV to BEV. Surgical aortic bioprostheses have generally exhibited a 10-year incidence of valvular failure between 10% and 40%. SVD requiring reoperation occurs in between 6% and 47% of patients, usually 12 to 20 years after surgical implantation. At 5 years, the incidence of structural failure is less than 5% and freedom from reoperation is greater than 95%.[66] Using the new definition of SVD, a weighted metanalysis of durability studies shows an incidence of severe SVD in THV of 1.3% at 5 to 8 years, and of BVF of 4.6% at 6 to 8 years. When specifically studying SEV, in high-risk patients, the incidence of moderate-severe SVD was 9.5% in TAVR and 26.6% in SAVR, predominantly drive by elevated mean gradients.[9] In low-risk patients, there was a similar pattern of moderate-severe SVD through 6 years, 24.0% in SAVR versus 4.8% in TAVR, which may be due to a higher incidence of PPM in the SAVR group.[67,68]

In the CHOICE Study, comparing durability between the two types of THVs, moderate to severe SVD was more frequent in those who received BEV (6.6%) compared to 0% in SEV patients, presumably because of their worse hemodynamic properties. The supra-annular design of the SEVs consistently sustains large EOAs and low mean gradients, which positively correlate to sustained durability and low rates of SVD, at least 6 to 8 years postimplantation.[22,38,69]

Most studies following patients after receiving THVs are currently limited to 8 to 9 years, so further data are needed to fully understand the durability of TAVR compared to SAVR. However, these initial findings dispelled fears of significantly higher SVD in THV and established optimism that THVs could match, and potentially exceed, durability of surgical valves.

SUMMARY

Self-expanding THVs have proven to be an excellent option for patients with severe AS, regardless of surgical risk. Compared with SAVR, in terms of overall mortality, quality of life and valve durability, TAVR with SEV compares favorably in most patient populations.

The journey of SEV from initial prototype to current model has included several modifications that correlate to improved clinical outcomes across the board, and future studies will continue to find ways to minimize risk and improve success in SEV TAVR.

VIDEO LOOPS FOR ONLINE

Live case of implantation
Animation of valve function
Animation of implantation

DISCLOSURE

Dr P.M. Grossman: Research support from Medtronic Cardiovascular and Edwards Lifesciences. Physician proctor for Medtronic TAVR and Edwards TAVR.

SUPPLEMENTARY DATA

Supplementary data related to this article can be found online at https://doi.org/10.1016/j.iccl.2021.06.004.

REFERENCES

1. Thaden JJ, Nkomo VT, Enriquez-Sarano M. The global burden of aortic stenosis. Prog Cardiovasc Dis 2014;56(6):565–71.
2. Otto CM, Prendergast B. Aortic-valve stenosis–from patients at risk to severe valve obstruction. N Engl J Med 2014;371(8):744–56.
3. Kapadia S, Stewart WJ, Anderson WN, et al. Outcomes of Inoperable Symptomatic Aortic Stenosis Patients Not Undergoing Aortic Valve Replacement: Insight Into the Impact of Balloon Aortic Valvuloplasty From the PARTNER Trial (Placement of AoRtic TraNscathetER Valve Trial). JACC Cardiovasc Interv 2015;8(2):324–33.
4. Cribier A, Eltchaninoff H, Bash A. Percutaneous transcatheter implantation of an aortic valve prosthesis for calcific aortic stenosis. ACC Curr J Rev 2003;12(2):95.
5. Leon MB, Smith CR, Mack M, et al. Transcatheter aortic-valve implantation for aortic stenosis in patients who cannot undergo surgery. N Engl J Med 2010;363(17):1597–607.
6. Smith CR, Leon MB, Mack MJ, et al. Transcatheter versus surgical aortic-valve replacement in high-risk patients. N Engl J Med 2011;364(23):2187–98.
7. O'Brien SM, Shahian DM, Filardo G, et al. The Society of Thoracic Surgeons 2008 cardiac surgery risk models: part 2–isolated valve surgery. Ann Thorac Surg 2009;88(1 Suppl):S23–42.
8. Barker CM, Reardon MJ. The CoreValve US pivotal trial. Semin Thorac Cardiovasc Surg 2014;26(3):179–86.

9. Gleason TG, Reardon MJ, Popma JJ, et al. 5-Year Outcomes of Self-Expanding Transcatheter Versus Surgical Aortic Valve Replacement in High-Risk Patients. J Am Coll Cardiol 2018;72(22):2687–96.
10. Leon MB, Smith CR, Mack MJ, et al. Transcatheter or Surgical Aortic-Valve Replacement in Intermediate-Risk Patients. N Engl J Med 2016; 374(17):1609–20.
11. Søndergaard L, Popma JJ, Reardon MJ, et al. Comparison of a Complete Percutaneous versus Surgical Approach to Aortic Valve Replacement and Revascularization in Patients at Intermediate Surgical Risk: Results from the Randomized SURTAVI Trial. Circulation 2019. https://doi.org/10.1161/CIRCULATIONAHA.118.039564.
12. Yakubov SJ, Van Mieghem NM, Reardon MJ, et al. Propensity-matched comparison of evolut-r transcatheter aortic valve implantation with surgery in intermediate-risk patients (from the SURTAVI Trial). Am J Cardiol 2020;131:82–90.
13. Choudhury T, Solomonica A, Bagur R. The Evolut R and Evolut PRO transcatheter aortic valve systems. Expert Rev Med Devices 2019;16(1):3–9.
14. Winter MP, Bartko P, Hofer F, et al. Evolution of outcome and complications in TAVR: a meta-analysis of observational and randomized studies. Sci Rep 2020;10(1):15568.
15. Popma JJ, Deeb GM, Yakubov SJ, et al. Transcatheter aortic-valve replacement with a self-expanding valve in low-risk patients. N Engl J Med 2019; 380(18):1706–15.
16. Mack MJ, Leon MB, Thourani VH, et al. Transcatheter aortic-valve replacement with a balloon-expandable valve in low-risk patients. N Engl J Med 2019;380(18):1695–705.
17. Bruschi G, De Marco F, Martinelli L, et al. CoreValve-transcatheter self-expandable aortic bioprosthesis. Expert Rev Med Devices 2013;10(1):15–26.
18. Páez JMG, Carrera A, Herrero EJ, et al. Influence of the selection of the suture material on the mechanical behavior of a biomaterial to be employed in the construction of implants. Part 2: Porcine pericardium. J Biomater Appl 2001;16(1):68–90.
19. Mahtta D, Elgendy IY, Bavry AA. From CoreValve to Evolut PRO: Reviewing the Journey of Self-Expanding Transcatheter Aortic Valves. Cardiol Ther 2017;6(2):183–92.
20. Claessen BE, Tang GHL, Kini AS, et al. Considerations for optimal device selection in transcatheter aortic valve replacement: a review. JAMA Cardiol 2021;6:102–12.
21. Abdel-Wahab M, Mehilli J, Frerker C, et al. Comparison of balloon-expandable vs self-expandable valves in patients undergoing transcatheter aortic valve replacement: the CHOICE randomized clinical trial. JAMA 2014;311(15):1503–14.
22. Abdel-Wahab M, Landt M, Neumann FJ, et al. 5-Year Outcomes After TAVR With Balloon-Expandable Versus Self-Expanding Valves: Results From the CHOICE Randomized Clinical Trial. JACC Cardiovasc Interv 2020;13(9):1071–82.
23. Abdelghani M, Allali A, Kaur J, et al. Impact of prosthesis-iteration evolution and sizing practice on the incidence of prosthesis-patient mismatch after transcatheter aortic valve replacement. Catheter Cardiovasc Interv 2019;93(5):971–9.
24. Hahn RT, Leipsic J, Douglas PS, et al. Comprehensive Echocardiographic Assessment of Normal Transcatheter Valve Function. JACC: Cardiovasc Imaging 2019;12(1):25–34.
25. Pasic M, Unbehaun A, Buz S, et al. Annular Rupture During Transcatheter Aortic Valve Replacement. JACC: Cardiovasc Interventions 2015;8(1):1–9.
26. Barbanti B. Avoiding Coronary Occlusion and Root Rupture in TAVI - the role of pre-procedural imaging and prosthesis selection. Interv Cardiol 2015;10(2):94–7.
27. Saad M, Seoudy H, Frank D. Challenging Anatomies for TAVR-Bicuspid and Beyond. Front Cardiovasc Med 2021;8:654554.
28. Barbanti M, Binder RK, Freeman M, et al. Impact of low-profile sheaths on vascular complications during transfemoral transcatheter aortic valve replacement. EuroIntervention 2013;9(8):929–35.
29. Abramowitz Y, Maeno Y, Chakravarty T, et al. Aortic angulation attenuates procedural success following self-expandable but not balloon-expandable TAVR. JACC Cardiovasc Imaging 2016;9(8):964–72.
30. Popma JJ, Reardon MJ, Yakubov SJ, et al. Safety and Efficacy of Self-Expanding TAVR in Patients With Aortoventricular Angulation. JACC: Cardiovasc Imaging 2016;9(8):973–81.
31. Veulemans V, Maier O, Bosbach G, et al. Novel insights on outcome in horizontal aorta with self-expandable new-generation transcatheter aortic valve replacement devices. Catheter Cardiovasc Interv 2020;96(7):1511–9.
32. van Rosendael PJ, Delgado V, Bax JJ. Pacemaker implantation rate after transcatheter aortic valve implantation with early and new-generation devices: a systematic review. Eur Heart J 2018;39(21):2003–13.
33. Ben-Shoshan J, Alosaimi H, Lauzier PT, et al. Double S-Curve Versus Cusp-Overlap Technique. JACC: Cardiovasc Interventions 2021;14(2):185–94.
34. Barbanti M, Costa G, Picci A, et al. Coronary cannulation after transcatheter aortic valve replacement: the RE-ACCESS study. JACC Cardiovasc Interv 2020;13(21):2542–55.
35. Diaz MA, Patton M, Valdes P, et al. A systematic review and meta-analysis of delayed coronary artery access for coronary angiography with or without

percutaneous coronary intervention (PCI) in patients who underwent transcatheter aortic valve replacement (TAVR). Cardiovasc Interv Ther 2021. https://doi.org/10.1007/s12928-020-00753-4.

36. Ahmed A, Levy KH. Valve-in-valve transcatheter aortic valve replacement versus redo surgical aortic valve replacement: A systematic review and meta-analysis. J Card Surg 2021;36(7):2486–95.

37. Edelman JJ, Khan JM, Rogers T, et al. Valve-in-Valve TAVR: State-of-the-Art Review. Innovations 2019;14(4):299–310.

38. Rogers T, Steinvil A, Gai J, et al. Choice of balloon-expandable versus self-expanding transcatheter aortic valve impacts hemodynamics differently according to aortic annular size. Am J Cardiol 2017; 119(6):900–4.

39. Sengupta A, Zaid S, Ahmad H, et al. Prosthesis-patient mismatch between transcatheter heart valves in TAVR using a computed tomography-derived comparative model. JACC Cardiovasc Interv 2020; 13(6):790–2.

40. Khan JM, Greenbaum AB, Babaliaros VC, et al. The BASILICA Trial: Prospective Multicenter Investigation of Intentional Leaflet Laceration to Prevent TAVR Coronary Obstruction. JACC Cardiovasc Interv 2019;12(13):1240–52.

41. Lederman RJ, Babaliaros VC, Rogers T, et al. Preventing coronary obstruction during transcatheter aortic valve replacement: from computed tomography to BASILICA. JACC Cardiovasc Interv 2019; 12(13):1197–216.

42. Goel SS, Ige M, Tuzcu EM, et al. Severe aortic stenosis and coronary artery disease-implications for management in the transcatheter aortic valve replacement era. J Am Coll Cardiol 2013;62(1):1–10.

43. Yudi MB, Sharma SK, Tang GHL, et al. Coronary angiography and percutaneous coronary intervention after transcatheter aortic valve replacement. J Am Coll Cardiol 2018;71(12):1360–78.

44. Abdelghani M, Landt M, Traboulsi H, et al. Coronary access after TAVR with a self-expanding bioprosthesis. JACC: Cardiovasc Interventions 2020; 13(6):709–22.

45. Alexis SL, Zaid S, Sengupta A, et al. Transcatheter aortic valve replacement aortic root orientation: implications for future coronary access and redo transcatheter aortic valve replacement. Ann Cardiothorac Surg 2020;9(6):502–4.

46. Tang GHL, Zaid S, Gupta E, et al. Impact of initial evolut transcatheter aortic valve replacement deployment orientation on final valve orientation and coronary reaccess. Circ Cardiovasc Interv 2019;12:e008044.

47. Tang GHL, Zaid S, Fuchs A, et al. Alignment of Transcatheter Aortic-Valve Neo-Commissures (ALIGN TAVR): Impact on Final Valve Orientation and Coronary Artery Overlap. JACC Cardiovasc Interv 2020;13(9):1030–42.

48. Grube E, Sinning J-M. The "big five" complications after transcatheter aortic valve replacement. JACC: Cardiovasc Interventions 2019;12(4):370–2.

49. Scarsini R, De Maria GL, Joseph J, et al. Impact of complications during transfemoral transcatheter aortic valve replacement: how can they be avoided and managed? J Am Heart Assoc 2019;8:e013801.

50. Khatri PJ, Webb JG, Rodés-Cabau J, et al. Adverse Effects Associated With Transcatheter Aortic Valve Implantation. Ann Intern Med 2013;158(1):35–46.

51. Carroll JD, Mack MJ, Vemulapalli S, et al. STS-ACC TVT Registry of Transcatheter Aortic Valve Replacement. Ann Thorac Surg 2021;111(2):701–22.

52. Buellesfeld L, Stortecky S, Heg D, et al. Impact of permanent pacemaker implantation on clinical outcome among patients undergoing transcatheter aortic valve implantation. J Am Coll Cardiol 2012; 60(6):493–501.

53. van der Boon RM, Nuis RJ, Van Mieghem NM, et al. New conduction abnormalities after TAVI–frequency and causes. Nat Rev Cardiol 2012;9(8):454–63.

54. Guetta V, Goldenberg G, Segev A, et al. Predictors and course of high-degree atrioventricular block after transcatheter aortic valve implantation using the CoreValve Revalving System. Am J Cardiol 2011; 108(11):1600–5.

55. Regueiro A, Abdul-Jawad Altisent O, Del Trigo M, et al. Impact of New-Onset Left Bundle Branch Block and Periprocedural Permanent Pacemaker Implantation on Clinical Outcomes in Patients Undergoing Transcatheter Aortic Valve Replacement: A Systematic Review and Meta-Analysis. Circ Cardiovasc Interv 2016;9(5):e003635.

56. Sinning JM, Hammerstingl C, Vasa-Nicotera M, et al. Aortic regurgitation index defines severity of peri-prosthetic regurgitation and predicts outcome in patients after transcatheter aortic valve implantation. J Am Coll Cardiol 2012;59(13):1134–41.

57. Reardon MJ, Van Mieghem NM, Popma JJ, et al. Surgical or Transcatheter Aortic-Valve Replacement in Intermediate-Risk Patients. N Engl J Med 2017;376(14):1321–31.

58. Grube E, Van Mieghem NM, Bleiziffer S, et al. Clinical Outcomes With a Repositionable Self-Expanding Transcatheter Aortic Valve Prosthesis: The International FORWARD Study. J Am Coll Cardiol 2017;70(7):845–53.

59. Généreux P, Head SJ, Van Mieghem NM, et al. Clinical outcomes after transcatheter aortic valve replacement using valve academic research consortium definitions. J Am Coll Cardiol 2012;59(25): 2317–26.

60. Power D, Schäfer U, Guedeney P, et al. Impact of percutaneous closure device type on vascular and

bleeding complications after TAVR: A post hoc analysis from the BRAVO-3 randomized trial. Catheter Cardiovasc Interv 2019;93(7):1374–81.

61. Jabbour RJ, Tanaka A, Finkelstein A, et al. Delayed Coronary Obstruction After Transcatheter Aortic Valve Replacement. J Am Coll Cardiol 2018; 71(14):1513–24.

62. Ribeiro HB, Webb JG, Makkar RR, et al. Predictive factors, management, and clinical outcomes of coronary obstruction following transcatheter aortic valve implantation: insights from a large multicenter registry. J Am Coll Cardiol 2013;62(17):1552–62.

63. Kostyunin AE, Yuzhalin AE, Rezvova MA, et al. Degeneration of Bioprosthetic Heart Valves: Update 2020. J Am Heart Assoc 2020;9:e018506.

64. Petronio AS, Giannini C. Developments in transcatheter aortic bioprosthesis durability. Expert Rev Cardiovasc Ther 2019;17(12):857–62.

65. Capodanno D, Petronio AS, Prendergast B, et al. Standardized definitions of structural deterioration and valve failure in assessing long-term durability of transcatheter and surgical aortic bioprosthetic valves: a consensus statement from the European Association of Percutaneous Cardiovascular Interventions (EAPCI) endorsed by the European Society of Cardiology (ESC) and the European Association for Cardio-Thoracic Surgery (EACTS). Eur Heart J 2017; 38(45):3382–90.

66. Barbanti M, Costa G, Zappulla P, et al. Incidence of Long-Term Structural Valve Dysfunction and Bioprosthetic Valve Failure After Transcatheter Aortic Valve Replacement. J Am Heart Assoc 2018;7: e008440.

67. Søndergaard L, Ihlemann N, Capodanno D, et al. Durability of transcatheter and surgical bioprosthetic aortic valves in patients at lower surgical risk. J Am Coll Cardiol 2019;73:546–53.

68. Thyregod HGH, Ihlemann N, Jørgensen TH, et al. Five-Year Clinical and Echocardiographic Outcomes from the Nordic Aortic Valve Intervention (NOTION) Randomized Clinical Trial in Lower Surgical Risk Patients. Circulation 2019. https://doi.org/10.1161/CIRCULATIONAHA.11 8.036606.

69. Barbanti M, Immè S, Ohno Y, et al. Prosthesis choice for transcatheter aortic valve replacement: Improved outcomes with the adoption of a patient-specific transcatheter heart valve selection algorithm. Int J Cardiol 2016;203:1009–10.

Conduction Disturbances and Pacing in Transcatheter Aortic Valve Replacement

Makoto Nakashima, MD, Hasan Jilaihawi, MD*

KEYWORDS

- Aortic stenosis • Transcatheter aortic valve replacement • Permanent pacemaker
- Conduction disturbances • Complete heart block • Membranous septum length
- Minimizing depth according to the membranous septum (MIDAS) approach • Cusp-overlap view

KEY POINTS

- Transcatheter aortic valve replacement (TAVR) is a rapidly emerging less invasive procedure for treatment of patients with aortic stenosis; however, postprocedural conduction disturbances are still a concern.
- A recent meta-analysis showed both new-onset left bundle branch block and new permanent pacemaker implantation were related to increased risk of all-cause mortality at 1 year after TAVR.
- Preprocedural computed tomography (CT) can highlight potential risk factors such as membranous septum length, device landing zone calcium, and the annulus size/degree of device oversizing.
- Preprocedural planning based on the CT findings is important to mitigate the risk of conduction disturbances after TAVR.

INTRODUCTION

The indications for transcatheter aortic valve replacement (TAVR) have been rapidly expanded to low–surgical risk patients with symptomatic severe aortic stenosis due to the improvement of TAVR devices and favorable trial results that compared TAVR with surgical aortic valve implantation (SAVR) in low–surgical risk patients.[1–5] However, the risk of permanent pacemaker implantation (PPMI) after TAVR was high at 6.7% to 38.0% compared with 2.4% to 8.9% for SAVR[1–6] (Table 1). The incidence of new PPMI can increase not only hospital cost and length of hospital stay but also the complications including traumatic, lead-related, pocket-related, generator problem and pacemaker-induced cardiomyopathy, which lead to the adverse long-term outcomes.[7–9]

The aim of this review article is to summarize the recent articles on the conduction disturbances (CDs), such as new high-degree atrioventricular block (HAVB)/complete heart block (CHB) that requires new PPMI and left bundle branch block (LBBB), and to clarify the incidences, predictors, and management of CDs high-risk patients.

THE MECHANISM OF CONDUCTION DISTURBANCES

In the SAVR procedure, conduction system injury can be caused by mechanical trauma associated with debriding the native valve and its annulus, deeply placed annular sutures, and placing a large bioprosthesis into a small aortic annulus. Fukuda and colleagues reported that the most common reason for conduction injury was

---

Heart Valve Center, NYU Langone Health, 530 1st Avenue, Suite 9V, New York, NY 10016, USA
* Corresponding author.
E-mail address: hasanjilaihawi@gmail.com

2211-7458/21/© 2021 Elsevier Inc. All rights reserved.

Table 1
The prevalence of new pacemaker implantation after procedure

Study, Year	At the Time of Evaluation	Patient Number (TAVR vs SAVR)	Pacemaker Rate (TAVR vs SAVR)
Leon et al,[1] 2016	1 y	1011 vs 1021	9.9% vs 8.9%
Reardon et al,[2] 2017	30 d	864 vs 796	25.9% vs 6.6%
Thyregod et al,[3] 2015	1 y	145 vs 135	38.0% vs 2.4%
Mack et al,[4] 2019	1 y	496 vs 454	7.5% vs 5.5%
Popma et al,[5] 2019	1 y	725 vs 678	19.4% vs 6.7%
Fadahunsi et al,[6] 2016	30 d	9785 (TAVR)	6.7% (TAVR)

Abbreviations: SAVR, surgical aortic valve replacement; TAVR, transcatheter aortic valve replacement.

traumatic injury from suture material as opposed to calcific infiltration or pressure from the prosthesis. In addition, the atrioventricular (AV) node and left bundle branch were the structures most commonly injured.[10,11] The mechanism of CDs after TAVR is also primarily caused by an injury to the conduction system with edema, hematoma, and ischemia related to the procedure with balloon, guidewire, and devices.[12] The AV node, located at the triangle of Koch, continues to the His bundle piercing the membranous septum (MS) and penetrating to the left ventricular bundle branch.[13–15] The left bundle branch run on the crest of the interventricular septum where the myocardial insulation is significantly less compared with the His bundle in the cardiac skeleton.[16] The left bundle branch and the interleaflet triangle, which separate the noncoronary and right coronary leaflets of the aortic valve, are closely related anatomically. Kawashima and Sasaki[17] reported that a so-called naked AV bundle passes within the MS in 21% of their investigated cases; this is in contrast to the typical path of the AV bundle that travels along the lower border of the MS in approximately 46.7% of cases and the AV bundle passing within the interventricular muscular septum in the remainder of patients. Both the naked AV bundle and shorter MS length, which may be measured by computed tomography (CT), may increase the risk of conduction system injury leading to new PPMI after TAVR.

PACEMAKER IMPLANTATION AFTER TRANSCATHETER AORTIC VALVE REPLACEMENT

The clinically important CDs after TAVR are HAVB/CHB and LBBB. In a recent meta-analysis, new-onset LBBB was observed more frequently in 22.7%.[18] Persistent CHB is the most frequent and standard cause of new PPMI. Most CDs usually occur immediately after or within 7 days after the procedure.[19,20] New PPMI between 30-days and 1-year after TAVR is not high at 1.9%.[21] Experts suggest at least 24- to 48-hour observation before device implant to determine reversibility from HABV/CHB. Bjerre and colleagues reported half of patients who seemed to have an absolute indication for PPMI showed resolution beyond the periprocedural period.[22]

A recent meta-analysis using 37 observational studies with 71,455 patients reported that overall incidence of PPMI after TAVR was 22%.[23] Three meta-analyses showed no significant association between periprocedural PPMI and the long-term outcomes.[24–26] On the other hand, a recent meta-analysis showed the increased risk of all-cause mortality with 21 studies (42,927) (relative risk [RR] 1.17, 95% confidence interval [CI] 1.11 to 1.25; $P<.001$; $I^2 = 21$%), however, no effect on cardiac death with 7 studies (RR 0.84, 95% CI 0.67–1.05; $P = .13$; $I^2 = 0$%).[18]

THE IMPACT OF LEFT BUNDLE BRANCH BROCK

The new-onset persistent LBBB is also a common conduction abnormality after TAVR. The presence of LBBB is a marker of poor long-term prognosis in the general population, especially in patients with cardiac disease.[27,28] The new-onset LBBB after TAVR arises a concern of HAVB/CHB, sudden cardiac death, or heart failure rehospitalization in the follow-up period. Notably, an injury to the left bundle branch with implanted prosthesis leads to complete AV block in patients with preexisting RBBB.

The incidence of new-onset LBBB has been investigated in many studies; however, there is a discordant about the impact on the mortality in each study.[29–40] Regueiro and colleagues showed an association between the new-onset

LBBB and cardiac death at 1 year using 5 pooled studies with 3554 patients with an RR of 1.39 (95% CI 1.04–1.86; P = .03; I^2 = 32%); however, they failed to show the increased risk of 1-year all-cause death using 8 studies with 4756 patients (RR, 1.21; 95% CI 0.98–1.50; P = .07; I^2 = 50%). The rate of new-onset LBBB at discharge ranged from 13.3% to 37%.[25] A larger meta-analysis recently published demonstrated an increased risk of all-cause death at 1 year in patients with new-onset LBBB (RR 1.32, 95% CI 1.17–1.49; P<.001; I^2 = 49%) from 12 studies (7792 patients) (Table 2). After pooling the results from 8 studies (5906 patients), the presence of new-onset LBBB post-TAVR was associated with a higher risk of 1-year cardiac death (RR 1.46, 95% CI 1.20–1.78; I^2 = 10%). Overall, 1-year all-cause death ranged from 6.3% to 27.8% and from 4.9% to 28.4% in patients with or without new-onset LBBB, respectively.[18]

The RR for 1-year heart failure hospitalization from 6 studies (3435 patients) was 1.35 (95% CI 1.05–1.72; P = .02; I^2 = 8%) in new-onset LBBB patients. The risk of new PPMI was also high at 1 year in new-onset LBBB patients (RR 1.89, 95% CI 1.58–2.27; P<.001; I^2 = 71%).[18]

RISK FACTORS FOR CONDUCTION DISTURBANCES AFTER TRANSCATHETER AORTIC VALVE REPLACEMENT

The type of self-expandable valve (SEV) has a significant effect on the incidence rate of PPMI. The rate of PPMI in SEV is 19.4% to 38.0%,[2,3,5] which is considerably higher compared with 4.3% to 9.9% for balloon-expandable valves (BEV)[1,4–6] (Table 3). Within the SEV devices, recent report showed Evolut R and PRO were associated with a tendency toward less PPMI compared with Corevalve in patients with conduction abnormalities (17% vs 19% vs 27%, P = .08) and lower PPMI in patients with normal conduction system (6% vs 11% vs 25%, P = .002).[41] A meta-analysis showed implantation of Medtronic SEV was associated with a 3.47-fold increased risk of new PPMI compared with BEV (odds ratio [OR] 3.47, 95% CI 1.75 to 6.88; P<.01; I^2 = 96%).[23] The Portico system trials also showed a relatively high PPMI rate at 15.4% to 27.7%.[42–44] Although it has been recently withdrawn for a delivery system issue, the new PPMI rate of the mechanically expanding LOTUS valve was very high at 22.5% to 41.7%.[41,44,45]

Mahajan and colleagues[23] revealed the demographic risk factors of new PPMI after TAVR in their meta-analysis, which include increased age (OR 1.15, 95% CI 1.01–1.32; P = .04; I^2 = 89%), diabetes mellitus (OR 1.08, 95% CI 1.03–1.11; P<.01; I^2 = 0%), and male gender (OR 1.29, 95% CI 1.23–1.35; P≤.01; I^2 = 0%) (Table 4). The risk factors for new PPMI regarding electrocardiography were presence of RBBB (OR 5.62, 95% CI 3.9–8.10; P<.01; I^2 = 82%), baseline AV block (OR 1.75, 95% CI 1.08–2.84; P = .02; I^2 = 91%), and left anterior fascicular block (OR 1.88, 95% CI 1.14–3.11; P = .01; I^2 = 7%). Regarding imaging and procedures, presence of high calcium volume extending into left ventricular outflow tract in the area below the left coronary cusp (LCC) (OR 4.21, 95% CI 1.90–9.31; P<.01; I^2 = 0%) and noncoronary cusp (NCC) (OR 3.15, 95% CI 1.26–7.88; P = .01; I^2 = 89%) were identified predictors for new PPMI. The device implantation depth (ID) (OR 1.24, 95% CI 1.11–1.40; P<.01; I^2 = 85%) and increased valve size/annulus size were also related to the increased risk (OR 1.14, 95% CI 1.02–1.27; P = .02; I^2 = 80%). Both predilatation and postimplant balloon dilation were identified as significant predictors with OR 2.32 (95% CI 1.56–3.44; P<.01; I^2 = 47%) and 1.76 (95% CI 1.10–2.82; P = .02; I^2 = 15%), respectively. Presence of postprocedural AVB was an important predictor (OR 3.08, 95% CI 1.34–7.10; P<.01; I^2 = 90%). There was no increased risk observed for patients with hypertension, chronic obstructive pulmonary disease, prior aortic valve procedure, prior percutaneous coronary intervention, logistic EuroSCORE, atrial fibrillation, LBBB, baseline interventricular conduction delay or change in QRS duration following procedure, presence of high calcium in the area below the right coronary cusp (RCC), or interventricular septal dimension.

Some studies investigated outcomes at 2-year follow-up and reported that new-onset LBBB was an independent predictor of all-cause mortality,[34,36,46] cardiovascular mortality, rehospitalization, and new PPMI.[34]

MEMBRANOUS SEPTUM ASSESSMENT IN PREPROCEDURAL COMPUTED TOMOGRAPHY

As mentioned earlier, short MS length may increase the risk of conduction system injury during the TAVR procedure. The MS length, measured by CT determining the thinnest part of interventricular septum, is also reported as an independent predictor of new CDs after TAVR for both SEV and BEV in several recent studies.[16,47–50] Given that implantation depth is modifiable, the combination of small MS length

Table 2
Prognostic implications of new-onset left bundle branch block

	New-onset LBBB, N	No New-onset LBBB, N	Risk Ratio
All-cause death	1770	6022	1.32
Cardiac death	1191	4715	1.46
Heart failure hospitalization	866	2569	1.35
Permanent pacemaker implantation	1363	5036	1.89

Abbreviations: LBBB, left bundle branch block; N, number.

and deep device implantation (MS length minus ID [ΔMSID]) has strong predictability for new PPMI after TAVR.[47,48,51]

There are 2 different methods currently used for measuring MS length: the coronal MS length and infraannular MS length (Fig. 1). The area under the curve of coronal ΔMSID and infraannular ΔMSID for predicting the occurrence of new PPMI or new LBBB within 30 days after TAVR were comparable (0.717 in coronal ΔMSID vs 0.708 in infraannular ΔMSID; $P = .761$). Although the cutoff value was larger in coronal-annular ΔMSID (3.2 mm) than infraannular ΔMSID (−0.2 mm), the correlation coefficient between coronal ΔMSID and infraannular ΔMSID was strong ($\rho = 0.834$; $P<.001$).[51] Caution must be taken for which measurement method used,

and further larger studies are required to evaluate the 2 methods.

The presence of calcium in the device landing zone is also reported as an independent risk of AV CDs in some reports.[48,52,53] This calcium distribution should also be taken into account in the preprocedural assessment.

MANAGEMENT OF PATIENTS AT HIGH ESTIMATED RISK OF PACEMAKER

Because new CDs were related to the adverse events such as all-cause mortality and heart failure hospitalization in the long-term, efforts to avoid those should be maximized as much as possible. Before the publication of Minimizing Depth According to the Membranous Septum (MIDAS)

Table 3
The incidences of new permanent pacemaker rate by device type after transcatheter artic replacement

Study	Device	Pacemaker Rate (%)
Reardon et al,[2] 2017	CoreValve/Evolut R	25.9
Thyregod et al,[3] 2015	CoreValve	38.0
Popma et al,[5] 2019	Medtronic CoreValve Revalving System	19.4
Kroon et al,[41] 2021	CoreValve/Evolut R/Evolut PRO[a]	27/17/19
Kroon et al,[41] 2021	CoreValve/Evolut R/Evolut PRO[b]	25/6/11
Fadahunsi et al,[6] 2016	Medtronic CoreValve Revalving System	25.1
Fadahunsi et al,[6] 2016	Edwards SAPIEN valve	4.3
Leon et al,[1] 2016	SAPIEN XT	9.9
Mack et al,[4] 2019	SAPIEN 3	7.5
Makkar et al,[42] 2020	Portico	27.7
Fontana et al,[43] 2020	Portico	15.4
Reardon et al,[44] 2019	LOTUS	41.7
Saito et al,[45] 2020	LOTUS	22.5

Abbreviation: TAVR, transcatheter aortic valve replacement.
[a] In patients with conduction abnormalities.
[b] In patients with normal conduction system.

Table 4
Risk factors for permanent pacemaker implantation after transcatheter aortic valve replacement

Demographic and Electrocardiographic Predictors	Odd Ratio
Age	1.15
Diabetes mellitus	1.08
Male gender	1.29
Preexisting RBBB	5.62
Preexisting LAFB	1.88
Preexisting atrioventricular block	1.75
Imaging predictors	
High LVOT calcium volume below LCC	4.21
High LVOT calcium volume below NCC	3.15
Short MS length	11.73[47]
Procedural predictors	
Self-expandable valve/mechanical valve implantation	3.47
Deep implantation depth in relation to MS length	1.24
Increase in valve size/annulus size ratio	1.14
Predilation and postimplant balloon	2.32
Postprocedure AVB	3.08

Abbreviations: AVB, atrioventricular block; LAFB, left anterior fascicular block; LCC, left coronary cusp; LVOT, left ventricular outflow tract; MS, membranous septum; NCC, noncoronary cusp; RBBB, right bundle branch block.

paper, the standardized approach for SEV was to implant in line with instructions for use of the device (3–5 mm), aiming for the higher range of the instructions for use (3–4 mm) in relation to the NCC and recapturing and repositioning the device when the device initially landed considerably lower than this target. The MIDAS approach, in which operators attempted to position the prosthesis at a prerelease depth in relation to the NCC of length smaller than that of the MS, significantly reduced the rate of new PPMI (3.0% vs 9.7%, P = .035) and new LBBB (9.0% vs 25.8%, P<.001) without valve embolization or a need of second valve.[47] A coplanar projection by overlapping the RCC and LCC (cusp-overlap view) offers several advantages in TAVR with SEV to achieve higher valve implantation with a low risk of device embolization in MIDAS approach.[54]

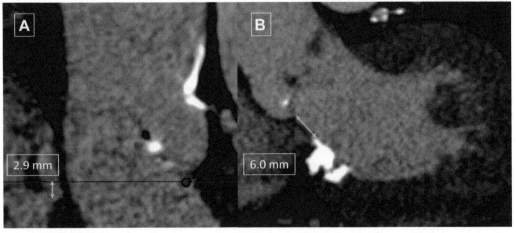

Fig. 1. The membranous septum length measurement by 2 different methods. (*A*) The membranous septum (MS) length was 2.9 mm by the infraannulus method. (*B*) The MS length of the same case was 6.0 mm by the coronal method.

The in-hospital management of new-onset LBBB patients is controversial. Rodés-Cabau and colleagues suggested a strategy depending on QRS and PR intervals. If LBBB persists without further progression of the duration of the QRS or PR interval is observed at day 1, temporary pacing can be discontinued. Patients with persistent LBBB at day 2 with QRS less than 150 ms and PR less than 240 ms can be discharged and implantation of continuous echocardiogram (ECG) monitoring (at least 2–4 weeks) could be considered. Patients with persistent LBBB with QRS greater than 150 ms or PR greater than 240 ms at day 2 are at increased risk of delayed HAVB/CHB requiring PPMI, and continuous ECG monitoring or electrophysiology (EP) studies may be considered to decide PPMI indication. If further prolongation of the QRS or PR interval (of at least 20 ms) is observed at day 1, the temporary pacing wire is recommended to be maintained for an additional 24 hours. If the prolongation of the QRS or PR intervals continues at day 2, additional evaluation with EP studies (followed by continuous ECG monitoring if no PPMI) or direct PPMI may be considered.[55]

Since the pacemaker dependency after TAVR was low in the previous studies, management of pacemaker setting and assessment of the risk of dependency are also important to reduce the dependency.[56,57] Meduri and colleagues reported preexisting RBBB (OR 3.46, 95% CI 1.70–7.06; $P = .0006$) and LVOT overstretch (OR 1.02, 95% CI 1.01–1.04; $P = .005$) were predictors of pacemaker dependency at 1 year after TAVR.[58] For the low–dependency risk patients, a percutaneous leadless pacemaker could be an optional choice, especially in old and patients with comorbidities.[59] Further study is warranted to attest the efficacy of leadless pacemakers in patients after TAVR.

SUMMARY

Postprocedural CDs were related to the adverse long-term outcomes. Preprocedural CT imaging can help identify risk factors for CDs such as MS length, device landing zone calcium, and annular size. Periprocedural planning based on the CT findings is important to mitigate the risk of CDs after TAVR.

CLINICS CARE POINTS

- Preprocedural risk stratification is important to predict CDs after TAVR. The MIDAS approach with cusp-overlap view should be considered in TAVR with SEV to reduce the CDs.
- Continuous ECG monitoring or EP studies may be useful to decide PPMI indication in patient with persistent LBBB (QRS>150 ms) or prolonged PR (> 240ms) at day 2.

DISCLOSURES

Dr Jilaihawi is a consultant to Boston Scientific, Edwards Lifesciences, and Medtronic Inc and has received grant/research support from Abbott Vascular, Bracco Inc, Edwards Lifesciences and Medtronic Inc.

HUMAN AND ANIMAL RIGHTS AND INFORMED CONSENT

This article does not contain any studies with human or animal subjects performed by any of the authors.

REFERENCES

1. Leon MB, Smith CR, Mack MJ, et al. Transcatheter or surgical aortic-valve replacement in intermediate-risk patients. N Engl J Med 2016; 374(17):1609–20.
2. Reardon MJ, Van Mieghem NM, Popma JJ, et al. Surgical or transcatheter aortic-valve replacement in intermediate-risk patients. N Engl J Med 2017; 376(14):1321–31.
3. Thyregod HG, Steinbrüchel DA, Ihlemann N, et al. Transcatheter versus surgical aortic valve replacement in patients with severe aortic valve stenosis: 1-year results from the all-comers NOTION randomized clinical trial. J Am Coll Cardiol 2015; 65(20):2184–94.
4. Mack MJ, Leon MB, Thourani VH, et al. Transcatheter aortic-valve replacement with a balloon-expandable valve in low-risk patients. N Engl J Med 2019;380(18):1695–705.
5. Popma JJ, Deeb GM, Yakubov SJ, et al. Transcatheter aortic-valve replacement with a self-expanding valve in low-risk patients. N Engl J Med 2019; 380(18):1706–15.
6. Fadahunsi OO, Olowoyeye A, Ukaigwe A, et al. Incidence, predictors, and outcomes of permanent pacemaker implantation following transcatheter aortic valve replacement: analysis from the U.S. Society of Thoracic Surgeons/American College of Cardiology TVT Registry. JACC Cardiovasc Interv 2016;9(21):2189–99.
7. Robich MP, Schiltz NK, Johnston DR, et al. Risk factors and outcomes of patients requiring a permanent pacemaker after aortic valve replacement in the United States. J Card Surg 2016;31(8):476–85.

8. Udo EO, Zuithoff NP, van Hemel NM, et al. Incidence and predictors of short- and long-term complications in pacemaker therapy: the FOLLOWPACE study. Heart Rhythm 2012;9(5):728–35.

9. Dreger H, Maethner K, Bondke H, et al. Pacing-induced cardiomyopathy in patients with right ventricular stimulation for >15 years. Europace 2012;14(2):238–42.

10. Fukuda T, Hawley RL, Edwards JE. Lesions of conduction tissue complicating aortic valvular replacement. Chest 1976;69(5):605–14.

11. Levack MM, Kapadia SR, Soltesz EG, et al. Prevalence of and risk factors for permanent pacemaker implantation after aortic valve replacement. Ann Thorac Surg 2019;108(3):700–7.

12. Moreno R, Dobarro D, López de Sá E, et al. Cause of complete atrioventricular block after percutaneous aortic valve implantation: insights from a necropsy study. Circulation 2009;120(5):e29–30.

13. Auffret V, Puri R, Urena M, et al. Conduction disturbances after transcatheter aortic valve replacement: current status and future perspectives. Circulation 2017;136(11):1049–69.

14. Piazza N, de Jaegere P, Schultz C, et al. Anatomy of the aortic valvar complex and its implications for transcatheter implantation of the aortic valve. Circ Cardiovasc Interv 2008;1(1):74–81.

15. Young Lee M, Chilakamarri Yeshwant S, Chava S, et al. Mechanisms of heart block after transcatheter aortic valve replacement - cardiac anatomy, clinical predictors and mechanical factors that contribute to permanent pacemaker implantation. Arrhythmia Electrophysiol Rev 2015;4(2):81–5.

16. Hamdan A, Guetta V, Klempfner R, et al. Inverse relationship between membranous septal length and the risk of atrioventricular block in patients undergoing transcatheter aortic valve implantation. JACC Cardiovasc Interv 2015;8(9):1218–28.

17. Kawashima T, Sasaki H. A macroscopic anatomical investigation of atrioventricular bundle locational variation relative to the membranous part of the ventricular septum in elderly human hearts. Surg Radiol Anat 2005;27(3):206–13.

18. Faroux L, Chen S, Muntané-Carol G, et al. Clinical impact of conduction disturbances in transcatheter aortic valve replacement recipients: a systematic review and meta-analysis. Eur Heart J 2020;41(29):2771–81.

19. Erkapic D, De Rosa S, Kelava A, et al. Risk for permanent pacemaker after transcatheter aortic valve implantation: a comprehensive analysis of the literature. J Cardiovasc Electrophysiol 2012;23(4):391–7.

20. Massoullié G, Bordachar P, Ellenbogen KA, et al. New-onset left bundle branch block induced by transcutaneous aortic valve implantation. Am J Cardiol 2016;117(5):867–73.

21. Nazif TM, Dizon JM, Hahn RT, et al. Predictors and clinical outcomes of permanent pacemaker implantation after transcatheter aortic valve replacement: the PARTNER (Placement of AoRtic TraNscathetER Valves) trial and registry. JACC Cardiovasc Interv 2015;8(1 Pt A):60–9.

22. Bjerre Thygesen J, Loh PH, Cholteesupachai J, et al. Reevaluation of the indications for permanent pacemaker implantation after transcatheter aortic valve implantation. J Invasive Cardiol 2014;26(2):94–9.

23. Mahajan S, Gupta R, Malik AH, et al. Predictors of permanent pacemaker insertion after TAVR: A systematic review and updated meta-analysis. J Cardiovasc Electrophysiol 2021. https://doi.org/10.1111/jce.14986.

24. Mohananey D, Jobanputra Y, Kumar A, et al. Clinical and echocardiographic outcomes following permanent pacemaker implantation after transcatheter aortic valve replacement: meta-analysis and meta-regression. Circ Cardiovasc Interv 2017;10(7). https://doi.org/10.1161/circinterventions.117.005046.

25. Regueiro A, Abdul-Jawad Altisent O, Del Trigo M, et al. Impact of new-onset left bundle branch block and periprocedural permanent pacemaker implantation on clinical outcomes in patients undergoing transcatheter aortic valve replacement: a systematic review and meta-analysis. Circ Cardiovasc Interv 2016;9(5):e003635.

26. Ueshima D, Nai Fovino L, Mojoli M, et al. The interplay between permanent pacemaker implantation and mortality in patients treated by transcatheter aortic valve implantation: A systematic review and meta-analysis. Catheter Cardiovasc Interv 2018;92(3):e159–67.

27. Zhang ZM, Rautaharju PM, Soliman EZ, et al. Mortality risk associated with bundle branch blocks and related repolarization abnormalities (from the Women's Health Initiative [WHI]). Am J Cardiol 2012;110(10):1489–95.

28. Zannad F, Huvelle E, Dickstein K, et al. Left bundle branch block as a risk factor for progression to heart failure. Eur J Heart Fail 2007;9(1):7–14.

29. El-Khally Z, Thibault B, Staniloae C, et al. Prognostic significance of newly acquired bundle branch block after aortic valve replacement. Am J Cardiol 15 2004;94(8):1008–11.

30. Khounlaboud M, Flecher E, Fournet M, et al. Predictors and prognostic impact of new left bundle branch block after surgical aortic valve replacement. Arch Cardiovasc Dis 2017;110(12):667–75.

31. Testa L, Latib A, De Marco F, et al. Clinical impact of persistent left bundle-branch block after transcatheter aortic valve implantation with CoreValve Revalving System. Circulation 2013;127(12):1300–7.

32. Urena M, Webb JG, Cheema A, et al. Impact of new-onset persistent left bundle branch block on late clinical outcomes in patients undergoing transcatheter aortic valve implantation with a balloon-expandable valve. JACC Cardiovasc Interv 2014; 7(2):128–36.

33. Sasaki K, Izumo M, Kuwata S, et al. Clinical impact of new-onset left bundle-branch block after transcatheter aortic valve implantation in the Japanese Population — A single high-volume center experience —. Circ J 2020;84(6):1012–9.

34. Nazif TM, Chen S, George I, et al. New-onset left bundle branch block after transcatheter aortic valve replacement is associated with adverse long-term clinical outcomes in intermediate-risk patients: an analysis from the PARTNER II trial. Eur Heart J 2019;40(27):2218–27.

35. Houthuizen P, Garsse LAFMV, Poels TT, et al. Left bundle-branch block induced by transcatheter aortic valve implantation increases risk of death. Circulation 2012;126(6):720–8.

36. Patrick H, Robert MAvdB, Urena M, et al. Occurrence, fate and consequences of ventricular conduction abnormalities after transcatheter aortic valve implantation. EuroIntervention 2014;9(10):1142–50.

37. Nazif TM, Williams MR, Hahn RT, et al. Clinical implications of new-onset left bundle branch block after transcatheter aortic valve replacement: analysis of the PARTNER experience. Eur Heart J 2013; 35(24):1599–607.

38. Franzoni I, Latib A, Maisano F, et al. Comparison of incidence and predictors of left bundle branch block after transcatheter aortic valve implantation using the CoreValve versus the edwards valve. Am J Cardiol 2013;112(4):554–9.

39. Carrabba N, Valenti R, Migliorini A, et al. Impact on left ventricular function and remodeling and on 1-year outcome in patients with left bundle branch block after transcatheter aortic valve implantation. Am J Cardiol 2015;116(1):125–31.

40. Muñoz-García AJ, Hernández-García JM, Jiménez-Navarro MF, et al. Changes in atrioventricular conduction and predictors of pacemaker need after percutaneous implantation of the CoreValve® aortic valve prosthesis. Rev Esp Cardiol 2010;63(12):1444–51.

41. Kroon HG, van Gils L, Ziviello F, et al. Impact of baseline and newly acquired conduction disorders on need for permanent pacemakers with 3 consecutive generations of self-expanding transcatheter aortic heart valves. Cardiovasc Revasc Med 2021. https://doi.org/10.1016/j.carrev.2021.01.025.

42. Makkar RR, Cheng W, Waksman R, et al. Self-expanding intra-annular versus commercially available transcatheter heart valves in high and extreme risk patients with severe aortic stenosis (PORTICO IDE): a randomised, controlled, non-inferiority trial. Lancet 2020;396(10252):669–83.

43. Fontana GP, Bedogni F, Groh M, et al. Safety profile of an intra-annular self-expanding transcatheter aortic valve and next-generation low-profile delivery System. JACC Cardiovasc Interv 2020;13(21): 2467–78.

44. Reardon MJ, Feldman TE, Meduri CU, et al. Two-Year outcomes after transcatheter aortic valve replacement with mechanical vs self-expanding valves: The REPRISE III Randomized Clinical Trial. JAMA Cardiol 2019;4(3):223–9.

45. Saito S, Hayashida K, Takayama M, et al. Clinical outcomes in patients treated with a repositionable and fully retrievable aortic valve - REPRISE Japan Study. Circ J 2020. https://doi.org/10.1253/circj.CJ-20-0064.

46. Schymik G, Tzamalis P, Bramlage P, et al. Clinical impact of a new left bundle branch block following TAVI implantation: 1-year results of the TAVIK cohort. Clin Res Cardiol 2015;104(4):351–62.

47. Jilaihawi H, Zhao Z, Du R, et al. Minimizing permanent pacemaker following repositionable self-expanding transcatheter aortic valve replacement. JACC Cardiovasc Interv 2019;12(18):1796–807.

48. Maeno Y, Abramowitz Y, Kawamori H, et al. A highly predictive risk model for pacemaker implantation after TAVR. JACC Cardiovasc Imaging 2017;10(10 Pt A):1139–47.

49. Zaid S, Sengupta A, Okoli K, et al. Novel anatomic predictors of new persistent left bundle branch block after evolut transcatheter aortic valve implantation. Am J Cardiol 2020;125(8):1222–9.

50. Miki T, Senoo K, Ohkura T, et al. Importance of pre-operative computed tomography assessment of the membranous septal anatomy in patients undergoing transcatheter aortic valve replacement with a balloon-expandable valve. Circ J 2020;84(2):269–76.

51. Chen YH, Chang HH, Liao TW, et al. Membranous septum length predicts conduction disturbances following transcatheter aortic valve replacement. J Thorac Cardiovasc Surg 2020. https://doi.org/10.1016/j.jtcvs.2020.07.072.

52. Oestreich BA, Mbai M, Gurevich S, et al. Computed tomography (CT) assessment of the membranous septal anatomy prior to transcatheter aortic valve replacement (TAVR) with the balloon-expandable SAPIEN 3 valve. Cardiovasc Revascularization Med 2018;19(5, Part B):626–31.

53. Latsios G, Gerckens U, Buellesfeld L, et al. "Device landing zone" calcification, assessed by MSCT, as a predictive factor for pacemaker implantation after TAVI. Catheter Cardiovasc Interv 2010;76(3):431–9.

54. Tang GHL, Zaid S, Michev I, et al. "Cusp-Overlap" view simplifies fluoroscopy-guided implantation of self-expanding valve in transcatheter aortic valve replacement. JACC Cardiovasc Interv 2018;11(16):1663–5.

55. Rodés-Cabau J, Ellenbogen KA, Krahn AD, et al. Management of conduction disturbances

associated with transcatheter aortic valve replacement: JACC scientific expert panel. J Am Coll Cardiol 2019;74(8):1086–106.

56. Miura M, Shirai S, Uemura Y, et al. Clinical impact of intraventricular conduction abnormalities after transcatheter aortic valve implantation with balloon-expandable valves. Am J Cardiol 2019;123(2):297–305.

57. Costa G, Zappulla P, Barbanti M, et al. Pacemaker dependency after transcatheter aortic valve implantation: incidence, predictors and long-term outcomes. EuroIntervention 2019; 15(10):875–83.

58. Meduri CU, Kereiakes DJ, Rajagopal V, et al. Pacemaker implantation and dependency after transcatheter aortic valve replacement in the REPRISE III Trial. J Am Heart Assoc 2019;8(21):e012594.

59. Tjong FVY, Knops RE, Udo EO, et al. Leadless pacemaker versus transvenous single-chamber pacemaker therapy: A propensity score-matched analysis. Heart Rhythm 2018;15(9):1387–93.

Mechanical Complications of Transcatheter Aortic Valve Replacement

Rory S. Bricker, MD[a], Joseph C. Cleveland Jr, MD[b],
John C. Messenger, MD[a],*

KEYWORDS

- Structural • Transcatheter aortic valve replacement • Embolization • Paravalvular leak
- Annular rupture • Pacemaker

KEY POINTS

- Life-threatening mechanical transcatheter aortic valve replacement complications are rare and result in a lack of individual institution and operator experience with management.
- Periodic review of strategies to manage these complications is critical for maintaining proficiency.
- Selecting prosthetic valve size based on computed tomography sizing has the competing risks of annular rupture versus paravalvular leak, and must be tailored to individual anatomy.
- Identifying high-risk features (anatomic and patient related) for complications and tailoring valve selection (balloon vs self-expanding) is essential.

Any landing you can walk away from is a good landing.
—*Aviation wisdom*

BACKGROUND

Transcatheter aortic valve replacement (TAVR) has rapidly gained popularity owing to its safety, efficacy, short hospital length of stay, and minimally invasive approach compared with surgical aortic valve replacement (SAVR). As of 2018, the volume of annual TAVRs exceeded SAVR in the United States as the primary treatment for severe aortic stenosis in all risk categories and there are now more than 700 active TAVR sites within the United States and its territories.[1]

Despite technological and technical advances, serious life-threatening mechanical complications still occur. These complications present challenges in acute management as well as difficulties for the training of new operators, because rare complications may go unencountered during training even at high-volume centers. It is the goal of this review to highlight some of the major life-threatening mechanical complications that can occur during TAVR and best practices in regard to prevention and management.

ANNULAR RUPTURE

Annular rupture is broadly defined as disruption of the aortic root, annulus, or left ventricular outflow tract (LVOT).[2] It is a rare, although potentially catastrophic, complication of TAVR that has been reported in less than 1% of TAVR procedures[3–5] and is associated with high morbidity and mortality.[3,5,6] The low observed rates of conversion to open surgery, now less than 0.25% of cases in contemporary

---

[a] Department of Medicine, Division of Cardiology, University of Colorado School of Medicine, 12631 East 17th Avenue, B130, Aurora, CO 80045, USA; [b] Department of Surgery, Division of Cardiothoracic Surgery, University of Colorado School of Medicine, 12631 East 17th Avenue, 6111, Aurora, CO 80045, USA
* Corresponding author. 12401 East 17th Avenue, Box B132, Aurora, CO 80045.
E-mail address: John.Messenger@CUAnschutz.edu

Intervent Cardiol Clin 10 (2021) 465–480
https://doi.org/10.1016/j.iccl.2021.06.007
2211-7458/21/© 2021 Elsevier Inc. All rights reserved.

US practice, suggests that the incidence of annular rupture is decreasing and management of cases are improving.[1] Annular rupture that is noncontained has been associated with a 7-fold increase in mortality within 30 days.[5] However, the clinical sequelae of annular rupture can vary widely from catastrophic hemodynamic collapse to a clinically silent event[6] based on the location and degree of acute injury.[3]

Risk Factors and Mechanism of Injury

The aortic annulus is not a true anatomic structure, but rather a "virtual ring" located at the nadirs of the aortic valve leaflet attachments at the junction of the LVOT and the aortic root.[2,4,7] Annular rupture occurs in the areas of the valve landing zone: the subannular LVOT, annulus, or supra-annular sinuses of Valsalva[3,4,8,9] (Fig. 1).[2]

Annular rupture is more common with balloon-expandable valves[10] than with self-expanding valves.[11] Several anatomic risk factors for annular rupture have been identified; however, understanding in whom and why annular rupture occurs remains a clinical challenge. Heavy LVOT calcification in combination with balloon oversizing by more than 10% to 20% of the annulus area has demonstrated a strong association of annular rupture with balloon-expandable valves.[2,6,10,12] Moderate to severe calcification in the LVOT alone, especially when present in the upper LVOT and extending below the noncoronary cusp, is also positively correlated with risk of annular rupture as well as paravalvular leak (PVL).[2,6,8,10,12] The presence of a PVL may necessitate additional post dilation, which has also been correlated with annular rupture.[2,6]

A subannular injury can involve the myocardial free wall, the fibrous continuation from the aortic leaflet attachment to the anterior mitral valve leaflet, or the interventricular septum.[2] Injury is hypothesized to occur from LVOT calcification being pressed into these structures during balloon inflation. Rupture of the free wall can vary in presentation from large volume bleeding into the pericardial space with rapid hemodynamic collapse, to a slower bleed that can develop into a subepicardial hematoma or a pseudoaneurysm with possibility of late rupture or coronary compression over time.[3,4] Acute coronary compression can also occur (Fig. 2) and successful management with stent placement has been reported.[13,14] Injury at the fibrous continuation below the NCC of the aortic valve can lead to a communication between the left ventricle to the left atrium, whereas interventricular septum rupture can create a fistula into the right-sided chambers. These traumatic shunts may lead to chronic heart failure over time.

Injury at the supra-annular level can involve the sinus of Valsalva, sinotubular junction (STJ), or the coronary ostia. These typically arise from balloon overdilation in a calcified aortic root with a small STJ diameter[4] during which the spines of the superior stent frame or a displaced calcified bulky leaflet can interact with the STJ, sinus of Valsalva, or coronary ostia with potential for perforation (Fig. 3). These injuries can present as a hematoma of the aortic wall, dissection, or frank bleeding into the pericardium or mediastinum.

Diagnosis

Rapid identification of annular injury is critical because there may be a therapeutic window to act before hemodynamic decompensation occurs. An assessment with echocardiography and aortography should be performed after each valve deployment and the diagnosis considered in cases where there is unexplained hemodynamic instability or failure of the myocardium to recover.[3] An echocardiographic assessment can identify a new pericardial effusion, subepicardial hematoma, periaortic hematoma, new aortic wall thickening, new valvular regurgitation, ventricular septal defect, or aortic dissection. If transthoracic views are not diagnostic, urgent conversion to a transesophageal echocardiogram is critical to diagnose the problem. Aortography can identify contrast extravasation owing to injury at the supra-annular or annular levels (see Fig. 3C), although small volume extravasation or a subannular injury may not be visualized. As such, an echocardiogram and aortography are both necessary and complementary for diagnosis.

Management of Annular Rupture

Acute management of annular rupture is guided by the location and severity of injury. A noncontained annular rupture is associated with high morbidity and mortality,[3,6] although if an early diagnosis is made, with emergent conversion to surgical repair, up to 50% of patients may survive.[3] In cases of hemodynamic instability, rapid insertion of a pericardial drain can stabilize the patient while converting to cardiopulmonary bypass, after which surgical exploration and repair should be considered. In cases where the patient is not suitable for surgery and conservative measures fail, a second valve-in-valve technique can be considered to seal the rupture site if the rupture does not extend above or below the skirt landing zone (see Fig. 2).[14] If

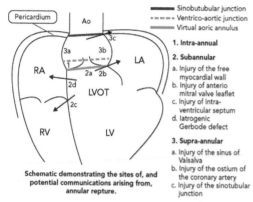

Sinobutubular junction
Ventrico-aortic junction
Virtual aoric annulus

Pericardium

Ao

RA

LA

LVOT

RV

LV

1. Intra-annual
2. Subannular
   a. Injury of the free myocardial wall
   b. Injury of anterio mitral valve leaflet
   c. Injury of intra-ventricular septum
   d. Iatrogenic Gerbode defect
3. Supra-annular
   a. Injury of the sinus of Valsalva
   b. Injury of the ostium of the coronary artery
   c. Injury of the sinotubular junction

Schematic demonstrating the sites of, and potential communications arising from, annular rupture.

Fig. 1. Location and communications arising from annular rupture. Ao, aorta; LA, left atrium; LV, left ventricle; LVOT, left ventricular outflow tract; RA, right atrium; RV, right ventricle. (*From*, Coughlan et. al. 2018,[2] Radcliffe Cardiology.)

these methods fail, successful sealing of the rupture site by coil embolization and vascular plugs has been reported as a final option.[15,16]

Some small aortic root ruptures can be successfully managed conservatively[3] (**Fig. 4**), although the data are limited as to which patients may best benefit from this strategy. After the detection of an effusion, a pericardial drain should be placed rapidly and anticoagulation reversed with protamine, with the goal of allowing a small defect to clot and seal. If a large volume of blood is being drained, autotransfusion can be considered as a temporizing measure by returning the aspirated pericardial blood back to the circulation with a large syringe.[17,18] If significant volume continues, surgical exploration should be considered. However, for those who remain hemodynamically stable with minimal or no ongoing bleeding after anticoagulation reversal, observation is a reasonable strategy to avoid sternotomy.[17,18] The long-term outcomes of this approach, however, are unknown.

Clinics care points

- Balloon oversizing in combination with moderate to severe annular calcium is a strong risk factor for annular rupture.
- Think of annular rupture in scenarios of unexplained hypotension (and/or bradycardia) after valve deployment. Conversion to transesophageal echocardiography may be required if using transthoracic echocardiography with conscious sedation.
- Preprocedural planning and accurate valve sizing are keys to prevention.

- Consider using self-expanding versus balloon-expandable valves in patients with risk factors identified on preprocedural computed tomography (CT) angiography

VALVE EMBOLIZATION

Prosthetic valve embolization is a rare but potentially catastrophic complication of transcatheter valve deployment. Although many cases are able to be managed percutaneously with favorable outcomes, embolization to the ventricle can require emergent conversion to open sternotomy and is associated with increased mortality.[19] The risk for valve embolization arises from anatomic, technical, and device-related factors.

Risk Factors and Mechanism of Injury
Anatomic features that increase the risk for valve embolization include a large annulus size, a small STJ, minimal annular or leaflet calcium, bulky calcified leaflets, a horizontal annulus, the presence of a prosthetic mitral valve, a bicuspid anatomy, and a small LVOT.[11,20–22] An undersized valve prosthesis may not achieve full apposition and is more prone to migration, particularly if no or minimal annular calcium is present to serve as an anchor.[11] A small LVOT or hypertrophied septum can lead to asymmetric expansion of the valve frame with a potential "watermelon seed" effect, particularly when there is minimal leaflet or annular calcium for anchoring. In addition, valve embolization has occurred during off-label use, such as for aortic insufficiency.

The most common technical errors that lead to embolization are misplacement of the valve too high in the annulus,[19,21] an inability to recognize the valve was not in a coaxial plane,[21] and interruptions in pacing.[11,19,21,23] Erroneously high valve placement can be caused by using an improper coplanar angle or calcium landmarks that are misidentified for valve positioning, especially in the presence of a bicuspid anatomy. Residual guidewire tension at time of deployment can also bias the valve toward the aorta during deployment, particularly if inflation is delayed or incomplete. A loss of pacing capture can lead to the valve being ejected during ventricular systole against the inflated balloon.[23] Pitfalls of pacing include unstable positioning of the right ventricular pacemaker lead and an insufficient pacing output or rate, as well as premature termination of pacing when the balloon remains inflated. In patients with mitral valve prosthesis, interaction of the distal inflated

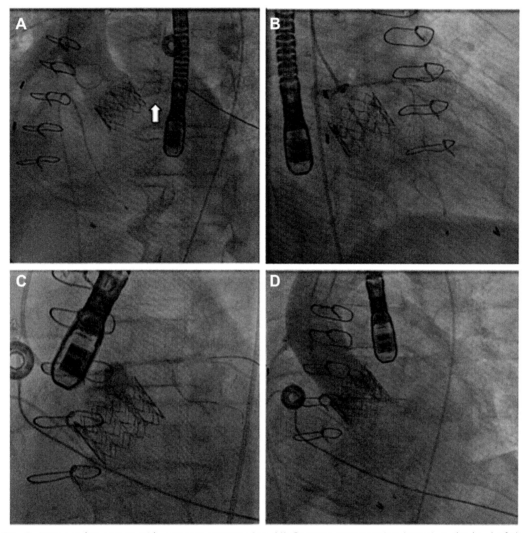

Fig. 2. Intra-annular rupture with coronary compression. (A) Contrast extravasation (arrow) at the level of the annulus after balloon-expanding valve deployment. Hematoma formation resulted in progressive coronary compression (B, C). Stent placement was attempted but unsuccessful (C). A second valve was placed with seal of the rupture (D).

balloon with mitral prosthetic strut has been reported with aortic displacement and embolization of the valve.[24]

Device-related factors can also lead to embolization and include interaction of the delivery system when retracting from the ventricle (Fig. 5), tabs failing to release from delivery catheter, or failure to retract the loader.[25]

Management

When an embolized valve is managed effectively, outcomes are favorable.[21] Optimal management of an embolized valve is determined by the direction of the embolization and hemodynamic stability. A valve that embolizes to the aortic root may often be retrieved and repositioned by percutaneous techniques if the patient is hemodynamically stable.[23] For a valve that has embolized to the ventricle, or in patients who are unstable, cardiopulmonary bypass and surgical retrieval will be required (Fig. 6).[11]

For either a self-expanding valve or balloon-expanding valve embolized to the aorta, the first critical step is to maintain the coaxial wire and valve position to stabilize the valve and avoid the valve flipping into an obstructive position.[11,26] Snare catheters, or in refractory cases, a bioptome, can be used to stabilize and reposition the valve to a more coaxial plane, often via the right or left radial arterial access site for valve stabilization.

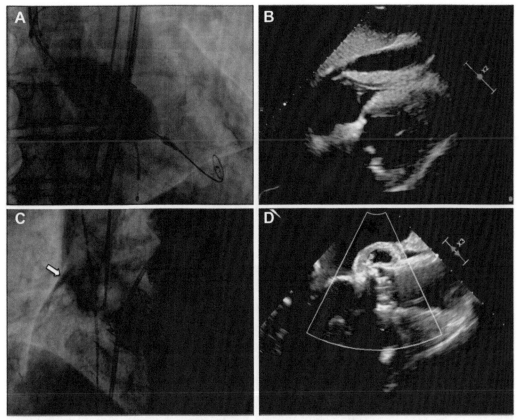

Fig. 3. Annular rupture at the sinus of Valsalva. (*A*) A 23-mm Edwards ultra balloon-expandable valve deployment demonstrates large stent frame size in relation to the STJ. (*B*) A transthoracic echocardiogram after clinical hypotension demonstrates new pericardial effusion. (*C*) A repeat aortogram demonstrates contrast reflux into the pericardial reflection. (*D*) A transesophageal echocardiogram demonstrates periaortic hematoma. Open sternotomy was emergently performed which confirmed perforation in the sinus of Valsalva above the noncoronary cusp.

For an aortic embolized balloon-expanding valve, a balloon can be readvanced through the valve to a point where the balloon nose is distal to the caudal edge of the stent frame (Fig. 7A). The balloon is then slowly inflated until it catches the valve, after which it can be carefully retracted to a safe area in the aorta for deployment, ideally in the descending aorta where it will not occlude major branch vessels (Fig. 7B–F). The regular practice of leaving the CT scan images open during the procedure can allow for rapid anatomic assessment in the event of an emergency to identify an area in the aorta that permits full apposition of the stent frame without obstructing branch vessels.

Embolization of self-expandable valves are reported more rarely.[11] Snare catheters can be used to reposition and retract the valve from the upper tabs to a safe location in the ascending aorta, while being cautious to avoid aortic injury in the process (see Fig. 5A–D). If the valve is unable to be stabilized, placement

of a second valve to pin the embolized valve is an alternative to surgery (see Fig. 5E–F).

After the valve has been deployed in a suitable alternate location, some advocate for the placement of a covered stent within the prosthesis to exclude the leaflets from the lumen and to further secure the valve to prevent future migration, particularly after patient ambulation. However, a functioning valve in the abdominal aorta has not been associated with significant adverse outcomes,[21] so stenting may not be required in cases in which the valve is well-seated and stable. Given the clinical equipoise, the practice patterns of placing covered stents vary by institution. After the embolized valve has been successfully stabilized, the mechanism of error should be reviewed to determine if this issue can be correctable before proceeding for a second attempt at transcatheter aortic valve implantation.

A ventricular embolization is typically not recoverable by percutaneous techniques.[11]

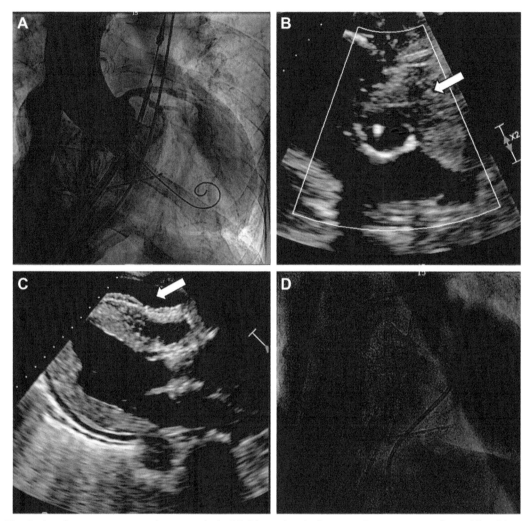

Fig. 4. Annular rupture managed conservatively. (*A*) After valve deployment, there was no angiographic evidence of annular injury, although the patient developed progressive unexplained hypotension. (*B, C*) Rapid assessment by transthoracic echocardiogram demonstrated hematoma and new pericardial effusion (*arrows*). (*D*) A pigtail drain was placed and anticoagulation was reversed. After 900 mL of bloody fluid was aspirated the drain slowed and was left in place. Drainage slowed and the drain was removed the following day without reaccumulation. The patient was discharged to home on postprocedure day 6, after a prolonged observation period.

Prompt placement on bypass and surgical retrieval with valve replacement is recommended.

Prevention

Preventing valve embolization requires meticulous attention to preprocedural CT imaging and procedural planning for valve sizing, selection of a predicted coplanar angle, and identifying anatomic factors that may increase the risk of embolization. An independent on-site CT scan analysis complements manufacturer analysis, particularly in cases with complex anatomy, imaging artifacts, in-between annulus sizes, and high-risk anatomic features.

In cases where the annulus area measurements are in between balloon-expandable valve sizes, it is our practice to choose the smaller of the 2 and expand above nominal, typically 1 to 3 mL depending on the size of valve selected. In this manner, the valve can be dilated up to achieve apposition, while minimizing the risk of annular injury that can occur with oversizing.[2,6,10,12] Very large annular areas that fall above the manufacturer's recommended sizing ranges present a unique challenge. Overinflation of a 29-mm Edwards valve has been performed successfully in some cases to achieve larger orifice sizes in this setting with good result,[27] although this technique should be

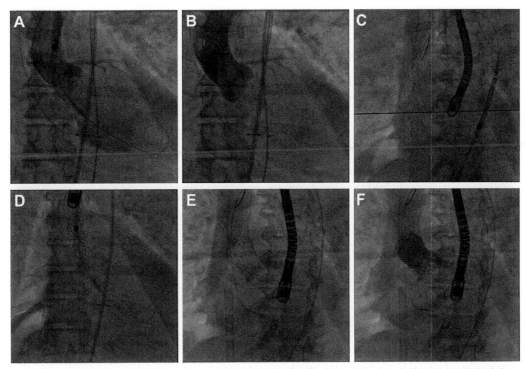

Fig. 5. Embolization of a self-expanding valve. (*A*) Initial uncomplicated Evolut deployment. (*B*) Inability to centralize the delivery catheter nose cone resulted in the catheter dragging across and embolizing the valve in aortic direction. (*C*) A gooseneck snare via the radial artery was unable to retract the valve to a more stable position. (*D*) The patient was felt to be a poor surgical candidate by the heart team, so a second valve was deployed in aortic position to treat native valve and "pin" the embolized valve. (*E*) Two valves in series, stable after pinning. (*F*) Final angiogram with mild to moderate PVL.

performed with caution, and the involvement of a manufacturer proctor can be a helpful resource for case selection. If inflation is performed above the nominal pressure, it is important to recognize greater shortening of the stent frame will occur from the caudal (ventricular) edge, which needs to be accounted for when positioning for deployment to avoid seating the valve and skirt too high.

Standardizing communication within the team and safety checks during predeployment and deployment sequences are critical to maintaining efficient and short pacing runs while ensuring safe and accurate valve deployment. Clear communication between operators during the pacing sequence with a repeat aortogram injection to confirm no valve migration, valve adjustments if needed, and full valve inflation are

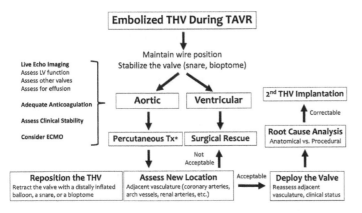

Fig. 6. ECMO, extracorporeal membrane oxygenation; THV, Tx,. (*From,* Alkhouli et al. 2019[11] with permission from Elsevier.)

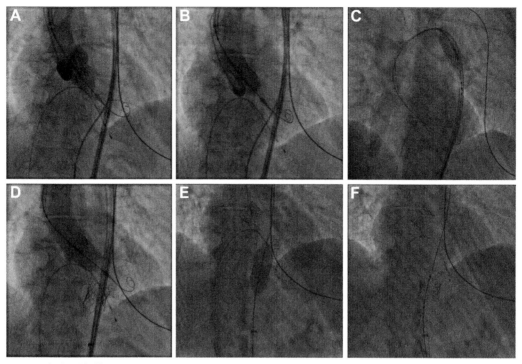

Fig. 7. Embolized balloon-expandable valve. (*A*) Initial position of a Sapien 3 valve during deployment. (*B*) Loss of capture with escape ventricular beat results in aortic embolization of the valve. (*C*) The balloon is stabilized and "captured" with an inflated balloon and retracted to the descending aorta. (*D*) A second valve is placed in the aortic position with uncomplicated deployment. (*E*) The embolized valve is fully deployed in the descending aorta. (*F*) The 2 valves in series are in stable position. The patient has had no clinical sequelae 2 years after the procedure.

critical.[11] Before deployment, we advocate a predeployment timeout or checklist be performed, which includes a brief review of the sequence of deployment, roles of operators in that sequence, confirming stable pacer capture, and ensuring contrast is filled in the injector. In our current era, when enhanced personal protective equipment may be in use, loud and clear communications should be emphasized. Rapid pacing runs must be efficient to minimize the duration of hypotension that occurs, while being of sufficient duration to allow full inflation and deflation of the delivery balloon to minimize balloon and valve interaction when pacing is terminated. For building programs, more routine use of balloon valvuloplasty may be useful to increase team repetitions and efficiency of this critical sequence. During post dilation of a valve, the same standardized sequence is followed, allowing for full deflation of the balloon before pacing termination to minimize interaction of the balloon and implanted valve.

Strategies have been proposed to improve pacing stability. The use of an active fixation temporary pacing lead (Tempo, Biotrace Medical, Menlo Park, CA) in the right ventricle has been shown to safe and effective and may safeguard against lead migration and may allow for earlier ambulation,[28,29] although larger trials are needed. Less common techniques have included pacing of the left ventricle directly via the stiff 0.035 delivery guidewire. This goal can be accomplished by attaching the pacemaker cathode to the distal wire with an alligator clip and attaching the anode to anesthetized skin in the groin with a second clip. In research settings, this procedure has been described as safe and effective when compared with right ventricular pacing while avoiding a second venous puncture and achieving decreased fluoroscopy time.[30,31] This technique has not been adopted widely in clinical practice and studies were underpowered to detect the effects of these strategies to prevent the rare occurrence of valve embolization, although it remains a promising area of investigation.

Clinics care points

- The most common technical errors that lead to embolization are deployment of the valve too high in the annulus, an

inability to recognize an inaccurate coaxial plane, and interruptions in pacing during deployment.
- Aortic embolized valves can often be managed percutaneously with good outcomes.

PARAVALVULAR LEAK

Traditionally, a major limitation of the stent mounted TAVR design has been greater rates of PVL when compared with SAVR in early trials.[32–38] The incidence of moderate to severe PVL has ranged widely between trials from 0% to 24%, largely owing to inconsistencies in detection and classification, which depend on the imaging modality, the timing of the assessment, and the grading scale used.[39,40] PVL is more common in bicuspid valve anatomy.[22] Multiple grading systems have been proposed,[40,41] although detection and standardization remain challenging owing to the complex nature of paravalvular regurgitant jets, which are often multiple, eccentric, and irregularly shaped with the assessment limited by acoustic shadows for spectral Doppler imaging.[38–40,42]

Iterative generations of valve designs have made changes to the stent frame and valve skirt in attempts to improve seal at the annulus.[43,44] With these design changes, and as these devices expanded to treat lower risk populations, the rates of moderate to severe PVL decreased significantly in both clinical trial[32–36] and registry settings. Moderate to severe PVL is now reported in fewer than 2% of cases in contemporary US practice.[1] The rates of trace and mild PVL have remained high,[1,32–36,39] although the clinical impact remains debated.[39,40] Despite improvements, PVL remains a major problem, because the presence of aortic regurgitation after valve intervention has been shown to be an independent predictor of long-term mortality for both surgical and transcatheter valves.[45,46] This association is more pronounced with greater degrees of regurgitation (≥2),[45] although present with mild regurgitation as well.[33]

Risk Factors and Mechanism
PVL after transcatheter valve implantation occurs from a low placed valve,[47,48] annular eccentricity,[49] undersizing of the device,[50–52] or irregular apposition with poor seal[38,53] owing to eccentric calcium distribution at the level of the annulus or LVOT. Bicuspid valves are associated with more irregularity of the annulus, as well as fibrotic and calcified leaflets, which likely

contribute to the observed higher rate of PVL after TAVR.[22]

Prevention
The use of multidetector computer tomography scans for accurate valve sizing has been shown to decrease the rate of significant PVL after implantation.[54] The degree of valve prosthesis oversizing to the native annulus by area and perimeter measured by CT scan has been shown to have an inverse relationship with moderate to severe paravalvular regurgitation with oversizing associated with less regurgitation.[55,56] This factor must be balanced with the converse risk of annular rupture and oversizing. CT scans can also be used to assess for anatomic factors such as ovoid shape or calcium nodules, which may result in incomplete seal and subsequent PVL. Although no direct comparative analysis has been performed between the most common commercial valve types (Edwards Lifesciences [Irvine, CA] balloon-expandable valve and the Medtronic [Dublin, Ireland] self-expandable CoreValve), self-expandable valves have been associated with higher rates of PVL.[39]

Diagnosis
After valve deployment, assessment for acute regurgitation is performed by an evaluation of hemodynamics, angiography, and echocardiography.[38,39,42] Aortic root angiography has the benefit of being able to performed immediately, although it is subject to the limitation of a single plane view. Angiographic insufficiency is graded by Seller criteria with a scale of 1 to 4 based on the time and density of contrast reflux into the ventricle.[40,57]

Hemodynamic tracings are also used to characterize the degree of insufficiency. An acute decrease in the aortic diastolic pressure or a narrowing of the difference between aortic and left ventricular diastolic pressures correlate with severity of aortic regurgitation.[39,42] The hemodynamic aortic regurgitation index, calculated as ([diastolic blood pressure − left ventricular end-diastolic pressure/systolic blood pressure) × 100, has been validated as an in-laboratory tool for semiquantitative measurement insufficiency that has prognostic significance, with lower index values being associated with increased regurgitation and associated one year mortality rate.[58]

The echo assessment with 2-dimensional and color Doppler should assess for both central and paravalvular origins as well as for total volume of regurgitation. A sweep of the aortic root should be performed to identify the origin of PVL with the possibility of multiple jets originating from different levels[42] and standardized criteria based on the American Society of Echocardiography should be used to grade a PVL[42] (Fig. 8). A wire or catheter across the valve may result in incomplete leaflet coaptation and overestimate the true degree of residual regurgitation, particularly if the wire is not centralized or if it is impairing leaflet coaptation.[38] The most accurate assessment and grading of residual regurgitation can be obtained with nothing across the valve, and, if a self-expanding valve is used, after sufficient time has allowed the system to completely expand.

Management

The acute management strategy for PVL depends on the mechanism and severity (Fig. 9).[40] If the degree of regurgitation is moderate or greater, and malapposition (or undersizing) is suspected, post dilation can be effective in decreasing the degree of regurgitation[38–40] and should be performed if risks of post dilation are low. The increased risks of annular rupture and stroke associated with post dilation, as well as the location of the prosthetic valve should be factored into this decision. Post dilation of a balloon-expandable valve will shorten the ventricular edge of the stent frame, and if a valve is highly seated with a poor seal, additional shortening may further worsen seal or lead to embolization. A valve with a poor seal as a result of being seated too low may require the placement of a valve in valve[40,47] in a higher position. Refractory moderate to severe PVL can be treated by conversion to surgery or the by use of percutaneous vascular plugs. This maneuver can be performed at the time of the procedure, or if stable, in a staged fashion with dedicated preprocedure planning. The consideration to proceed with plugging must account for the stability of the prosthesis, because passing additional equipment and plugs around an unstable valve may increase the risk of valve embolization. Patients with residual PVL should be monitored closely with aggressive blood pressure control, serial monitoring for clinically significant hemolysis, and follow-up echocardiographic assessment.

LEFT VENTRICULAR OUTFLOW TRACT OBSTRUCTION WITH SUICIDE LEFT VENTRICLE

Long-standing pressure overload with a fixed valvular obstruction will lead to left ventricular remodeling with asymmetric septal hypertrophy as an adaptive mechanism.[59] Sudden relief of that outflow obstruction with a rapid decrease in the left ventricular afterload can unmask an underlying dynamic outflow tract gradient in predisposed individuals with the potential for acute hemodynamic decompensation.[60–62] Acute improvement in left ventricular systolic function can be seen as early 30 minutes after aortic valve replacement, which may further exacerbate the dynamic gradient.[63]

This hemodynamic decompensation after TAVR or SAVR has been termed the "suicide left ventricle"[60] or "ASH crash," and has been well-described in the surgical literature.[61] In individuals with increased basal hypertrophy (sigmoid septum) at time of aortic valve replacement, a concomitant myectomy may be performed as a preventative strategy.[61]

Risk Factors and Mechanism

Dynamic outflow obstruction after TAVR has been hypothesized to be due to the complex interplay between septal hypertrophy and increased flow velocity across the septum, with anterior displacement of the mitral valve causing outflow obstruction.[62,64] This outflow obstruction is highly sensitive to left ventricular loading conditions.[65]

Prevention

Preprocedural provocative testing of outflow tract hypertrophy is limited in the setting of concomitant severe aortic stenosis and data to predict patients who may develop post-valve dynamic interventricular gradient is unfortunately limited. Therefore, preprocedural risk stratification is reliant on CT scans and echocardiographic imaging to identify anatomic features that may increase risk for developing outflow tract obstruction, such as hypertrophied septum and small left ventricular cavity size with low stroke volume. A greater angulation of the aorta and left ventricular outflow axis has also shown an associated with increased LVOT gradient at baseline.[66]

Similar to preemptive surgical myectomy before SAVR, preemptive alcohol septal ablation in patients with increased septal thickness has been described in a small series to be a feasible concept in managing ASH before TAVR[67]; however, the limited data are hypothesis generating only, and a randomized trial is needed to assess benefit and appropriate patient selection.

Management

The acute management of dynamic intraventricular gradient with hemodynamic compromise focuses on rapid identification and optimizing

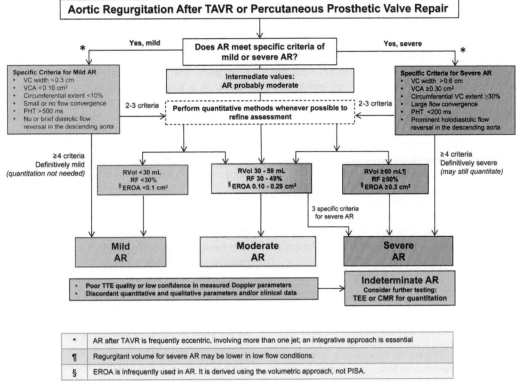

Aortic Regurgitation After TAVR or Percutaneous Prosthetic Valve Repair

Fig. 8. Suggested algorithm to guide implementation and integration of multiple parameters of aortic regurgitation severity after TAVR or prosthetic aortic valve repair. A good-quality echocardiographic imaging and complete data acquisition are assumed. If imaging is technically difficult, consider transesophageal echocardiography or cardiac MR imaging. Aortic regurgitation severity may be indeterminate owing to poor image quality, technical issues with data, internal inconsistency among echocardiographic findings, or discordance with clinical findings. (*From*, Zoghbi et al. 2019,[42] with permission from Elsevier.)

loading conditions: maintaining preload of the left ventricle by intravascular volume resuscitation, slowing of the heart rate to maximize diastolic filling time, use of negative inotropic agents, and maintenance of sinus rhythm.[60,62] Pharmacologic agents with positive inotropic or afterload reducing effects can worsen the dynamic outflow obstruction and should be avoided if possible.[60] If a vasopressor is required, an alpha agonist is preferred to avoid adding to the hypercontractile state.

In the event of severe LVOT obstruction refractory to medical therapies, bail-out emergent alcohol septal ablation has been described.[68] In less severe cases, the septal wall thickness has been shown to often regress spontaneously

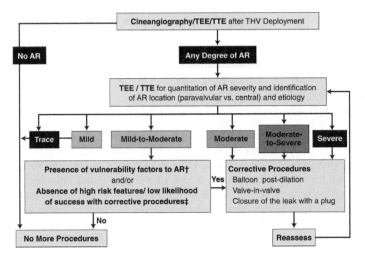

Fig. 9. Algorithm for diagnosis and management of PVL. AR, atrial regurgitation; TEE, transesophageal echocardiography; TTE, transthoracic echocardiography. (*From*, Pibarot et al. 2015,[40] with permission from Elsevier.)

over time[59] as the ventricle remodels in response to decreased chronic left ventricular pressure. Septal hypertrophy from primary hypertrophic cardiomyopathy, however, will unlikely regress. For such cases of refractory symptoms owing to LVOT obstruction with a septal hypertrophy greater than 15 mm and a suitable septal perforator anatomy, alcohol septal ablation can be an effective approach. Surgical myectomy is complicated by the presence of the prosthetic aortic valve.[62] Those treated with alcohol septal ablation and TAVR are at very high risk for pacemaker, because the risk for left bundle branch block in TAVR can be 10% to 25%, whereas the risk for patients with right bundle branch block with ablation is up to 60%.[62]

Clinics care point

- Management of an LVOT obstruction after valve deployment focuses on prompt recognition by echocardiographic imaging, optimization of left ventricular loading conditions, and avoidance of agents known to worsen the condition.

VENTRICULAR PERFORATION

Left ventricular perforation is a rare mechanical complication during TAVR. Trauma can occur as a linear laceration of the ventricle from delivery wires or perforation from blunt injury of a distal delivery catheter nosecone,[69] the consequences of which can range from delayed left ventricular pseudoaneurysm formation to acute hemodynamic collapse.[14,70] Although outcomes data are limited, mortality from left ventricular perforation is high,[14,69,70] with a combined mortality rate from left ventricular injury or annular rupture of up to 50%.

Right ventricular perforation is most commonly the result of injury to the right ventricular free wall from a temporary pacemaker. The risk factors for right ventricular perforation increase in the presence of recent oral steroid use, the use of screw in leads, and in elderly patients with a thinner right ventricle free wall.[69,71]

Management
Diagnosis of left ventricle perforation can be suspected by new effusion by echocardiogram, left ventriculography demonstrating contrast extravasation into the pericardium, or by surgical exploration for ongoing bleeding despite pericardiocentesis.[69] The management of left ventricular free wall injury is similar to free annular

rupture and is directed by extent of injury. A free-flowing left ventricular perforation with hemodynamic instability will nearly always require emergent surgical exploration and ventricle repair. In a patient who is not a candidate for emergent surgery, percutaneous repair has been reported.[72] A hemodynamically stable perforation that develops into a pseudoaneurysm can be initially managed conservatively and later repaired nonemergently by surgical approach or percutaneously with a vascular plug.[14,70,73]

Right ventricular perforation typically can be managed conservatively with reversal of anticoagulation, removal of the temporary pacemaker, and pericardial drainage. Most patients will not require surgical intervention.[69]

Prevention
The risk of left ventricular perforation can be minimized by shaping a broad curve or coil on the tip of the delivery wire to decrease direct pressure against the ventricle with wire movement during valve delivery. Careful attention to wire manipulation and stored wire tension is critical, particularly during balloon inflation[70] and valve deployment, when attention may be diverted away from the distal wire.[69] Device advancement across a restrictive valve should be performed with caution, with the possibility of the nosecone to "jump" deep into the ventricle.

Techniques have been adopted to further cushion the stiff wire tip against the ventricle, including spiral type tip bends, or attempts to create a cushioned stiff wire by fashioning a cut pigtail catheter coil onto the distal wire with sutures, which must be exchanged through a 6F sheath, to act as both a cushion at the contact zone of the wire and ventricle and as a bumper against nose cone advancing too far distally.[69] Such techniques, although limited in efficacy data, highlight the ingenuity of the field and how necessity is the mother of innovation as we await advances in wire technology.

MITRAL VALVE INJURY

Mitral valve disruption is a rare complication that results from a direct injury of the papillary muscles or avulsion of the mitral chordal apparatus from balloons and catheters being delivered behind mitral chordae. Such injuries can lead to acute mitral regurgitation.[26] In addition, direct physical interaction between the prosthetic valve frame and the anterior mitral valve leaflet can result in direct leaflet injury or restricted mobility with acute mitral dysfunction.[38,74]

Prevention

Mitral valve injury can be prevented by visually ensuring the wire is free in its course when crossing the aortic valve to the apex and not entrapped behind chordal structures that may become injured during balloon inflation. Freeing the delivery wire by advancing a pigtail catheter to the apex and confirming the absence of any tethering before repositioning the wire in the apex can avoid subsequent mitral apparatus injury. Marked ectopy or new mitral regurgitation detected by echocardiography after the valve has been crossed can be signs that there is interaction with the mitral apparatus and that the wire should be repositioned.

Preprocedural CT imaging can be used to assess the distance between the annulus and anterior leaflet of the native mitral valve, or in cases of mitral prosthesis the potential for interaction of a valve strut. By nature of stent design, the self-expanding Core valve has a greater landing zone within the LVOT[74] by traditional implant technique and care should be taken to avoid low implantation that has the potential to interact with the mitral valve.

Management

The management of acute mitral regurgitation depends on the degree of insufficiency. Rarely are cases severe enough to require surgical removal of the implanted prosthesis. Lesser degrees of mitral regurgitation can be managed medically, although the long-term outcomes are not known.[26]

Iatrogenic Ventricular Septal Defect

Iatrogenic ventricular septum defect is a very rare complication after TAVR, with only 20 cases from 2002 to 2015 identified in the largest series.[75] The majority of cases have involved the membranous or perimembranous septum near the valve landing zone, although this complication can occur anywhere along the septum, which communicates with the right ventricle, including the ventricular apex or atrioventricular septum.[75] The mechanism of injury is poorly understood, although direct trauma at the time of valve implantation and delayed scar rupture from a periprocedural injury with transapical approach,[76] as well as changes in the tensile forces across the ventricle after valve implantation have all been hypothesized.[14,75] Balloon-expandable valve use was more commonly reported (85%), as well as pre or post dilation, in the reported cases of an iatrogenic ventricular septal defect.[75]

Timing to diagnosis can range from immediate, to up to a year after valve implantation, with the median time of 7 days following the procedure. Clinical presentations vary from asymptomatic to symptomatic heart failure.[14,75]

Management is guided by the presence of absence of symptoms. Asymptomatic ventricular septal defects can often be managed conservatively. In symptomatic patients, closure can be performed and appears safe from a limited series.[75] For repair, percutaneous closure has been performed more often than surgery and is presumed to be related to the high risk nature of the TAVR population.[14,75]

SUMMARY

Mechanical complications after TAVR are fortunately rare with the current generation of devices. Unfortunately, life-threatening complications will occur and it is the responsibility of operators to be familiar with strategies to prevent and manage these challenging scenarios. Because these cases do not occur often, it is important for us to highlight and talk about those that do occur, to learn best practices in how to manage and prevent them going forward. We can learn much from each other's good crash landings.

DISCLOSURE

None.

REFERENCES

1. Carroll JD. STS-ACC TVT registry of transcatheter aortic valve replacement. J Am Coll Cardiol 2020; 76(21):25.
2. Coughlan J, Kiernan T, Mylotte D, et al. Annular rupture during transcatheter aortic valve implantation: predictors, management and outcomes. Interv Cardiol Rev 2018;13(3):140.
3. Pasic M, Unbehaun A, Dreysse S, et al. Rupture of the device landing zone during transcatheter aortic valve implantation: a life-threatening but treatable complication. Circ Cardiovasc Interv 2012;5(3): 424–32.
4. Pasic M. Annular rupture during transcatheter aortic valve replacement. 2015;8(1):9.
5. Walther T, Hamm CW, Schuler G, et al. Perioperative results and complications in 15,964 transcatheter aortic valve replacements. J Am Coll Cardiol 2015;65(20):2173–80.
6. Barbanti M, Yang T-H, Rodès Cabau J, et al. Anatomical and procedural features associated with aortic root rupture during balloon-expandable transcatheter aortic valve replacement. Circulation 2013;128(3):244–53.

7. Hoffman J, Fullerton D. Surgical anatomy of the aortic and mitral valves. In: Transcatheter heart valve handbook: a surgeon's and interventional council review. Washington, DC: American College of Cardiology; 2018.

8. John D, Buellesfeld L, Yuecel S, et al. Correlation of device landing zone calcification and acute procedural success in patients undergoing transcatheter aortic valve implantations with the self-expanding CoreValve prosthesis. JACC Cardiovasc Interv 2010;3(2):233–43.

9. Pasic M. Annular rupture during TAVR. JACC Cardiovasc Interv 2020;13(15):1800–2.

10. Okuno T, Asami M, Heg D, et al. Impact of left ventricular outflow tract calcification on procedural outcomes after transcatheter aortic valve replacement. JACC Cardiovasc Interv 2020;13(15):1789–99.

11. Alkhouli M, Sievert H, Rihal CS. Device embolization in structural heart interventions. JACC Cardiovasc Interv 2019;12(2):113–26.

12. Hansson NC, Nørgaard BL, Barbanti M, et al. The impact of calcium volume and distribution in aortic root injury related to balloon-expandable transcatheter aortic valve replacement. J Cardiovasc Comput Tomogr 2015;9(5):382–92.

13. Kim RJ, McGehee E, Mack MJ. Left main occlusion secondary to aortic root rupture following transcatheter aortic valve replacement managed by left main stenting: LM occlusion after TAVR. Catheter Cardiovasc Interv 2014;83(1):E146–9.

14. Langer NB, Hamid NB, Nazif TM, et al. Injuries to the aorta, aortic annulus, and left ventricle during transcatheter aortic valve replacement: management and outcomes. Circ Cardiovasc Interv 2017; 10(1). https://doi.org/10.1161/CIRCINTERVENTIONS.116.004735.

15. Alkhouli M, Carpenter E, Tarabishy A, et al. Annular rupture during transcatheter aortic valve replacement: novel treatment with Amplatzer vascular plugs. Eur Heart J 2018;39(8):714–5.

16. Azarrafiy R, Albuquerque FN, Carrillo RG, et al. Coil embolization to successfully treat annular rupture during transcatheter aortic valve replacement. Catheter Cardiovasc Interv 2018;92(6):1205–8.

17. Vannini L, Andrea R, Sabaté M. Conservative management of aortic root rupture complicated with cardiac tamponade following transcatheter aortic valve implantation. World J Cardiol 2017;9(4):391.

18. Fiocca L, Cereda AF, Bernelli C, et al. Autologous blood reinfusion during iatrogenic acute hemorrhagic cardiac tamponade: safety and feasibility in a cohort of 30 patients. Catheter Cardiovasc Interv 2019;93(1):E56–62.

19. Ibebuogu UN, Giri S, Bolorunduro O, et al. Review of reported causes of device embolization following trans-catheter aortic valve implantation. Am J Cardiol 2015;115(12):1767–72.

20. Nagabandi AK, Panchal H, Srivastava R, et al. When prosthetic valves compete for space: a case of transcatheter aortic valve embolization due to prosthetic mitral valve. Cureus 2019. https://doi.org/10.7759/cureus.4299.

21. Tay ELW, Gurvitch R, Wijeysinghe N, et al. Outcome of patients after transcatheter aortic valve embolization. JACC Cardiovasc Interv 2011;4(2):228–34.

22. Mylotte D, Lefevre T, Søndergaard L, et al. Transcatheter aortic valve replacement in bicuspid aortic valve disease. J Am Coll Cardiol 2014;64(22):2330–9.

23. Vendrik J, van den Boogert TPW, Koch KT, et al. Balloon-expandable TAVR prosthesis dislocates into the ascending aorta. JACC Case Rep 2019; 1(2):101–4.

24. Ali AMA, Altwegg L, Horlick EM, et al. Prevention and management of transcatheter balloon-expandable aortic valve malposition. Catheter Cardiovasc Interv 2008;72(4):573–8.

25. Moreno-Samos JC, Vidovich MI. Device embolization in transcatheter aortic valve procedures. JACC Case Rep 2019;1(2):105–7.

26. Masson J-B. Transcatheter aortic valve implantation. Transcatheter Aortic Valve Implant 2009;2(9):10.

27. Mathur M, McCabe JM, Aldea G, et al. Overexpansion of the 29 mm SAPIEN 3 transcatheter heart valve in patients with large aortic annuli (area > 683 mm^2): A case series. Catheter Cardiovasc Interv 2018;91(6):1149–56.

28. Nazif T, Sanchez C, Whisenant B, et al. Analysis of the initial United States experience WITH the Biotrace Tempo temporary pacing lead in transcatheter aortic valve replacement (TAVR) and other cardiac procedures. J Am Coll Cardiol 2018; 71(11):A1285.

29. Webster M, Pasupati S, Lever N, et al. Safety and feasibility of a novel active fixation temporary pacing lead. J Invasive Cardiol 2018;30(5):163–7.

30. Faurie B, Souteyrand G, Staat P, et al. Left ventricular rapid pacing via the valve delivery guidewire in transcatheter aortic valve replacement. JACC Cardiovasc Interv 2019;12(24):2449–59.

31. Faurie B, Abdellaoui M, Wautot F, et al. Rapid pacing using the left ventricular guidewire: reviving an old technique to simplify BAV and TAVI procedures: LV guidewire for rapid pacing during BAV and TAVI. Catheter Cardiovasc Interv 2016;88(6):988–93.

32. Leon MB, Svensson LG, Makkar RR, et al. Transcatheter aortic-valve implantation for aortic stenosis in patients who cannot undergo surgery. N Engl J Med 2010;363(17):1597–607.

33. Leon MB, Svensson LG, Miller DC, et al. Transcatheter or surgical aortic-valve replacement in intermediate-risk patients. N Engl J Med 2016; 374(17):1609–20.

34. Mack MJ, Leon MB, Thourani VH, et al. Transcatheter aortic-valve replacement with a balloon-expandable valve in low-risk patients. N Engl J Med 2019;380(18):1695–705.

35. Mack MJ, Leon MB, Smith CR, et al. 5-year outcomes of transcatheter aortic valve replacement or surgical aortic valve replacement for high surgical risk patients with aortic stenosis (PARTNER 1): a randomised controlled trial. Lancet 2015; 385(9986):2477–84.

36. Makkar RR, Thourani VH, Mack MJ, et al. Five-year outcomes of transcatheter or surgical aortic-valve replacement. N Engl J Med 2020; 382(9):799–809.

37. Sponga S, Perron J, Dagenais F, et al. Impact of residual regurgitation after aortic valve replacement. Eur J Cardiothorac Surg 2012;42(3):486–92.

38. Holmes DR, Mack MJ, Kaul S, et al. 2012 ACCF/AATS/SCAI/STS expert consensus document on transcatheter aortic valve replacement. J Am Coll Cardiol 2012;59(13):1200–54.

39. Gä P. Paravalvular leak after transcatheter aortic valve replacement. Minerva Cardioangiol 2013; 61(11):12.

40. Pibarot P, Hahn RT, Weissman NJ, et al. Assessment of paravalvular regurgitation following TAVR. JACC Cardiovasc Imaging 2015;8(3): 340–60.

41. Kappetein AP, Head SJ, Blackstone EH, et al. Updated standardized endpoint definitions for transcatheter aortic valve implantation: The Valve Academic Research Consortium-2 consensus document. Eur Heart J 2012;33(19):2403–18.

42. Zoghbi WA, Asch FM, Bruce C, et al. Guidelines for the evaluation of valvular regurgitation after percutaneous valve repair or replacement. J Am Soc Echocardiogr 2019;32(4):431–75.

43. Welle GA, El-Sabawi B, Thaden JJ, et al. Effect of a fourth-generation transcatheter valve enhanced skirt on paravalvular leak. Catheter Cardiovasc Interv 2020. https://doi.org/10.1002/ccd.29317. ccd.29317.

44. Forrest JK, Kaple RK, Tang GHL, et al. Three generations of self-expanding transcatheter aortic valves. JACC Cardiovasc Interv 2020;13(2):170–9.

45. Kodali SK, Williams MR, Smith CR, et al. Two-year outcomes after transcatheter or surgical aortic-valve replacement. N Engl J Med 2012;366(18): 1686–95.

46. Tamburino C, Capodanno D, Ramondo A, et al. Incidence and predictors of early and late mortality after transcatheter aortic valve implantation in 663 patients with severe aortic stenosis. Circulation 2011;123(3):299–308.

47. Eggebrecht H, Doss M, Schmermund A, et al. Interventional options for severe aortic regurgitation after transcatheter aortic valve implantation:

48. balloons, snares, valve-in-valve. Clin Res Cardiol 2012;101(6):503–7.

48. Latib A, Michev I, Laborde J-C, et al. Post-implantation repositioning of the CoreValve percutaneous aortic valve. JACC Cardiovasc Interv 2010;3(1): 119–21.

49. Unbehaun A, Pasic M, Dreysse S, et al. Transapical aortic valve implantation. J Am Coll Cardiol 2012; 59(3):211–21.

50. Détaint D, Lepage L, Himbert D, et al. Determinants of significant paravalvular regurgitation after transcatheter aortic valve implantation. JACC Cardiovasc Interv 2009;2(9):821–7.

51. Buzzatti N, Maisano F, Latib A, et al. Computed tomography-based evaluation of aortic annulus, prosthesis size and impact on early residual aortic regurgitation after transcatheter aortic valve implantation. Eur J Cardiothorac Surg 2013;43(1): 43–51.

52. Schultz CJ, Tzikas A, Moelker A, et al. Correlates on MSCT of paravalvular aortic regurgitation after transcatheter aortic valve implantation using the Medtronic CoreValve prosthesis. Catheter Cardiovasc Interv 2011. https://doi.org/10.1002/ccd. 22993.

53. Block PC. Leaks and the "great ship" TAVI. Catheter Cardiovasc Interv 2010;75(6):873–4.

54. Jilaihawi H, Zhao Z, Du R, et al. Minimizing permanent pacemaker following repositionable self-expanding transcatheter aortic valve replacement. JACC Cardiovasc Interv 2019;12(18):1796–807.

55. Popma JJ, Reardon MJ, Khabbaz K, et al. Early clinical outcomes after transcatheter aortic valve replacement using a novel self-expanding bioprosthesis in patients with severe aortic stenosis who are suboptimal for surgery. JACC Cardiovasc Interv 2017;10(3):8.

56. Blanke P. Computed tomography-based oversizing degrees and incidence of paravalvular regurgitation of a new generation. Transcatheter Heart Valve 2017;10(8):11.

57. Nishimura RA, Carabello BA. Hemodynamics in the cardiac catheterization laboratory of the 21st century. Circulation 2012;125(17):2138–50.

58. Vasa-Nicotera M, Sinning J-M, Chin D, et al. Impact of paravalvular leakage on outcome in patients after transcatheter aortic valve implantation. JACC Cardiovasc Interv 2012;5(8):858–65.

59. Hess OM, Schneider J, Turina M, et al. Asymmetric septal hypertrophy in patients with aortic stenosis: An adaptive mechanism or a coexistence of hypertrophic cardiomyopathy. J Am Coll Cardiol 1983; 1(3):783–9.

60. Suh WM, Witzke CF, Palacios IF. Suicide left ventricle following transcatheter aortic valve implantation. Catheter Cardiovasc Interv 2010;76(4): 616–20.

61. Kayalar N, Schaff HV, Daly RC, et al. Concomitant septal myectomy at the time of aortic valve replacement for severe aortic stenosis. Ann Thorac Surg 2010;89(2):459–64.

62. Sorajja P, Booker JD, Rihal CS. Alcohol septal ablation after transaortic valve implantation: the dynamic nature of left outflow tract obstruction: ASA after TAVI. Catheter Cardiovasc Interv 2013; 81(2):387–91.

63. Jin XY, Pepper JR, Brecker SJ, et al. Early changes in left ventricular function after aortic valve replacement for isolated aortic stenosis. Am J Cardiol 1994;74(11):1142–6.

64. Nishimura RA, Ommen SR. Hypertrophic cardiomyopathy: the search for obstruction. Circulation 2006;114(21):2200–2.

65. Schwartzenberg S, Sorajja P. Cardiac tamponade or normal respiratory variation? An illustrative case of septal ablation for obstructive hypertrophic cardiomyopathy. Catheter Cardiovasc Interv 2010; 76(6):901–6.

66. Kwon DH, Smedira NG, Popovic ZB, et al. Steep left ventricle to aortic root angle and hypertrophic obstructive cardiomyopathy: study of a novel association using three-dimensional multimodality imaging. Heart 2009;95(21):1784–91.

67. Khan AA, Tang GHL, Engstrom K, et al. Aortic stenosis with severe asymmetric septal hypertrophy. JACC Cardiovasc Interv 2019;12(21):2228–30.

68. Krishnaswamy A, Tuzcu EM, Svensson LG, et al. Combined transcatheter aortic valve replacement and emergent alcohol septal ablation. Circulation 2013; 128(18). https://doi.org/10.1161/CIRCULATIONAHA. 112.000470.

69. Rezq A, Basavarajaiah S, Latib A, et al. Incidence, management, and outcomes of cardiac tamponade during transcatheter aortic valve implantation. JACC Cardiovasc Interv 2012;5(12):1264–72.

70. Ksiazcyzk M, Walczak A, Jegier B, et al. Rare case of enormous left ventricular pseudoaneurysm complicating transcatheter aortic valve implantation. Circ Cardiovasc Imaging 2020;13(5):3. https://doi.org/ 10.1161/CIRCIMAGING.119.010263.

71. Mahapatra S, Bybee KA, Bunch TJ, et al. Incidence and predictors of cardiac perforation after permanent pacemaker placement. Heart Rhythm 2005; 2(9):907–11.

72. Bhatia N, Kaiser CA, Fredi JL. Emergent percutaneous closure of left ventricular free wall perforation during transcatheter aortic valve replacement. JACC Cardiovasc Interv 2018;11(15): 1534–5.

73. Foerst J. Percutaneous repair of left ventricular wire perforation complicating transcatheter aortic valve replacement for aortic regurgitation. JACC Cardiovasc Interv 2016;9(13):1410–1.

74. Cozzarin A, Cianciulli TF, Guidoin R, et al. CoreValve prosthesis causes anterior mitral leaflet perforation resulting in severe mitral regurgitation. Can J Cardiol 2014;30(9):1108.e11-3.

75. Ando T, Holmes AA, Taub CC, et al. Iatrogenic ventricular septal defect following transcatheter aortic valve replacement: a systematic review. Heart Lung Circ 2016;25(10):968–74.

76. Massabuau P, Dumonteil N, Berthoumieu P, et al. Left-to-right interventricular shunt as a late complication of transapical aortic valve implantation. JACC Cardiovasc Interv 2011;4(6):710–2.

Risk and Mitigation of Coronary Obstruction in Transcatheter Aortic Valve Replacement

Giorgio A. Medranda, MD[a], Toby Rogers, MD, PhD[a,b,*]

KEYWORDS

- TAVR • Transcatheter aortic valve replacement • BASILICA • Valve-in-valve
- Coronary obstruction

KEY POINTS

- Coronary artery obstruction is a rare but devastating complication of transcatheter aortic valve replacement.
- Risk factors for coronary obstruction include low coronary heights, bulky calcified leaflets, small sinus of Valsalva, valve-in-valve transcatheter aortic valve replacement with either externally mounted leaflet or stentless bioprosthesis, and transcatheter aortic valve replacement prosthesis used for the case.
- Snorkel stenting, while relatively simple to perform, carries risks of challenging coronary re-access, stent thrombosis or stent compression from the frame of the transcatheter aortic valve replacement and sinotubular junction.
- BASILICA (Bioprosthetic or native Aortic Scallop Intentional Laceration to prevent Iatrogenic Coronary Artery obstruction) is a more physiologic way of preventing coronary obstruction.

INTRODUCTION

As indications for transcatheter heart valve replacement (TAVR) have expanded to include younger patients, there is an even stronger impetus to focus on prevention of complications.[1] Iatrogenic coronary obstruction during TAVR remains rare but devastating complication, associated with extremely high mortality.[2–7] The purpose of this review is to summarize the incidence, risk factors, mitigation strategies, and management of coronary obstruction during TAVR through a systemic review of the published literature.

WHAT DEFINES CORONARY OBSTRUCTION, AND HOW OFTEN DOES IT OCCUR?

Coronary obstruction is angiographic or echo-cardiographic evidence of a new—partial or complete—obstruction of a coronary ostium, either by the transcatheter valve prosthesis itself, the displaced leaflets of the failing native or bioprosthetic aortic valve, calcifications, dissection, or debris/thrombus embolization that occurs during or after the TAVR procedure.[8–15] Acute coronary obstruction occurs immediately after valve deployment. The most

[a] Section of Interventional Cardiology, MedStar Washington Hospital Center, 110 Irving Street NW, Suite 4B1, Washington, DC 20010, USA; [b] Cardiovascular Branch, Division of Intramural Research, National Heart, Lung and Blood Institute, National Institutes of Health, Bethesda, MD, USA
* Corresponding author. MedStar Washington Hospital Center, 110 Irving Street NW, Suite 4B1, Washington, DC 20010.
E-mail address: toby.rogers@medstar.net

Intervent Cardiol Clin 10 (2021) 481–490
https://doi.org/10.1016/j.iccl.2021.05.004
2211-7458/21/© 2021 Elsevier Inc. All rights reserved.

common mechanisms of acute coronary obstruction are displacement of the diseased leaflets of the failing native or bioprosthetic aortic valve over the coronary ostium, or the occlusion of the coronary ostium by the covered skirt portion of the TAVR valve.[16]

Delayed coronary obstruction is defined as obstruction of the coronary artery occurring after a patient has completed the TAVR procedure in stable condition and requires diagnosis by contrast-enhanced computed tomography scan, invasive angiography, surgery, or autopsy, assuming that the event was not solely related to progression of preexisting coronary artery disease or in-stent restenosis.[5–7] Delayed coronary obstruction after TAVR can be further categorized as early (0–7 days after TAVR) or late (>7 days after TAVR).[5] The proposed mechanisms for early delayed coronary obstruction include continued valve expansion, dissection, or expanding hematoma.[5–7] Late delayed coronary obstruction may be due to thrombus, valve endothelization, or late valve expansion.[5]

The incidence of acute coronary obstruction has been reported to be less than 1%. The pivotal US TAVR trials reported their incidence of coronary obstruction after TAVR to be between 0% and 0.9%.[8–15] Subsequent real-world experience has confirmed this finding, with an incidence of less than 1% for native valve TAVR using initial generations of valves.[2,3,17] Registry data from patients undergoing valve-in-valve (ViV) TAVR, however, have demonstrated a higher rate of up to 3.5%.[18] Data on delayed coronary obstruction remains sparse, but 1 study of 17,092 patients across 18 centers in the United States, Europe, and the Middle East between 2005 and 2016 reported an overall incidence of 0.18% in native valve TAVR and 0.89% in ViV TAVR[5] (Table 1).

The initial experience using earlier generation valves in a native valve TAVR reported that coronary obstruction involved the ostium of the left main (LM) in 88% of patents.[2] Coronary occlusion in ViV TAVR involves the ostium of the LM in up to 91.7% of cases, either alone or with right coronary artery occlusion.[4] In 1 study from the VIVID registry (Valve-in-Valve International Data), 58.3% of cases occurred immediately after valve deployment with an additional 36.1% occurring in the days that followed[4] (see Table 1).

WHICH PATIENTS ARE AT RISK FOR CORONARY OBSTRUCTION?

According to the literature, the mean age (76.7–83.1 years) of patients with acute coronary obstruction does not seem to differ much from the general population of TAVR trials.[2–4] The same is reported in patients with delayed coronary obstruction.[5] However, female sex does seem to be a risk factor for coronary obstruction in both acute (54.1%–84.1%) and delayed (74.3%) presentations.[2–5] The most important factors when attempting to identify patients at risk for coronary obstruction are the aortic root anatomy, the type of aortic valve present, and the type of implant.

Aortic root anatomy is best defined using pre-TAVR computed tomography scans. Alternative imaging using 3-dimensional transesophageal echocardiography often underestimates the annular size and offers only a limited evaluation of the rest of the aortic root, including the coronary ostia.[19,20] There are certain anatomic features detected on a computed tomography scan that are considered to be high risk for coronary obstruction. The first is a low LM ostial height (<10 mm), which is defined as the distance between the LM ostium and the aortic annulus.[16] Several studies have reported mean LM ostial heights between 9.5 and 10.6 mm in patients with acute coronary obstruction after TAVR.[2–4] The second is the virtual valve-to-coronary distance that, if less than 4 mm, places a patient at high risk for acute coronary obstruction in ViV TAVR.[4] In the VIVID registry, patients with acute coronary obstruction after a ViV TAVR had a mean virtual valve-to-coronary distance of 3.24 mm in the left and 3.90 mm in the right.[4] Another high-risk finding for the ostia of the LM is the presence of severe aortic valve thickening and calcification with bulky calcium nodules in the left cusp (Fig. 1).[16] Significant ostial LM disease (≥50% angiographic stenosis, a minimal luminal area of ≤6 mm^2 on intravascular ultrasound examination, or a previous LM ostial stent), sinus width and sinotubular junction height are also contributing risk factors (Table 2).[16]

The type of aortic valve present before TAVR plays a role in assessing risk as well. There is clearly an increased risk of coronary obstruction in patients undergoing TAVR for failing bioprosthetic valves.[16] In particular, stentless bioprosthetic (eg, Freestyle, Medtronic, Minneapolis, MN) and pericardial surgical valves with leaflets sutured outside the stent posts (eg, Mitroflow, Sorin, Milan, Italy, or Trifecta, St. Jude Medical, St. Paul, MN) are considered high risk because the leaflets are unconstrained by the commissural suture posts and are more prone to bulging outward during TAVR.[18,21]

Finally, a major consideration is the type of valve to be used during TAVR. One review

Table 1
Summary of published data on acute coronary obstruction after TAVR

Study	Incidence	Patients with Coronary Obstruction	Balloon Expandable Valve	Left Main Involvement	PCI Attempted	PCI Successful	Conversion to Open Heart Surgery	Inpatient Mortality
Native Valve TAVR								
PARTNER Trial,[9] 2011	0%							
Khatri et al,[17] 2013	0.8%	21	71.4%					
Ribeiro et al,[2] 2013		24	87.5%	87.5%	95.8%	91.3%	8.3%	8.3%
Ribeiro et al,[3] 2013		44	84.1%	95.5%	75.0%	81.8%	6.1%	40.9%
CoreValve Trial,[10] 2014	0.5%	2	0%				100%	
PARTNER 2 Trial,[12] 2016	0.4%	4	100%					
Low Risk TAVR Trial,[38] 2018	0.5%	1					100%	0%
PARTNER 3 Trial,[14] 2019	0.2%	1	100%					
Evolut Low Risk Trial,[15] 2019	0.9%							
ViV TAVR								
Dvir et al,[18] 2012	3.5%	7	42.9%	100%			57.1%	57.1%
Ribeiro et al,[4] 2018	2.3%	37	32.4%	91.7%	77.8%	64.3%	9.7%	22.2%

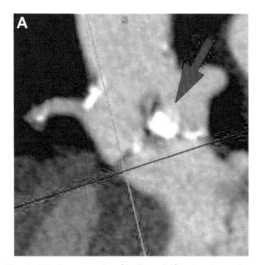
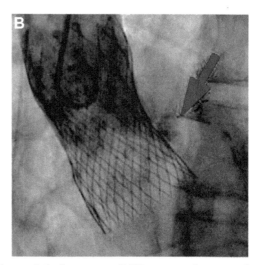

Fig. 1. (*A*) An example of bulky calcification (*arrow*) on native aortic leaflet on a pre-TAVR computed tomography scan, which resulted in (*B*) coronary obstruction (*arrow*) after deployment of the TAVR valve.-

demonstrated that 88% of cases of coronary obstruction occurred in patients receiving a balloon expandable valve.[2] According to a multi-center registry of 6688 using earlier generation valves, for native valve TAVR, the coronary obstruction rate was more than twice as high using a balloon-expandable valve compared with a self-expanding valve (0.81% vs 0.34%; P = .023).[3] The fundamental differences in valve design and the mechanism of deployment may explain this disparity, which is particularly important in the fourth-generation balloon-expandable SAPIEN 3 Ultra (Edwards Lifesciences, Irving, CA), which now contains a textured polyethylene terephthalate skirt at its base that is 40% taller.[22] Balloon-expandable valves are also more likely to flare outward at the outflow in the aorta, particularly if inflated at higher pressures, which pushes the displaced native or bioprosthetic valve leaflet further outward toward the coronary ostia. However, it is also likely that certain native valve anatomic characteristics, such as coronary height, play a role in valve selection for operators, leading to selection bias in patients at high risk for acute coronary obstruction to preferentially receive a lower profile balloon-expandable valve. In contrast, data on delayed coronary obstruction in native valve TAVR, reports it to be more frequently associated with the use of self-expanding bioprostheses (0.36% vs 0.11%; P<.001), which could be explained by ongoing expansion of the self-expanding Nitinol frame after deployment.[5] For ViV TAVR, coronary occlusion occurs more frequently using self-expanding TAVR valves as well (76.9% of the time in 1 study),[4]

but this difference could be explained by selection bias in patients with small surgical bioprostheses and operator preference for supra-annular self-expanding transcatheter valves to optimize hemodynamics. Also of concern with all contemporary transcatheter heart valves is the inability to guarantee where the commissural suture posts will land with respect to the coronary ostia. Commissural malalignment is likely a contributor to coronary occlusion in some patients, because the otherwise open cells of the transcatheter heart valve frames are either fully or partially covered at the commissures.

HOW CAN WE MITIGATE THE RISK OF CORONARY OBSTRUCTION?

First, prevention is better than a cure. The anatomic, device, and procedural risk factors should be assessed in every patient to identify those at high risk for coronary obstruction and assist in procedural planning. For low surgical risk patients with significant risk factors for acute coronary obstruction, a robust heart team discussion is essential, because surgical aortic valve replacement may be a more appropriate treatment strategy. However, many patients deemed to be at risk for acute coronary obstruction are high or prohibitive surgical risks and their only option is TAVR.[1–5] For these patients, several techniques have been described in the literature aimed at mitigating the risk for acute coronary obstruction after TAVR.

The so-called coronary protection, in which a guidewire with a premounted coronary stent is

Table 2
Key computed tomography variable that impact risk of coronary obstruction during TAVR

	Controls (n = 90)	Coronary Obstruction (n = 20)	P Value
Surgical frame mean diameter (mm)	20.6 ± 2.6	21.1 ± 3.3	.39
Surgical frame area (cm²)	3.37 ± 0.85	3.59 ± 1.25	.35
Sinus of Valsalva width (mm)	32.55 ± 3.98	27.44 ± 4.05	<.001
Sinotubular junction height (mm)	19.25 ± 3.97	20.01 ± 7.58	.52
LCA height to annulus distance (mm)	9.69 ± 4.12	9.48 ± 2.67	.82
RCA height to annulus distance (mm)	11.17 ± 4.33	11.97 ± 2.52	.43
LCA originates above posts	5/86 (5.8)	0 (0)	.27
RCA originates above posts	14/86 (16.3)	0 (0)	.05
VTC to LCA (mm)	6.30 ± 2.34	3.24 ± 2.22	<.001
VTC to RCA (mm)	6.08 ± 2.43	3.90 ± 3.49	.002

Values are expressed as mean ± SD.

Abbreviations: LCA, left coronary artery; RCA, right coronary artery; SD, standard deviation; SOV, sinus of Valsalva; STJ, sinotubular junction; VTC, distance between a virtual transcatheter ring at a size of the implanted device at the level of each coronary ostium.

(Reproduced from Ribeiro and colleagues.[4])

positioned in the at-risk coronary artery before the transcatheter valve is deployed, has been widely used. In the event of acute coronary obstruction after valve deployment, the stent is deployed.[3,16,23–27] There are 2 predominant stenting techniques described in the literature. The first is the more traditional ostial stenting technique in which the stent is deployed just protruding into the aorta but this remains unproven in TAVR.[16,23] The second is the snorkel stenting technique, in which the stent is implanted in the ostia, then snorkeled up alongside the TAVR valve into the aorta.[25–27] The International Chimney Registry described 60 cases of snorkel stenting during TAVR.[25] In this retrospective, multicenter study, 44 patients underwent prophylactic placement of a guidewire and stent in the proximal left anterior descending in anticipation of acute coronary obstruction.[25] Stent failure was reported in 2 cases with a median follow-up of 612 days.[25] The CORPROTAVR (CORonary PROtection during TAVR) study, was another multicenter retrospective study of 236 patients deemed to be at risk for acute coronary obstruction who received preemptive coronary protection.[27] In this study, 143 patients received stenting, of which 79.9% underwent snorkel stenting and the remaining 20.1% received ostial stenting.[27] Outcomes at 3 years were generally favorable, with cardiac

mortality occurring in just 7.8% of patients and stent thrombosis is just 0.9% of patients.[27] Nonetheless, there remains concern regarding the long-term outcomes of the snorkel stenting technique. Stent protrusion into the aorta risks thrombosis, and interaction with the metallic transcatheter heart valve frame risks stent failure. Snorkeled stents can also be compressed between the metallic frame of the transcatheter heart valve and the aortic wall (Fig. 2). Additionally, the optimal duration and intensity of antiplatelet therapy has not been studied using this stenting technique. This point is particularly important when considering the population at risk for coronary obstruction, and their increased bleeding risk. Finally, future coronary reaccess in these patients is expected to be extremely challenging after snorkel stenting. With all of these factors in mind, the snorkel stenting technique remains unproven, with numerous technical and mechanical concerns and should, in our opinion, remain a bailout option and not a first-line preventative strategy.

A more physiologic approach to prevent coronary obstruction is the bioprosthetic or native aortic scallop intentional laceration to prevent coronary artery obstruction (BASILICA) procedure.[28–35] The BASILICA procedure was inspired by the electrosurgical leaflet laceration of the LAMPOON procedure, in which catheters are

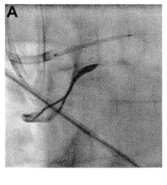
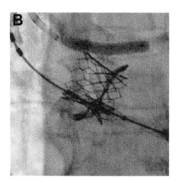
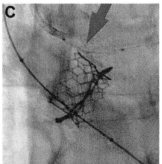
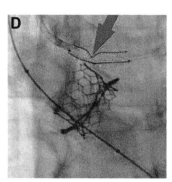

Fig. 2. A complication of snorkel stent during TAVR with a balloon expandable valve. (A) Prophylactic placement of a coronary stent before TAVR. (B) Stent deployment after TAVR deployment resulting in (C/D) compression of the stent between the balloon-expandable transcatheter heart valve frame and the aortic wall.

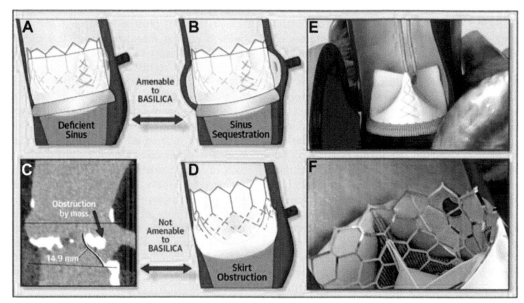

Fig. 3. The BASILICA procedure. (A) In a deficient sinus of Valsalva, the outwardly displaced leaflets directly obstruct the coronary artery ostium. (B) In a low sinus of Valsalva and narrow sinotubular junction, the outwardly displaced leaflets indirectly obstruct the coronary artery ostium by sequestering the sinus. (C) A bulky leaflet mass can directly obstruct the coronary ostium. (D) In a low coronary ostium, the fabric-covered frame or skirt can directly obstruct the coronary artery ostium. (E) An electrified BASILICA guidewire lacerates the prior aortic valve leaflets. (F) A TAVR implant splays the lacerated leaflets and ensures inflow to the threatened coronary ostium after BASILICA. (Reproduced with permission from Khan J. et al. JACC, 2019, 12(13):1240-52.)

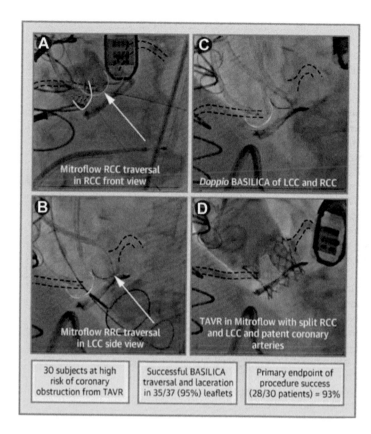

Fig. 4. Key findings from the BASILICA trial. (*A*) The guidewire traverses the right coronary cusp (RCC). (*B*) The guidewire traverses the left coronary cusp (LCC) into a snare in the left ventricular outflow tract. (*C*) BASILICA guidewire loops are formed through the base of both right and left cusps, ready for radiofrequency-assisted laceration. (*D*) Aortic root angiography demonstrates flow to both coronaries through the split Mitroflow leaflets after TAVR with a SAPIEN 3 valve. (*Reproduced with permission from Khan J. et al. JACC, 2019, 12(13):1240-52.*)

used to split the anterior mitral valve leaflet to prevent left ventricular outflow tract obstruction after transcatheter mitral valve intervention.[36,37] Laceration of the offending aortic valve leaflet is an effective approach for preventing coronary obstruction by creating a split in the leaflet that widens into a splay when the transcatheter heart valve is implanted, and that provides a channel to maintain coronary flow. In the BASILICA procedure, a guide catheter is positioned at the scallop hinge point using angiographic (and/or echocardiographic) guidance, with a second catheter positioned in the left ventricular outflow tract with a snare.[31] Through the first catheter, a guidewire sheathed in an insulating polymer jacket is electrified and advanced through the target leaflet and into the left ventricular outflow tract, then snared by the second catheter.[31] Then, while applying tension at both ends of the guidewire, using a burst of radiofrequency energy, the aortic leaflet is lacerated using a flying V cutting edge[31] (**Figs. 3 and 4**). The initial experience in the BASILICA Trial was encouraging in both native aortic valves and surgical bioprosthetic aortic valves.[32] In fact, specialized catheters (pachyderm-shaped guiding catheters) have been designed specifically

for the BASILICA procedure, decreasing the time to traversal.[34] This procedure may offer additional benefits in improving sinus and neosinus flow patterns after TAVR.[28,29] Further data are needed to determine whether BASILICA is effective for TAV-in-TAV procedures.[30] If snorkel stenting fails to protect the coronary artery, then emergent open heart surgery is usually the only option; if BASILICA results in suboptimal leaflet laceration or partial coronary obstruction from leaflet remnants, then this condition can usually be treated with orthotopic stenting (ie, through the open cells of the transcatheter heart valve and into the coronary ostium, rather than a long stent trapped behind the valve frame as with snorkel stenting). In our opinion, BASILICA offers a more physiologic approach compared with the previously described stenting techniques for patients at risk for coronary obstruction during TAVR.

WHAT IS THE CLINICAL PRESENTATION OF AND HOW CAN WE MANAGE CORONARY OBSTRUCTION?

Acute severe hypotension and ST-elevation on the electrocardiogram after valve deployment in TAVR are the most common presentations of acute coronary occlusion and should prompt immediate investigation using echocardiography and angiography.[2–4] As described elsewhere in this article, delayed coronary obstruction can present in the days to weeks that follow TAVR and is manifested by signs and symptoms of ischemia and/or acute coronary syndrome.[5–7] Electrocardiography will demonstrate ischemic ST-segment changes in approximately 50% of cases, with 25% experiencing ventricular arrythmias.[2–4] The in-patient mortality for acute coronary obstruction in native valve TAVR remains exceedingly high and has been reported to be between 8.3% and 40.9%.[2,3] For patients undergoing ViV TAVR, in-patient mortality after acute coronary obstruction was even higher, between 22.2% and 57.1%[4,18] (see Table 1).

If acute coronary obstruction occurs, first-line therapy usually involves emergent percutaneous coronary intervention (PCI), mechanical circulatory support, snaring the transcatheter heart valve, and intentionally embolizing it into the ascending aorta. If all else fails, then open heart surgery should be considered. In the international Chimney Registry, 16 of the 60 cases of chimney stenting during TAVR occurred as a bailout procedure with acceptable short-term and mid-term outcomes.[25] PCI is attempted in most, but not all, patients with acute coronary obstruction, ranging from 75.0% to 95.8% of patients.[2–4] Unfortunately, bailout PCI is not always successful, with ViV TAVR seeing the lowest rates of success (64.3%).[4] For patients in whom PCI is unsuccessful, conversion to open heart surgery is the only remaining option, carrying the highest mortality.[2–4]

SUMMARY

Coronary obstruction, albeit extremely rare, remains a devastating complication of TAVR and is associated with an extremely high mortality rate. Those at greatest risk seem to be females, with low coronary heights, with small aortic annuli, and with failing aortic valve bioprostheses. The identification of patients at high risk of obstruction is critical and a prevention strategy with BASILICA or snorkel stenting should be planned before TAVR. Management options if coronary obstruction occurs are limited, with PCI and emergent surgery both associated with a high mortality rate. In the future, enhanced transcatheter heart valve designs and deployment techniques that guarantee anatomic commissural alignment should also help to further mitigate the risk of coronary obstruction in TAVR.

CLINICS CARE POINTS

- Acute coronary artery occlusion is a rare but devastating complication of transcatheter aortic valve replacement.
- The key factors that identify patients at risk for coronary obstruction are aortic root anatomy, type of aortic valve present (native vs. bioprosthetic) and type of transcatheter heart valve to be implanted.
- Coronary obstruction can be prevented using intentional leaflet laceration with BASILICA and stenting techniques, however bailout stenting can be challenging and conversion to emergent open-heart surgery may be required, both of which are associated with high morbidity and mortality.

ACKNOWLEDGMENTS

The authors thank Drs Adam Greenbaum, Vasilis Babaliaros, and John Lisko from Emory University Hospital Midtown for the images in Fig. 2.

REFERENCES

1. Arnold SV, Manandhar P, Vemulapalli S, et al. Impact of short-term complications of TAVR on longer-term outcomes: results from the STS/ACC transcatheter valve therapy registry. European Heart Journal - Quality of Care and Clinical Outcomes 2021;7:208–13.
2. Ribeiro HB, Nombela-Franco L, Urena M, et al. Coronary obstruction following transcatheter aortic valve implantation: a systematic review. JACC Cardiovasc Interv 2013;6(5):452–61.
3. Ribeiro HB, Webb JG, Makkar RR, et al. Predictive factors, management, and clinical outcomes of coronary obstruction following transcatheter aortic valve implantation: insights from a large multicenter registry. J Am Coll Cardiol 2013;62(17):1552–62.
4. Ribeiro HB, Rodes-Cabau J, Blanke P, et al. Incidence, predictors, and clinical outcomes of coronary obstruction following transcatheter aortic valve replacement for degenerative bioprosthetic surgical valves: insights from the VIVID registry. Eur Heart J 2018;39(8):687–95.
5. Jabbour RJ, Tanaka A, Finkelstein A, et al. Delayed coronary obstruction after transcatheter aortic valve replacement. J Am Coll Cardiol 2018;71(14):1513–24.
6. Spiro J, Nadeem A, Doshi SN. Delayed left main stem obstruction following successful TAVI with an Edwards SAPIEN XT valve: successful resuscitation and percutaneous coronary intervention using

a non-invasive automated chest compression device (AutoPulse). J Invasive Cardiol 2012;24(5): 224–8.

7. Kukucka M, Pasic M, Dreysse S, et al. Delayed subtotal coronary obstruction after transapical aortic valve implantation. Interact Cardiovasc Thorac Surg 2011;12(1):57–60.

8. Leon MB, Smith CR, Mack M, et al. Transcatheter aortic-valve implantation for aortic stenosis in patients who cannot undergo surgery. N Engl J Med 2010;363(17):1597–607.

9. Smith CR, Leon MB, Mack MJ, et al. Transcatheter versus surgical aortic-valve replacement in high-risk patients. N Engl J Med 2011;364(23):2187–98.

10. Adams DH, Popma JJ, Reardon MJ, et al. Transcatheter aortic-valve replacement with a self-expanding prosthesis. N Engl J Med 2014;370(19):1790–8.

11. Popma JJ, Adams DH, Reardon MJ, et al. Transcatheter aortic valve replacement using a self-expanding bioprosthesis in patients with severe aortic stenosis at extreme risk for surgery. J Am Coll Cardiol 2014;63(19):1972–81.

12. Leon MB, Smith CR, Mack MJ, et al. Transcatheter or surgical aortic-valve replacement in intermediate-risk patients. N Engl J Med 2016; 374(17):1609–20.

13. Reardon MJ, Van Mieghem NM, Popma JJ, et al. Surgical or transcatheter aortic-valve replacement in intermediate-risk patients. N Engl J Med 2017; 376(14):1321–31.

14. Mack MJ, Leon MB, Thourani VH, et al. Transcatheter aortic-valve replacement with a balloon-expandable valve in low-risk patients. N Engl J Med 2019;380(18):1695–705.

15. Popma JJ, Deeb GM, Yakubov SJ, et al. Transcatheter aortic-valve replacement with a self-expanding valve in low-risk patients. N Engl J Med 2019; 380(18):1706–15.

16. Abramowitz Y, Chakravarty T, Jilaihawi H, et al. Clinical impact of coronary protection during transcatheter aortic valve implantation: first reported series of patients. EuroIntervention 2015;11(5):572–81.

17. Khatri PJ, Webb JG, Rodes-Cabau J, et al. Adverse effects associated with transcatheter aortic valve implantation: a meta-analysis of contemporary studies. Ann Intern Med 2013;158(1):35–46.

18. Dvir D, Webb J, Brecker S, et al. Transcatheter aortic valve replacement for degenerative bioprosthetic surgical valves: results from the global valve-in-valve registry. Circulation 2012;126(19):2335–44.

19. Prihadi EA, van Rosendael PJ, Vollema EM, et al. Feasibility, accuracy, and reproducibility of aortic annular and root sizing for transcatheter aortic valve replacement using novel automated three-dimensional echocardiographic software: comparison with multi-detector row computed tomography. J Am Soc Echocardiogr 2018;31(4):505–14.e3.

20. Hafiz AM, Medranda GA, Kakouros N, et al. Is intra-procedure three-dimensional transesophageal echocardiogram an alternative to preprocedure multidetector computed tomography for the measurement of the aortic annulus in patients undergoing transcatheter aortic valve replacement? Echocardiography 2017;34(8):1195–202.

21. Dvir D, Leipsic J, Blanke P, et al. Coronary obstruction in transcatheter aortic valve-in-valve implantation: preprocedural evaluation, device selection, protection, and treatment. Circ Cardiovasc Interv 2015;8(1).

22. Solomonica A, Choudhury T, Bagur R. Newer-generation of Edwards transcatheter aortic valve systems: SAPIEN 3, Centera, and SAPIEN 3 Ultra. Expert Rev Med Devices 2019;16(2):81–7.

23. Chakravarty T, Jilaihawi H, Nakamura M, et al. Pre-emptive positioning of a coronary stent in the left anterior descending artery for left main protection: a prerequisite for transcatheter aortic valve-in-valve implantation for failing stentless bioprostheses? Catheter Cardiovasc Interv 2013;82(4):E630–6.

24. Yamamoto M, Shimura T, Kano S, et al. Impact of preparatory coronary protection in patients at high anatomical risk of acute coronary obstruction during transcatheter aortic valve implantation. Int J Cardiol 2016;217:58–63.

25. Mercanti F, Rosseel L, Neylon A, et al. Chimney stenting for coronary occlusion during TAVR: insights from the chimney registry. JACC Cardiovasc Interv 2020;13(6):751–61.

26. Rosseel L, Rosseel M, Hynes B, et al. Chimney stenting during transcatheter aortic valve implantation. Interv Cardiol 2020;15:e09.

27. Palmerini T, Chakravarty T, Saia F, et al. Coronary protection to prevent coronary obstruction during TAVR: a multicenter international registry. JACC Cardiovasc Interv 2020;13(6):739–47.

28. Hatoum H, Maureira P, Lilly S, et al. Impact of leaflet laceration on transcatheter aortic valve-in-valve washout: BASILICA to solve neosinus and sinus stasis. JACC Cardiovasc Interv 2019;12(13):1229–37.

29. Hatoum H, Maureira P, Lilly S, et al. Impact of BASILICA on sinus and neo-sinus hemodynamics after valve-in-valve with and without coronary flow. Cardiovasc Revasc Med 2020;21(3):271–6.

30. Khan JM, Bruce CG, Babaliaros VC, et al. TAVR roulette: caution regarding BASILICA laceration for TAVR-in-TAVR. JACC Cardiovasc Interv 2020;13(6): 787–9.

31. Khan JM, Dvir D, Greenbaum AB, et al. Transcatheter laceration of aortic leaflets to prevent coronary obstruction during transcatheter aortic valve replacement: concept to first-in-human. JACC Cardiovasc Interv 2018;11(7):677–89.

32. Khan JM, Greenbaum AB, Babaliaros VC, et al. The BASILICA trial: prospective multicenter investigation of intentional leaflet laceration to prevent

TAVR coronary obstruction. JACC Cardiovasc Interv 2019;12(13):1240–52.

33. Lederman RJ, Babaliaros VC, Rogers T, et al. Preventing coronary obstruction during transcatheter aortic valve replacement: from computed tomography to BASILICA. JACC Cardiovasc Interv 2019; 12(13):1197–216.

34. Lisko JC, Babaliaros VC, Lederman RJ, et al. Pachyderm-shape guiding catheters to simplify BASILICA leaflet traversal. Cardiovasc Revasc Med 2019;20(9): 782–5.

35. Zhingre Sanchez JD, Iles TL, Dvir D, et al. Direct visualisation of the BASILICA technique post TAVR to enhance coronary flow. EuroIntervention 2020; 16(8):680–1.

36. Khan JM, Rogers T, Schenke WH, et al. Intentional laceration of the anterior mitral valve leaflet to prevent left ventricular outflow tract obstruction during transcatheter mitral valve replacement: pre-clinical findings. JACC Cardiovasc Interv 2016;9(17):1835–43.

37. Babaliaros VC, Greenbaum AB, Khan JM, et al. Intentional percutaneous laceration of the anterior mitral leaflet to prevent outflow obstruction during transcatheter mitral valve replacement: first-in-human experience. JACC Cardiovasc Interv 2017; 10(8):798–809.

38. Waksman R, Rogers T, Torguson R, et al. Transcatheter aortic valve replacement in low-risk patients with symptomatic severe aortic stenosis. J Am Coll Cardiol 2018;72(18):2095–105.

Valve-in-Valve Transcatheter Aortic Valve Replacement, with Present-Day Innovations and Up-to-Date Techniques

Salem A. Salem, MD, Jason R. Foerst, MD*

KEYWORDS

- Valve-in-valve TAVR • Bioprosthetic • Valve • SAPIEN • Evolut • Basilica • Coronary height
- Coronary obstruction

KEY POINTS

- Valve-in-Valve (ViV) TAVR is an alternative to open surgical intervention for patients with failing bioprosthetic aortic valves.
- ViV TAVR should be performed by highly skilled operators at high volume centers for optimal results.
- Careful patient selection and thorough preoperative planning is one key for successful ViV TAVR.
- When compared with native aortic valve TAVR, ViV TAVR has increased residual trans-aortic valve gradients, and heightened risk for coronary artery obstruction, with lower risk for need for permanent pacemaker implantation.

INTRODUCTION

Severe valvular heart disease has traditionally been treated with surgical valve replacement with either a bioprosthetic or a mechanical valve (Table 1).[1–8] Over the past 2 decades, there has been a shift toward greater bioprosthetic valve utilization.[6,7] This is attributed to morbidity and mortality associated with mechanical valves from thromboembolism or anticoagulant use,[8] improved newer generation bioprosthetic surgical valves,[9–11] and patients' preference to avoid long-term anticoagulation.[8] Bioprosthetic valves have been shown to have higher rate of reoperation due to structural deterioration[8,12,13] and, despite this, many younger patients are undergoing implantation of bioprosthetic valves.[6]

Moreover, young patients who are recipients of bioprosthetic surgical valves have an accelerated degeneration process compared with older counterparts.[6,8,14,15] Although some patients are candidates for reoperation, many others are at increased, if not prohibitive risk for surgery.[8,16–18] Since the inception of the Transcatheter Valve Therapeutics (TVT) Registry, the rate of valve-in-valve transcatheter aortic valve replacement (ViV TAVR) has ranged from 4.6% to 6.7% of cases, and at last count nearly 4900 cases were performed in 2019.[1–3] The first clinical ViV TAVR was performed in 2007 in an 80-year-old man with severe bioprosthetic aortic valve insufficiency.[17] In 2010, Azadani and colleagues[19,20] illustrated the potential long-term feasibility of ViV TAVR through ex vivo

All authors take responsibility for all aspects of the reliability and freedom from bias of the data presented and their discussed interpretation. The authors report no financial relationships or conflicts of interest regarding the content herein.

Structural and Interventional Cardiology, Virginia Tech Carilion School of Medicine, Carilion Clinic, 1906 Belleview Avenue SE, Roanoke, VA 24014, USA
* Corresponding author.
E-mail address: JRFoerst@Carilionclinic.org

2211-7458/21/© 2021 Elsevier Inc. All rights reserved.

Table 1
Computed tomography data, according to the occurrence of coronary obstruction following transcatheter aortic valve replacement

Anatomical parameters	Controls (n = 90)	Coronary Obstruction (n = 20)	P Value
Surgical frame mean diameter, mm	20.6 ± 2.6	21.1 ± 3.3	.39
Surgical frame area, cm^2	3.37 ± 0.85	3.59 ± 1.25	.35
SOV width, mm	32.55 ± 3.98	27.44 ± 4.05	<.001
STJ height, mm	19.25 ± 3.97	20.01 ± 7.58	.52
LCA height to annulus distance, mm	9.69 ± 4.12	9.48 ± 2.67	.82
RCA height to annulus distance, mm	11.17 ± 4.33	11.97 ± 2.52	.43
LCA originates above the posts	5/86 (5.8)	0 (0)	.27
RCA originate above the posts	14/86 (16.3)	0 (0)	.05
VTC to LCA, mm	6.30 ± 2.34	3.24 ± 2.22	<.001
VTC to RCA, mm	6.08 ± 2.43	3.90 ± 3.49	.002

Abbreviations: LCA, left coronary artery; RCA, right coronary artery; STJ, sinotubular junction; SOV, sinus of valsalva; VTC, heart valve to coronary distance.

From: (Ribeiro, H. B., Rodes-Cabau, J., Blanke, P., Leipsic, J., Kwan Park, J., Bapat, V., . . . Dvir, D. (2018). Incidence, predictors, and clinical outcomes of coronary obstruction following transcatheter aortic valve replacement for degenerative bioprosthetic surgical valves: insights from the VIVID registry. *Eur Heart J, 39*(8), 687-695. https://doi.org/10.1093/eurheartj/ehx455). Reprinted with Permission.

hemodynamic profiles of balloon-expandable transcatheter heart valve (THV) implanted into Carpentier-Edwards PERIMOUNT (Edwards Lifescience, Irvine, CA) surgical valves. The US Food and Drug Administration (FDA) approved ViV TAVR with the commercially available self-expanding THV in 2015 and balloon-expandable valve in 2017 for patients with failed surgical valves who are at high risk of reoperation.[4–6] ViV TAVR appears deceptively simple, but the attendant risks of ViV TAVR, such as coronary artery obstruction and patient-prosthesis mismatch, have prompted significant focus to the nuances of the procedure.[21]

BIOPROSTHETIC SURGICAL VALVE STRUCTURE

Crucial to ViV TAVR is the understanding of the type, size, and structure of the bioprosthetic surgical valve, and mechanism of failure. Stented bioprosthetic surgical valves contain a base ring, from which 3 struts arise at right angles to suspend the valve leaflets. The base ring can be either circular or saddle shaped. The ring and the stent are made of a variety of components, including metallic alloys, silicone, rubber, synthetic polymers, or stainless steel. The stent is covered with a covering cloth, usually made of Dacron,

pericardium, polytetrafluoroethylene, or some other polyester fabric. The base ring and covering cloth are also known as the "suture ring." Valve leaflets can be of xenograft (porcine aortic valve or bovine pericardium), or less commonly, of homograft origin[14] (Fig. 1). Valve leaflets are treated with anticalcification agents and are either sewn internal or external to the stent (see Fig. 1).

The inner stent diameter (the inner base ring diameter) is the internal diameter of the base ring. The outer stent diameter (the outer base ring diameter) is the outer diameter of the base ring, excluding the covering cloth. The external valve diameter (the outer suture ring diameter) includes the base ring and the sewing cuff[14] (see Fig. 1). The outer suture ring diameter reflects the commercial size of the bioprosthetic surgical valve that corresponds to the native aortic valve annular size as measured by preoperative computed tomography (CT) or by the operating surgeon at the time of implant using manufacturer-specific sizing tools. Bioprosthetic surgical valve selection can be influenced by various factors, including availability, expertise, philosophy, and technical and/or anatomic variables. The most pertinent dimension for ViV TAVR is the inner base ring diameter, where the THV anchors.[22] Valve labeling of size is inconsistent among manufacturers,

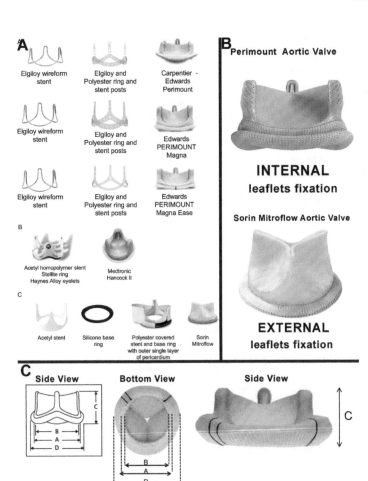

Fig. 1. (A) Stented bioprosthetic valves consist of a base ring and stent with supporting posts. (B) Leaflet fixation relative to bioprosthetic aortic valve stent. External leaflet fixation suspends leaflets to the inner edge of stent strut. Internal leaflet fixation suspends leaflets to the outer edge of the stent strut. (C) Dimensions of stented bioprosthetic valves. A: outer stent diameter, B: inner stent diameter, C: prosthesis height, D: outer sewing ring diameter. (From: (Piazza, N., Bleiziffer, S., Brockmann, G., Hendrick, R., Deutsch, M. A., Opitz, A., . . . Lange, R. (2011). Transcatheter aortic valve implantation for failing surgical aortic bioprosthetic valve: from concept to clinical application and evaluation (part 1). JACC Cardiovasc Interv, 4(7), 721-732. https://doi.org/10. 1016/j.jcin.2011.03.016). Reprinted with permission.)

thus hemodynamic outcomes of "similar" labeled valve sizes from different valve manufacturers may vary.[14] Different valve types have various radiopaque elements that can help align the THV for accurate depth and positioning.[8] Different dimensions, leaflet mounting, durability, radiographic appearance, valve frame compliance, and many more useful parameters are available by various industry sources but must always be measured by CT imaging.[8]

SAFETY OF VALVE-IN-VALVE TRANSCATHETER AORTIC VALVE REPLACEMENT

The earliest data to evaluate ViV TAVR have been the Valve-in-Valve International Data (VIVID) and Society of Thoracic Surgeons (STS)/American College of Cardiology (ACC) TVT registries.[10,15,23,24] Overall mortality at 30 days was 2.1% in 1150 patients in the TVT Registry,[24] and 4.6% of 1168 patients undergoing ViV TAVR who were included in the VIVID Registry.[25] Aortic stenosis, but not regurgitation, and presence of a small bioprosthetic

surgical valve ($\leq$23 mm) was associated with increased mortality in the VIVID Registry.[23] When compared with native valve TAVR, ViV TAVR had higher residual mean gradients (16 mm Hg vs 9 mm Hg), but lower rate of paravalvular leak (PVL) (3.5% vs 6.6%), lower rate of stroke, or need for new pacemaker (3%).[24] There are no randomized data comparing the risk of ViV TAVR with redo SAVR. The largest scale long-term assessment of ViV TAVR to date (2020) concluded that survival was lower at 8 years in patients with small-failed bioprostheses (internal diameter [ID] $\leq$20 mm) compared with those with large-failed bioprostheses (ID >20 mm) (33.2% vs 40.5%, $P = .01$). Another independent correlate for long-term mortality was nontransfemoral access.[26]

PREOPERATIVE PLANNING FOR VALVE-IN-VALVE TRANSCATHETER AORTIC VALVE REPLACEMENT

Detailed history taking, physical examination, and thorough discussion with a multidisciplinary team of ViV TAVR versus SAVR is important.

Surgical risk stratification, including SAVR risk, should be clearly discussed with the patient. Acquisition and meticulous analysis of high-quality gated CT scan using standardized protocols for optimal assessment of the valve is fundamental. Detailed knowledge of the type and size of bioprosthetic valve, internal ring diameter, year of implantation, mode of failure (stenosis vs regurgitation), and susceptibility to fracture is crucial in planning ViV TAVR. The CT scan is not only needed to corroborate the manufacturer measurements but also assess for risks of coronary obstruction.

Radiographic and angiographic analysis of feasibility of transfemoral access, and optimal coplanar angle for implantation should be performed. ViV TAVR carries heightened risks for coronary ostial obstruction, hence, more variables need to be assessed preoperatively. Coronary ostia heights, sinus of Valsalva width, sinotubular junction height, and virtual THV to coronary distance (VTC) should be carefully analyzed[27] (Fig. 2). VTC is obtained by identifying the basal ring plane and the geometric center of the surgical valve. Then, a virtual cylinder with the estimated nominal size of the anticipated THV leads to a cylinder with the same height of the THV and is placed in the middle of the basal ring. The centers of the basal ring and of the cylinder are aligned. Finally, the horizontal distance between the edge of the cylinder and the ostia of the coronary arteries is measured with a caliper measurement tool of the CT imaging software (Fig. 3). A VTC cutoff value of 4 mm best identified those patients at higher risk for coronary obstruction.[21]

VALVE-IN-VALVE APP

A commonly used compendium of bioprosthetic valve information is the Valve-in-Valve App, available free-of-charge. Developed by Dr Vinayak Bapat, and in collaboration with UBQO (a software developing company), the application provides comprehensive bioprosthetic surgical and THV valve details pertinent to performing ViV TAVR. If the valve type is unknown, the App also provides a method for determining the surgical valve via fluoroscopic signature. The App remains a vital source of information for performing ViV procedures and is widely recommended (Fig. 4).[28]

PROCEDURAL TECHNIQUE

Crossing of the surgical prosthesis can be more challenging than a native valve, especially if the

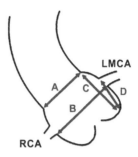

A: Sinotubular Junction diameter
B: Sinus of Valsalva diameter
C: Sinus of Valsalva height
D: Coronary Ostia Height

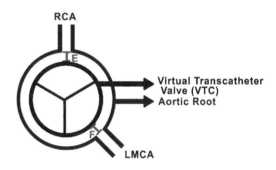

E: Virtual Transcatheter Distance to Right Coronary Artery

F: Virtual Transcatheter Distance to Left Main Coronary Artery

Fig. 2. Illustration showing various measurable parameters useful in risk stratification of post-TAVR coronary obstruction.

sinuses are large or there is critical stenosis. Standard techniques for valve crossing are implemented with Judkins right or Amplatz left catheters and straight wires. In rare circumstances, retrograde crossing of a severely stenotic bioprosthetic aortic valve may not be possible. In this scenario, an antegrade-retrograde technique is performed by transseptal puncture and exchange for a deflectable sheath into the left atrium. By using a deflectable sheath, a balloon-tipped catheter is inserted into the left ventricle and floated antegrade through the prosthetic valve to enable crossing of the stenotic prosthesis with an exchange length wire. Then, the wire is snared in the aorta to facilitate retrograde crossing of a catheter.[29] Once retrograde catheter access is established, the ViV TAVR may proceed in usual fashion.

Currently, there are 2 commercially available THVs that are approved for ViV TAVR. The self-expanding valve (Medtronic CoreValve/Evolut)

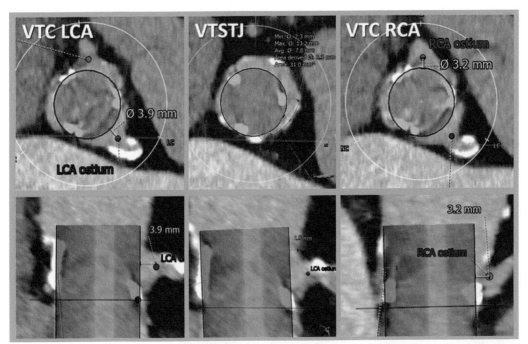

Fig. 3. Virtual valve to coronary distance and virtual valve-to-sinotubular junction. The virtual VTC distance is measured in 2 orthogonal planes (top, axial; bottom, longitudinal). Representative VTC distance measurement for a right coronary artery (RCA) and left coronary artery (LCA). The valve-to-sinotubular junction (VTSTJ) distance is measured in orthogonal planes: axial (*upper*) and longitudinal (*lower*), when the sinotubular junction is lower than the height of the transcatheter aortic valve replacement device. (*From*: (Lederman, R. J., Babaliaros, V. C., Rogers, T., Khan, J. M., Kamioka, N., Dvir, D., & Greenbaum, A. B. (2019). Preventing Coronary Obstruction During Transcatheter Aortic Valve Replacement: From Computed Tomography to BASILICA. *JACC Cardiovasc Interv, 12*(13), 1197-1216. https://doi.org/10.1016/j.jcin.2019.04.052). Reprinted with permission.)

and balloon-expandable valve (Edwards SAPIEN XT or S3 valve) have both been approved by the FDA for aortic ViV procedures in patients who are at high or extreme risk for SAVR.[4–6] Each THV type has its advantages and disadvantages when used for ViV TAVR. Only SAPIEN could be used for transapical ViV TAVR, as it could be mounted in either direction on the propriety delivery system. This delivery system is steerable, allowing for easier crossing and delivery, especially with more tortuous or angulated aortas. CoreValve/Evolut implants in a "supra-annular" position relative to the bioprosthetic valve neoannulus, which has the potential for improved postoperative hemodynamics and decreased residual transvalvular gradients. SAPIEN THV, on the other hand, implants in an "intra-annular" position, requires rapid pacing for deployment, and cannot be recaptured for adjustment once deployed (Fig. 5).[8] Most ViV TAVRs are performed using the smaller to medium size THVs (23 mm or 26 mm SAPIEN, 26 mm or 29 mm for CoreValve/Evolut) due to the limits imposed by the internal ring diameter of the bioprosthesis valve.[14] Oversizing of the THV relative

to the inner diameter of the prosthetic surgical valve can lead to underexpansion of THV and allows for leaflet redundancy and increased leaflet stresses that may impact durability and transvalvular regurgitation. On the other hand, an undersized THV valve increases risk for valve embolization or PVL.[14]

Midha and colleagues[30] studied optimal positioning of THV in ViV TAVR. ViV TAVR was simulated in a physiologic left heart simulator by deploying a 23-mm SAPIEN, and 23-mm and 26-mm CoreValve within a 23-mm Edwards PERIMOUNT surgical bioprosthesis. Each THV was deployed into 5 different positions: normal (inflow of THV was juxtaposed with inflow of surgical bioprosthesis), −3 and −6 mm subannular, and +3 and + 6 mm supra-annular. The optimal deployment location for ViV in a 23 PERIMOUNT surgical bioprosthesis was at a +6 mm supra-annular position for a 23-mm SAPIEN valve and at the normal position for both the 23-mm and 26-mm CoreValves.[30]

The recommended percentage depth of implantation for SAPIEN valve should be targeted no less than 80% aortic, 20% ventricular for

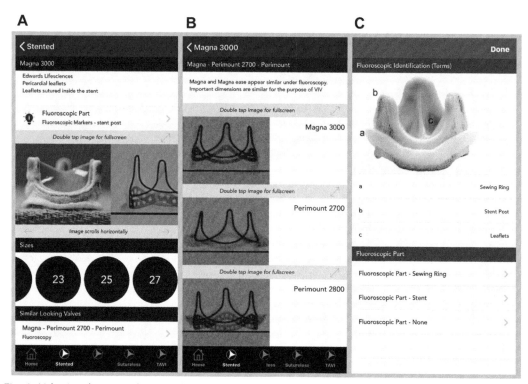

Fig. 4. Valve-in-valve smartphone application. (*A*) Identification and available sizes of different valves. (*B*) Fluoroscopic identification of various bioprosthetic valves. (*C*) Gross identification of the valve, highlighting different parts. (*Images are Courtesy of:* Dr. Vinayak Bapat, M.D. (Bapat, V. (2014). Valve-in-valve apps: why and how they were developed and how to use them. *EuroIntervention, 10 Suppl U*, U44-51. https://doi.org/10.4244/EIJV10SUA7).)

optimal results. Most operators are now aiming for 95:5 implant using the radiolucent line on the inflow portion of the frame. This positions the SAPIEN valve at the upper border of the neo-annulus, while reducing risk for embolization or PVL (**Fig. 6**).[31] For optimal results, the operator may choose to align the radiolucent line on the bottom of SAPIEN valve with the radiopaque ring to achieve high deployment position (>90% aortic), to decrease postoperative gradients and rate of permanent pacemaker. Ramanathan and colleagues[32] evaluated this novel technique on 50 patients (mean age of 81.5 years). Success rate was 100% (50 of 50), with 0% permanent pacemaker rate. There was no instance of valve embolization, coronary obstruction, or postprocedural death.[32] Operators need to be mindful, however, of the height of the sinotubular junction when using this technique, to minimize the risk of coronary obstruction. In stented valves, radiopaque components are the best landmarks to identify the perfect landing zone. The fluoroscopic viewing angle for valve positioning and deployment should be perpendicular to the base ring (bioprosthetic valve coplanar angle), which is often determined by preoperative CT scan or angiography but could also be easily obtained intraoperatively. Repeat supravalvular aortograms, transesophageal echocardiography (TEE), and the position of pigtail catheter are other adjunct methods of ViV TAVR implantation but are often not required when a radiopaque bioprosthetic ring is present. In stentless bioprosthetic valves, or in stented bioprosthetic valves without radiopaque markers, those positioning methods are vital for optimal ViV TAVR positioning.

According to the ACC/American Heart Association and European Society of Cardiology valvular heart disease guidelines, percutaneous balloon interventions are contraindicated in the therapy of stenotic left-sided bioprostheses.[33,34] Those guidelines have been published and practiced before increased spread of ViV TAVR. Hence, practice patterns vary significantly between operators. In native valve TAVR, balloon aortic valvuloplasty (BAV) is used in select patients to predilate and facilitate crossing of critically stenosed valves. BAV within degenerated bioprosthesis carries the risk of friable material embolization.[14] Despite that, there are few reported cases of uneventful BAV of ViV

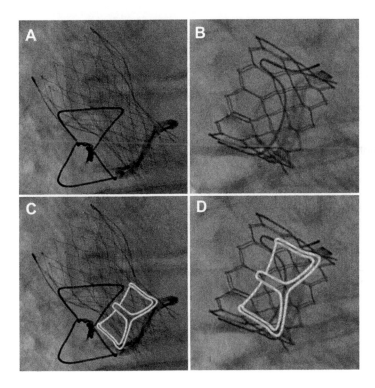

Fig. 5. Fluoroscopic examples of ViV TAVR. Medtronic CoreValve Evolut R (*A*) and Edwards SAPIEN 3 (*B*) THVs deployed within bioprosthetic aortic valves. (*C*) Illustrates supra-annular position of the bioprosthetic valve in CoreValve system, in comparison with intra-annular position in SAPIEN (*D*). (*Adapted from*: (Murdoch, D. J., & Webb, J. G. (2018). Transcatheter valve-in-valve implantation for degenerated surgical bioprostheses. *J Thorac Dis*, *10*(Suppl 30), S3573-S3577. https://doi.org/10.21037/jtd.2018.05.66). Reprinted with permission.)

bioprosthetic valve 1 year after ViV TAVR.[35] Moreover, high-pressure BAV before or after ViV TAVR is used in select patients to fracture the degenerated bioprosthetic valve or to achieve optimal expansion after ViV TAVR. Simultaneous aortography and BAV is a technique used by some operators in native valve TAVR to assess risk for coronary obstruction,[36] or size the THV.[37] Although this strategy seems attractive to assess heightened risk of coronary obstruction in ViV TAVR, there are no reports or studies in the literature to justify its use. Obtaining final invasive gradients across the newly deployed THV are important in determining the risk of patient-prosthesis mismatch and the need for bioprosthetic valve fracture.

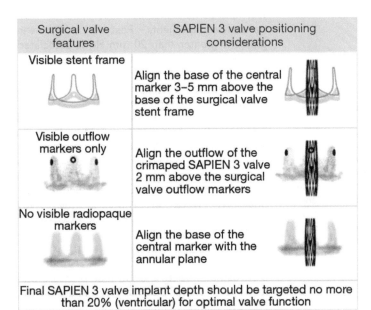

Surgical valve features	SAPIEN 3 valve positioning considerations	
Visible stent frame	Align the base of the central marker 3–5 mm above the base of the surgical valve stent frame	
Visible outflow markers only	Align the outflow of the crimaped SAPIEN 3 valve 2 mm above the surgical valve outflow markers	
No visible radiopaque markers	Align the base of the central marker with the annular plane	
Final SAPIEN 3 valve implant depth should be targeted no more than 20% (ventricular) for optimal valve function		

Fig. 6. Recommended positioning of the SAPIEN 3 valve inside the bioprosthetic valve. (*From*: (Murdoch, D. J., & Webb, J. G. (2018). Transcatheter valve-in-valve implantation for degenerated surgical bioprostheses. *J Thorac Dis*, *10*(Suppl 30), S3573-S3577. https://doi.org/10.21037/jtd.2018.05.66).Reprinted with permission.)

COMPLICATIONS

Stented ViV TAVR carries lower rates of PVL, aortic root rupture, and need for permanent pacemaker when compared with native aortic valve TAVR, but considerable risk for patient-prosthesis mismatch and coronary artery obstruction. Many complications of ViV TAVR occur at similar rates as those for native valve TAVR (bleeding, access site complications, major adverse cardiac events, need for blood transfusion or urgent surgical intervention). However, some complications are uniquely more frequent in ViV TAVR and relevant to the bioprosthetic valve architecture. The risk for needing a permanent pacemaker after ViV TAVR is low (3%) because the ViV THV is implanted inside the ring, and the myocardium is shielded from the THV.[24] It is not currently fully known whether surgical bioprosthetic valve fracture or remodeling alters the rates of new permanent pacemaker implantation. However, data from small clinical studies showed no new permanent pacemaker following bioprosthetic valve fracture or remodeling.[38,39]

Stentless ViV TAVR carries greater periprocedural complications (initial device malposition, second THV, coronary obstruction, paravalvular leak) than stented ViV TAVR, but no difference in 30-day and 1-year outcome (Fig. 7).[40] Duncan and colleagues[40] performed large comprehensive analysis of ViV TAVR for failed stentless bioprostheses between 2007 and 2016 (n = 1598; 291 stentless, 1307 stented bioprostheses). Compared with stented ViV TAVR, stentless ViV TAVR has higher rates of initial device malposition (10.3% vs 6.2%; P = .014), second THV (7.9% vs 3.4%), coronary obstruction (6.0% vs 1.5%), and PVL (all P<.001). Hospital stay duration (median 7 days) was no different, and 30-day (6.6% vs 4.4%; P = .12) and 1-year mortality rate (15.8% vs 12.6%; P = .15) was numerically higher, but not statistically different, after stentless ViV TAVR.[40] Those outcomes were attributed to lack of fluoroscopic markers, and guidance for device sizing, with increased rates of PVL, coronary obstruction, and malposition (Fig. 8).[40] In certain stentless valves (Freestyle; Medtronic, St. Paul, MN) without radiopaque landmarks, operators must target Dacron sewing ring for a firm anchor. Surgical implantation methods (full root or subcoronary), as well as variations in surgical technique introduce heterogeneity in the implantation position, which represents a technical challenge.

TRANSVALVULAR GRADIENT FOLLOWING VALVE-IN-VALVE TRANSCATHETER AORTIC VALVE REPLACEMENT

Various factors influence high gradients after ViV TAVR. The type and size of the original bioprosthetic valve, implantation technique, the size and morphology of the native aortic annulus, degree of leaflet and annular calcification, the type, size, and implant depth of THV, presence of PVL around bioprosthetic valve or THV are some variables responsible for final transvalvular gradients.[8] Post ViV TAVR, mean gradient greater than 20 mm Hg is associated with worse clinical outcomes and decreased 1-year survival.[23] Moreover, THV may not fully expand inside the bioprosthetic valve, resulting in high shear forces on the leaflets, hence, accelerated structural deterioration.[41] Small surgical bioprosthetic valves ≤21 mm yield poor results after ViV TAVR due to persistently high gradients.[23] Severe patient-prosthesis mismatch is present when the indexed effective orifice area (EOA) ≤0.65 cm^2/m^2 and this was found to occur post VIV TAVR in 31.8% in the VIVID Registry.[23,42]

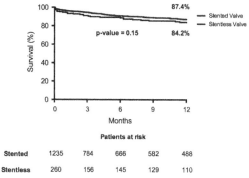

Fig. 7. Kaplan-Meier survival curves by bioprosthetic valve type. Kaplan-Meier survival curves up to 1 year showing no difference in 1-year mortality between ViV TAVR for stentless versus stented failing aortic valve bioprostheses. (*From*: (Duncan, A., Moat, N., Simonato, M., de Weger, A., Kempfert, J., Eggebrecht, H., . . . Dvir, D. (2019). Outcomes Following Transcatheter Aortic Valve Replacement for Degenerative Stentless Versus Stented Bioprostheses. *JACC Cardiovasc Interv*, 12(13), 1256-1263. https://doi.org/ 10.1016/j.jcin.2019.02.036). Reprinted with permission.)

BIOPROSTHETIC VALVE FRACTURE

Bioprosthetic fracture using high-pressure balloons to allow for optimal THV expansion can improve hemodynamics and decrease patient-

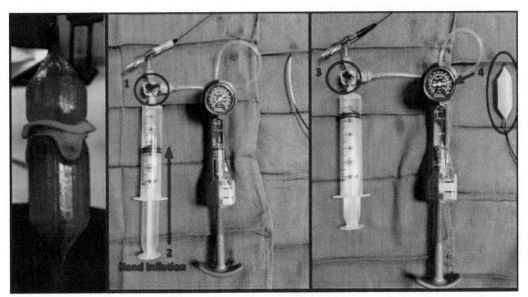

Challenges in aortic valve-in-valve

Stentless

Stented

- Lack of fluoroscopic markers
- More failure with regurgitation
- Malposition
- Paravalvular leakage
- Coronary obstruction

- More failure with stenosis
- Prosthesis-patient mismatch
- Residual stenosis

Fig. 8. Comparison of challenges in ViV stented versus stentless valves. There are several challenges involved in aortic ViV and these are distributed differently across surgical valve types. (*From*: (Duncan, A., Moat, N., Simonato, M., de Weger, A., Kempfert, J., Eggebrecht, H., . . . Dvir, D. (2019). Outcomes Following Transcatheter Aortic Valve Replacement for Degenerative Stentless Versus Stented Bioprostheses. *JACC Cardiovasc Interv*, *12*(13), 1256-1263. https://doi.org/10.1016/j.jcin.2019.02.036). Reprinted with permission.)

prosthesis mismatch.[4] The technique was described after 2 published series describing bench testing for commercially available surgical bioprosthetic valves, and response to high-pressure, noncompliant balloon valvuloplasty expansion[4] (**Fig. 9**). Typically, the balloons used are the True Dilation and VIDA Balloons (Bard, Tempe, AZ). Valvuloplasty balloons were selected 1 mm larger in diameter than the labeled surgical bioprosthetic valve intended for fracture. Successful fracture may be evident by an audible click, and/or sudden decrease in inflation pressure with visible release of balloon waist (**Figs. 10** and **11**).

Fig. 9. Technique of high-pressure balloon inflation to perform bioprosthetic valve fracture. 1: A high-pressure stopcock connects the valvuloplasty balloon to a syringe of dilute contrast and an indeflator. 2: The syringe is used to inflate the balloon manually. 3: The stopcock is turned so that the syringe is off and the indeflator is on. 4: The indeflator is dialed to the desired pressure, until the bioprosthetic valve fractures or the balloon ruptures. (*From:*(Saxon, J. T., Allen, K. B., Cohen, D. J., & Chhatriwalla, A. K. (2018). Bioprosthetic Valve Fracture During Valve-in-valve TAVR: Bench to Bedside. *Interv Cardiol*, *13*(1), 20-26. https://doi.org/10.15420/icr.2017:29:1). Reprinted with permission.)

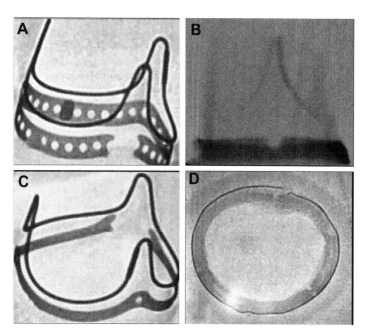

Fig. 10. Fluoroscopic examples of surgical valve fracture. (*A*) Edwards Magna. (*B*) Edwards MagnaEase. (*C*) Sorin Mitrlfow. (*D*) St Jude Biocor Epic. (*Adapted from:* (Saxon, J. T., Allen, K. B., Cohen, D. J., & Chhatriwalla, A. K. (2018). Bioprosthetic Valve Fracture During Valve-in-valve TAVR: Bench to Bedside. *Interv Cardiol*, *13*(1), 20-26. https://doi.org/10.15420/icr.2017:29:1). Reprinted with permission.)

Sudden decrease in indeflator pressure with deflation of the balloon is consistent with balloon rupture and is considered unsuccessful surgical valve fracture. All valves are susceptible to fracture, except Hancock II and Trifecta valves, which are modifiable but fracture resistant.[4] Fracture or modification of bioprosthetic valve may lead to improved hemodynamics and

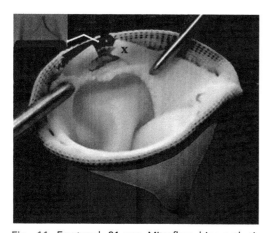

Fig. 11. Fractured 21-mm Mitroflow bioprosthetic valve. The Dacron sewing cuff has been partially removed to display the single separation of the polymer ring. x indicates the surgical ring that has been fractured. (*From:* (Saxon, J. T., Allen, K. B., Cohen, D. J., & Chhatriwalla, A. K. (2018). Bioprosthetic Valve Fracture During Valve-in-valve TAVR: Bench to Bedside. *Interv Cardiol*, *13*(1), 20-26. https://doi.org/10.15420/icr.2017:29:1). Reprinted with Permission.)

decreased valvular gradients (**Fig. 12**). The timing or fracturing before or after ViV TAVR is a somewhat controversial, but recent ex vivo hydrodynamic testing of ViV showed that post-THV implantation fracturing led to improved hemodynamics and THV expansion.[43] A major concern about pre-THV implant fracture is causing hemodynamic instability and inadequate THV expansion. Conversely, the long-term implications of subjecting THV leaflets to high-pressure dilation is unclear, histologic and long-term outcomes are pending. In a large multicenter series, surgical valve fracture was safely performed in conjunction with both balloon- and self-expanding THVs and resulted in significantly lower final transvalvular residual gradients and increased valve EOA.[38] In addition, 1-year follow-up demonstrates sustained low gradients, no signal for THV injury, and improved survival compared with historical controls.[44] However, long-term impact on clinical outcomes and THV durability, either positive or negative, requires further study.

RISK OF CORONARY OBSTRUCTION FOLLOWING VALVE-IN-VALVE TRANSCATHETER AORTIC VALVE REPLACEMENT

Coronary artery obstruction following ViV TAVR is a catastrophic complication, with a more than 50% mortality rate.[36] It is 4 times more common in ViV TAVR than with native valve

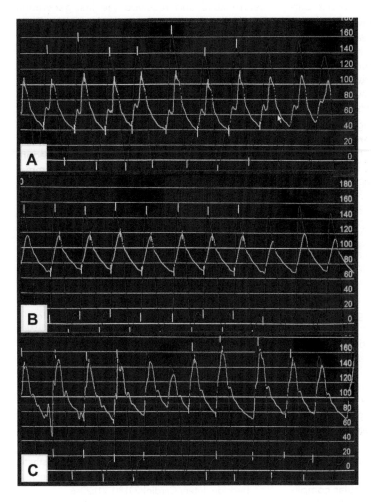

Fig. 12. Hemodynamics during ViV TAVR. Severe bioprosthetic aortic valve regurgitation with moderate bioprosthetic stenosis of a 23-mm Mitroflow surgical valve. (A) Hemodynamics before ViV TAVR showing 27 mm Hg pressure gradient across the surgical valve (stenosis), with equalization of aortic and left ventricular end diastolic pressures (regurgitation) (B) Post ViV TAVR with 23-mm SAPIEN S3 Valve, with resolution of regurgitation but with unacceptably high transvalvular residual gradient of 22 mm Hg. (C) Post ViV remodeling of bioprosthetic valve with 24-mm non-compliant balloon, resulted in reduction of transvalvular gradient to 12 mm Hg.

TAVR.[45] Displacement of surgical valve leaflets outward during THV implantation obstructs flow to the coronary arteries either directly by covering the coronary ostia or sequestering the entire sinus of Valsalva. The left coronary artery is more frequently impacted (72%), followed by bilateral coronary obstruction (20%), and isolated right coronary artery (8%) rarely occurs.[6] Stented surgical valves with externally mounted leaflets (ie, MITROFLOW [Sorin Group USA, Inc., Arvada, CO] and Trifecta [St. Jude Medical, St. Paul, MN]) (see Fig. 1) are associated with a nearly eightfold increased hazard of coronary obstruction during ViV TAVR.[21] Stentless aortic valves also exhibit high risk for coronary obstruction (3.7%) when compared with native valve TAVR.[21,46] Other risk factors for coronary obstruction are bicuspid native aortic valve, lower height of the coronary ostium above the valve annulus, narrow sinuses of Valsalva, narrow or low sinotubular junction, tall or bulky leaflets, and VTC

less than 4 mm.[21] The most common sign of coronary obstruction is hypotension with cardiogenic shock (68.2%).[45] Management of coronary obstruction is with either emergency percutaneous coronary intervention or emergency coronary artery bypass graft, but carries very high mortality rates of 36.4% and 50.0%, respectively.[45] Hence, meticulous preoperative planning and identification of patients at risk for coronary obstruction will help further risk-stratify patients for redo SAVR or ViV TAVR with protective measures. If the patient is still deemed at high or prohibitive risk for redo SAVR, then ViV TAVR with coronary protective measures could be pursued. Preemptive coronary protection, with a guidewire, with or without a coronary balloon or stent prepositioned down the coronary artery, is variably successful.[36] Another technique, often termed "chimney stenting" or "Snorkel technique" involves stent implantation from the coronary ostium at high risk of obstruction to the aorta within the space between the valve frame and the aortic wall. This technique creates complex valve/stent configuration that can hinder repeat coronary interventions.[47] A novel technique (bioprosthetic or native aortic scallop intentional laceration to prevent coronary artery obstruction [BASILICA]) offers a promising alternative to "chimney" stenting to provide durable prevention against coronary obstruction from ViV TAVR.[36]

PRE–VALVE-IN-VALVE TRANSCATHETER AORTIC VALVE REPLACEMENT LEAFLET MODIFICATION TECHNIQUE (BIOPROSTHETIC OR NATIVE AORTIC SCALLOP INTENTIONAL LACERATION TO PREVENT CORONARY ARTERY OBSTRUCTION)

BASILICA is a novel technique that allows for ViV TAVR in patients otherwise ineligible for any therapy because of a high risk of valve leaflet-induced coronary artery obstruction. Detailed analysis of the technical details are discussed separately.[36]

The BASILICA trial enrolled 30 patients between February 2018 and July 2018. Primary success was met in 28 (93%) subjects. BASILICA traversal and laceration was successful in 35 (95%) of 37 attempted leaflets. There was 100% freedom from coronary obstruction and reintervention. Primary safety was met in 21 (70%), driven by 6 (20%) major vascular complications related to TAVR but not BASILICA. There was 1 death at 30 days. There was 1 (3%) disabling stroke and 2 (7%) nondisabling strokes. Transient hemodynamic compromise was rare (7%) and resolved promptly with TAVR.[48] BASILICA technique offers a promising alternative to prophylactic complex techniques to prevent coronary obstruction after ViV TAVR. BASILICA is limited by its complexity and lack of dedicated catheters to facilitate leaflet traversal.

CONTROVERSIES AND FUTURE PERSPECTIVES

Lifelong management of aortic stenosis now requires a thorough heart team discussion weighing the merits of initial SAVR versus TAVR based on anatomic considerations and the potential for subsequent ViV TAVR. ViV TAVR is associated with patient-prosthesis mismatch and patients with small bioprostheses are found to have lower survival, prompting consideration of a randomized head-to-head comparison of

ViV TAVR with redo SAVR.[26,49] Although bioprosthetic valve fracture/modification has proven effective and feasible, we need a better understanding of the long-term impact of high-pressure inflations on fresh THV leaflets. Finally, novel tools for leaflet modification will be required to mitigate the risk of coronary artery obstruction with ViV TAVR. Regardless, nearly 5000 patients underwent ViV TAVR in 2019 and as transcatheter heart valves begin to degenerate, operators will face yet another dilemma, the complexities of performing ViV in failed THVs. Clearly, growth in transcatheter heart valves will continue to break new ground in the coming years.

REFERENCES

1. Carroll JD, Mack MJ, Vemulapalli S, et al. STS-ACC TVT registry of transcatheter aortic valve replacement. J Am Coll Cardiol 2020;76(21):2492–516.
2. Hammermeister K, Gulshan KS, Henderson WG, et al. Outcomes 15 years after valve replacement with a mechanical versus a bioprosthetic vavle: final report of the veterans affairs randomized trial. J Am Coll Cardiol 2000;36:1152–8.
3. Kalra A, Raza S, Hussain M, et al. Aortic valve replacement in bioprosthetic failure: insights from the Society of Thoracic Surgeons National Database. Ann Thorac Surg 2020;110(5):1637–42.
4. Saxon JT, Allen KB, Cohen DJ, et al. Bioprosthetic valve fracture during valve-in-valve TAVR: bench to bedside. Interv Cardiol 2018;13(1):20–6.
5. Deeb GM, Chetcuti SJ, Reardon MJ, et al. 1-Year results in patients undergoing transcatheter aortic valve replacement with failed surgical bioprostheses. JACC Cardiovasc Interv 2017;10(10):1034–44.
6. Edelman JJ, Khan JM, Rogers T, et al. Valve-in-valve TAVR: state-of-the-art review. Innovations (Phila) 2019;14(4):299–310.
7. Otto CM, Nishimura RA, Bonow RO, et al. 2020 ACC/AHA guideline for the management of patients with valvular heart disease: a report of the American College of Cardiology/American Heart Association Joint Committee on Clinical Practice Guidelines. Circulation 2020;143(5):e72–227.
8. Reul RM, Ramchandani MK, Reardon MJ. Transcatheter aortic valve-in-valve procedure in patients with bioprosthetic structural valve deterioration. Methodist Debakey Cardiovasc J 2017;13(3):132–41.
9. McClure RS, Narayanasamy N, Wiegerinck E, et al. Late outcomes for aortic valve replacement with the Carpentier-Edwards pericardial bioprosthesis: up to 17-year follow-up in 1,000 patients. Ann Thorac Surg 2010;89(5):1410–6.

10. Johnston DR, Soltesz EG, Vakil N, et al. Long-term durability of bioprosthetic aortic valves: implications from 12,569 implants. Ann Thorac Surg 2015;99(4):1239–47.

11. Bourguignon T, Lhommet P, El Khoury R, et al. Very long-term outcomes of the Carpentier-Edwards Perimount aortic valve in patients aged 50-65 years. Eur J Cardiothorac Surg 2016;49(5):1462–8.

12. Chan V, Jamieson WR, Germann E, et al. Performance of bioprostheses and mechanical prostheses assessed by composites of valve-related complications to 15 years after aortic valve replacement. J Thorac Cardiovasc Surg 2006;131(6):1267–73.

13. Chiang YP, Chikwe J, Moskowitz AJ, et al. Survival and long-term outcomes following bioprosthetic vs mechanical aortic valve replacement in patients aged 50 to 69 years. JAMA 2014;312(13):1323–9.

14. Piazza N, Bleiziffer S, Brockmann G, et al. Transcatheter aortic valve implantation for failing surgical aortic bioprosthetic valve: from concept to clinical application and evaluation (part 1). JACC Cardiovasc Interv 2011;4(7):721–32.

15. Banbury MK, Cosgrove DM 3rd, White JA, et al. Age and valve size effect on the long-term durability of the Carpentier-Edwards aortic pericardial bioprosthesis. Ann Thorac Surg 2001;72(3):753–7.

16. Chan V, Lam BK, Rubens FD, et al. Long-term evaluation of biological versus mechanical prosthesis use at reoperative aortic valve replacement. J Thorac Cardiovasc Surg 2012;144(1):146–51.

17. Wenaweser P, Buellesfeld L, Gerckens U, et al. Percutaneous aortic valve replacement for severe aortic regurgitation in degenerated bioprosthesis: the first valve in valve procedure using the Corevalve Revalving system. Catheter Cardiovasc Interv 2007;70(5):760–4.

18. Kirsch M, Nakashima K, Kubota S, et al. The risk of reoperative heart valve procedures in octogenarian patients. J Heart Valve Dis 2004;13(6):991–6 [discussion: 996].

19. Azadani AN, Jaussaud N, Matthews PB, et al. Transcatheter aortic valves inadequately relieve stenosis in small degenerated bioprostheses. Interact Cardiovasc Thorac Surg 2010;11(1):70–7.

20. Azadani AN, Tseng EE. Transcatheter valve-in-valve implantation for failing bioprosthetic valves. Future Cardiol 2010;6(6):811–31.

21. Ribeiro HB, Rodes-Cabau J, Blanke P, et al. Incidence, predictors, and clinical outcomes of coronary obstruction following transcatheter aortic valve replacement for degenerative bioprosthetic surgical valves: insights from the VIVID registry. Eur Heart J 2018;39(8):687–95.

22. Christakis GT, Buth KJ, Goldman BS, et al. Inaccurate and misleading valve sizing: a proposed standard for valve size nomenclature. Ann Thorac Surg 1998;66(4):1198–203.

23. Dvir D, Webb JG, Bleiziffer S, et al. Valve-in-Valve International Data Registry, I., Transcatheter aortic valve implantation in failed bioprosthetic surgical valves. JAMA 2014;312(2):162–70.

24. Tuzcu EM, Kapadia SR, Vemulapalli S, et al. Transcatheter aortic valve replacement of failed surgically implanted bioprostheses: the STS/ACC Registry. J Am Coll Cardiol 2018;72(4):370–82.

25. Pibarot P, Simonato M, Barbanti M, et al. Impact of pre-existing prosthesis-patient mismatch on survival following aortic valve-in-valve procedures. JACC Cardiovasc Interv 2018;11(2):133–41.

26. Bleiziffer S, Simonato M, Webb JG, et al. Long-term outcomes after transcatheter aortic valve implantation in failed bioprosthetic valves. Eur Heart J 2020;41(29):2731–42.

27. Dvir D, Webb JG, Bleiziffer S, et al. Transcatheter aortic valve implantation in failed bioprosthetic surgical valves. JAMA 2014;312(2):162–70.

28. Bapat V. Valve-in-valve apps: why and how they were developed and how to use them. EuroIntervention 2014;10(Suppl U):U44–51.

29. Wong I, Bieliauskas G, Sondergaard L, et al. The antegrade-retrograde technique applied in uncrossable valve-in-valve TAVR: a step-by-step guide. JACC Cardiovasc Interv 2020;14(2):227–9.

30. Midha PA, Raghav V, Condado JF, et al. Valve type, size, and deployment location affect hemodynamics in an in vitro valve-in-valve model. JACC Cardiovasc Interv 2016;9(15):1618–28.

31. Murdoch DJ, Webb JG. Transcatheter valve-in-valve implantation for degenerated surgical bioprostheses. J Thorac Dis 2018;10(Suppl 30):S3573–7.

32. Ramanathan PK, Nazir S, Elzanaty AM, et al. Novel method for implantation of balloon expandable transcatheter aortic valve replacement to reduce pacemaker rate—line of lucency method. Struct Heart 2020;4(5):427–32.

33. American College of Cardiology/American Heart Association Task Force on Practice, G.; Society of Cardiovascular, A.; Society for Cardiovascular, A.; Interventions; Society of Thoracic, S., Bonow RO, Carabello BA, Kanu C, et al. ACC/AHA 2006 guidelines for the management of patients with valvular heart disease: a report of the American College of Cardiology/American Heart Association Task Force on Practice Guidelines (writing committee to revise the 1998 Guidelines for the Management of Patients With Valvular Heart Disease): developed in collaboration with the Society of Cardiovascular Anesthesiologists: endorsed by the Society for Cardiovascular Angiography and Interventions and the Society of Thoracic Surgeons. Circulation 2006;114(5):e84–231.

34. Vahanian A, Baumgartner H, Bax J, et al, Task Force on the Management of Valvular Hearth Disease of the European Society of, C.. Guidelines, E. S. C. C. f. P., Guidelines on the management of valvular heart disease: The Task Force on the Management of Valvular Heart Disease of the European Society of Cardiology. Eur Heart J 2007;28(2):230–68.

35. Badami A, Lushaj EB, Jacobson K, et al. Recurrent severe aortic stenosis one year after transcatheter aortic valve-in-valve implantation: successful treatment with balloon aortic valvuloplasty. J Cardiol Cases 2016;14(2):35–7.

36. Khan JM, Dvir D, Greenbaum AB, et al. Transcatheter laceration of aortic leaflets to prevent coronary obstruction during transcatheter aortic valve replacement: concept to first-in-human. JACC Cardiovasc Interv 2018;11(7):677–89.

37. Barbanti M, Sgroi C, Imme S, et al. Usefulness of contrast injection during balloon aortic valvuloplasty before transcatheter aortic valve replacement: a pilot study. EuroIntervention 2014;10(2):241–7.

38. Allen KB, Chhatriwalla AK, Saxon JT, et al. Bioprosthetic valve fracture: technical insights from a multicenter study. J Thorac Cardiovasc Surg 2019; 158(5):1317–1328 e1.

39. Hamandi M, Nwafor I, Hebeler KR, et al. Bioprosthetic valve fracture during valve-in-valve transcatheter aortic valve replacement. Proc (Bayl Univ Med Cent) 2020;33(3):317–21.

40. Duncan A, Moat N, Simonato M, et al. Outcomes following transcatheter aortic valve replacement for degenerative stentless versus stented bioprostheses. JACC Cardiovasc Interv 2019;12(13): 1256–63.

41. Sathananthan J, Sellers S, Barlow AM, et al. Valve-in-valve transcatheter aortic valve replacement and bioprosthetic valve fracture comparing different transcatheter heart valve designs: an ex vivo bench study. JACC Cardiovasc Interv 2019;12(1):65–75.

42. Rahimtoola SH. The problem of valve prosthesis-patient mismatch. Circulation 1978;58(1):20–4.

43. Janarthanan S, Rob F, Hoda H, et al. A bench test study of bioprosthetic valve fracture performed before versus after transcatheter valve-in-valve intervention. EuroIntervention 2020;15(16):1409–16.

44. Allen KB, Chhatriwalla AK, Saxon JT, et al. Bioprosthetic valve fracture to facilitate valve-in-valve transcatheter aortic valve repair. Ann Cardiothorac Surg 2020;9(6):528–30.

45. Ribeiro HB, Webb JG, Makkar RR, et al. Predictive factors, management, and clinical outcomes of coronary obstruction following transcatheter aortic valve implantation: insights from a large multicenter registry. J Am Coll Cardiol 2013;62(17): 1552–62.

46. Vriesendorp MD, de Lind van Wijngaarden RAF, Rao V, et al. An in vitro comparison of internally versus externally mounted leaflets in surgical aortic bioprostheses. Interact Cardiovasc Thorac Surg 2020;30(3):417–23.

47. Burzotta F, Kovacevic M, Aurigemma C, et al. An "orthotopic" snorkel-stenting technique to maintain coronary patency during transcatheter aortic valve replacement. Cardiovasc Revasc Med 2020. https://doi.org/10.1016/j.carrev.2020.12.013.

48. Khan JM, Greenbaum AB, Babaliaros VC, et al. The BASILICA trial: prospective multicenter investigation of intentional leaflet laceration to prevent TAVR coronary obstruction. JACC Cardiovasc Interv 2019;12(13):1240–52.

49. Sá MPBO, Van den Eynde J, Simonato M, et al. Valve-in-valve transcatheter aortic valve replacement versus redo surgical aortic valve replacement: an updated meta-analysis. JACC: Cardiovasc Interv 2021;14(2):211–20.

Alternative Access for Transcatheter Aortic Valve Replacement
A Comprehensive Review

Marvin H. Eng, MD[a],*, Mohammed Qintar, MD, MSc[b],
Dmitrios Apostolou, MD[c], William W. O'Neill, MD[d]

KEYWORDS

- TAVR • Transcarotid • Transcaval • Transaxillary • Antegrade • Direct apical • Direct aortic
- Alternative access

KEY POINTS

- Alternative access is used in a minority of cases and is associated with higher rates of morbidity and mortality because of patient and technical factors.
- Transthoracic access is associated with higher rates of mortality and postprocedure atrial fibrillation.
- A myriad of choices is available, but centers should focus on 1 to 2 techniques to optimize proficiency in alternative access.
- Transaxillary access is popular and widely used but associated with higher rates of stroke as compared with other alternative access techniques.

INTRODUCTION

Transcatheter aortic valve replacement (TAVR) has rapidly become the treatment of choice as an alternative to surgical aortic valve replacement in patients at high, intermediate, and low procedural risk patients.[1–3] Iterative advances in technology results in increasingly lower profile sheaths, enabling broad use of transfemoral access. Despite these improvements, alternative access is still recommended in up to 21% of patients[4] because of iliofemoral disease, tortuosity, severe calcification, aneurysms, mural thrombus, or previous vascular surgery, hence the continued need for alternative access to avoid

vascular complications and their associated morbidity and mortality.[5,6] Recently, an analysis of TAVR procedures from 2015 to 2017 revealed that 15.3% of cases used alternative access, and an inverse relationship between operator volume and 30-day mortality was seen in the transcatheter valve therapy (TVT) registry.[7] Given the 19.45% relative reduction of 30-day mortality between the highest and lowest volume operators, expertise is a major determinate of outcomes.[7] The differential in knowledge and experience prompts this comprehensive review of the technique and outcomes of the following nonfemoral artery alternative access routes: antegrade, transapical (TA), transaortic (TAo),

Funding sources. None.

Disclosure of potential conflicts of interest: M.H. Eng is a clinical proctor for Edwards Lifesciences and Medtronic. W.W. O'Neill is a consultant to Abiomed, Medtronic, and Boston Scientific.

[a] Division of Cardiology, Banner- University Medical Center Phoenix, 1111 East McDowell Road, Phoenix, AZ 85006, USA; [b] Division of Cardiology, Sparrow Hospital, 1215 East Michigan Avenue, Lansing, MI 48912, USA; [c] Division of Cardiothoracic Surgery, Department of Surgery, Henry Ford Health System, 2799 West Grand Boulevard, Detroit, MI 48202, USA; [d] Division of Cardiology, Center for Structural Heart Disease, Henry Ford Health System, 2799 West Grand Boulevard, Detroit, MI 48202, USA

* Corresponding author.

E-mail addresses: Marvin.eng@bannerhealth.com; engm@arizona.edu

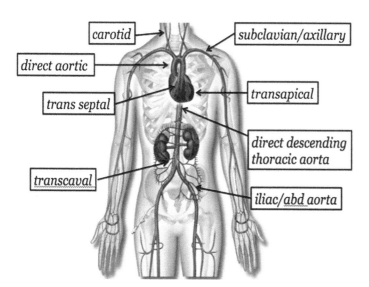

Fig. 1. Comprehensive list of non-transfemoral access previously used to perform TAVR. abd, abdomen.

Labels in figure: carotid, direct aortic, trans septal, transcaval, subclavian/axillary, transapical, direct descending thoracic aorta, iliac/abd aorta

suprasternal, transaxillary (TAx), transcarotid (TC), and transcaval (TCav) access (Fig. 1).

ANTEGRADE (TRANSSEPTAL) ACCESS

The progenitor balloon expandable valve required using a 24F sheath, but a retrograde delivery catheter had not yet been designed; therefore, first-in-man TAVR used antegrade, transseptal access (Fig. 2). The initial description of TAVR was a 6-patient series of transseptal antegrade transcatheter heart valve (THV) delivery by Dr Alain Cribier and colleagues in 2004.[8,9] The procedure was successful in 5 patients, but mitral valve injury prevented the widespread adoption of the technique; TAVR did not disseminate until the engineering of a retrograde delivery system.[10,11] This technique is seldom used, There are few with the expertise to use antegrade access, and despite venous access for the large-bore sheath, major bleeding occurred in nearly half of the small series.[12]

TRANSTHORACIC (APICAL [TRANSAPICAL] AND DIRECT AORTIC [TRANSAORTIC]) ACCESS

First-generation Sapien valve (Edwards Lifesciences, Irvine, CA, USA) delivery systems required 22 to 24F sheaths for transfemoral access, and transthoracic alternative access were commonly used.

Transapical

First described by Lichtenstein and colleagues,[13] TA access experienced its highest utilization during PARTNER I and the first-generation Edwards

SAPIEN commercial roll-out. TA access begins with a limited thoracotomy, and apical exposure is followed by horizontal mattress pledgeted suture placement surrounding the intended area of access, typically lateral to the true apex (Fig. 3). After puncturing with an 18-gauge needle, most operators take the approach of minimizing sheath exchanges in the heart. Following apical puncture, the apex is cannulated with a small sheath and then exchanged for a stiff wire in the descending aorta. After the large delivery sheath (24–33F Ascendra or Acendra II, Edwards Lifesciences, Irvine, CA) is placed over the stiff wire, valve delivery ensues (see Fig. 3). Hemostasis is achieved by first lowering the blood pressure using rapid pacing, sheath withdrawal, and pledget tightening with care not to overtension the sutures. A chest tube is left in place, and the thoracotomy is closed. Avoid systemic hypertension and undue stress to the repaired apex with antihypertensive medications if necessary. Apical tissue integrity is sometimes unpredictable, and cases have been aborted because of degeneration of apical tissue architecture or copious apical adiposity causing ambiguity during pledget placement.

During the PARTNER I trial, 42% of patients underwent TA access and experienced an increased rates of in-hospital death, renal failure, bleeding, and longer lengths of stay relative to transfemoral procedures.[12] Moreover, data show that TA access was associated with increased myocardial injury compared with other access routes.[14] Patients with chronic lung disease are easily compromised by apical exposure because of thoracic pain and the presence of a chest tube. Moreover, patients with chronic

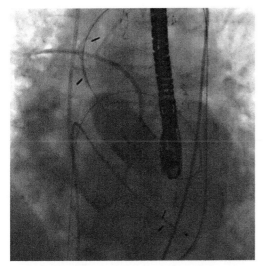

Fig. 2. Antegrade, transseptal TAVR performed using an arterial-venous loop.

obstructive pulmonary disease have longer post-procedural ventilation times when treated via TA relative to TF TAVR, indicating that TA should be avoided in such individuals.[15] The use of apical access declined in the PARTNER II trial to 8.5%, and a newer, smaller-caliber delivery sheath (Ascendra II 24F) was introduced at this time.[2] Although technology improved, thoracic access (both TA and TAo) was still associated with increased death, stroke, vascular complications, and new atrial fibrillation (Table 1). Currently, the Sapien 3/Ultra balloon expandable valves (Edwards Lifesciences, Irvine, CA) use the Certitude delivery system (Edwards Lifesciences, Irvine, CA) that has an internal diameter of 18 to 21F depending on the valve size used.

After concerns with myocardial injury and comfort with limited sternotomy or aortic cannulation, TAo access was developed by Bapat and colleagues.[16] TAo access is feasible so long as the aorta is not excessively calcified and there is at least 6.5 to 7 cm of length between the proposed entry side and the aortic annulus to allow for valve preparation. Aortic access is achieved using J-sternotomy or right lateral thoracotomy, depending on the position of the aorta (Fig. 4). After placing pledgeted sutures at the access site, direct puncture is performed with an 18-gauge needle (see Fig. 4). A small sheath should be inserted to facilitate crossing the stenotic aortic valve and exchanged for a stiff wire that enables large-sheath delivery. Following THV implantation, the pledgeted sutures are tightened for hemostatic control and the thorax closed in the usual fashion. Some surgeons prefer TAo over TA access because of less surgical site pain, minimal myocardial injury, and freedom from concerns about apical tissue integrity. Rare complications of dissections or intramural hematomas occur, and convalescence is still prolonged.[17] The use of TAo access in the PARTNER II trial was only 3.05%,[2] and US registry data show that TAo is associated with an 8% in-hospital mortality, 40% rate of renal failure with the minority of patients able to be discharged home (see Table 1).

Intuitively, thoracic invasion for THV implantation is less preferred. Tsuyoshi Kaneko and colleagues[18] give credence to this notion by showing higher rates of mortality, blood transfusion, atrial fibrillation, and intensive care unit length of stay when using transthoracic access. Moreover, new-onset atrial fibrillation is significantly increased in thoracic access, especially TA, compared with any extrathoracic access.[19] As such, transthoracic access is declining, and TA/TAo access accounts for less than 2.8% of all Sapien TAVR cases in the US TVT registry between 2015 and 2018.[20]

SUPRASTERNAL ACCESS

In 2018, Codner and colleagues[21] described suprasternal access using the dedicated Aegis

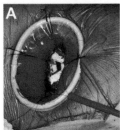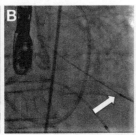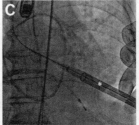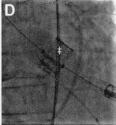

Fig. 3. TA access. (A) Surgical exposure of the myocardial apex using a soft tissue retractor and pericardial stay stitches. Pledgeted horizontal mattress sutures have been embedded in the periapical area in preparation for apical puncture. (B) Puncture of the apex with an 18-gauge needle (arrow) and a 0.035" J-tipped wire is inserted. (C) An Ascendra sheath (asterisk) (Edwards Lifesciences) is advanced over a stiff wire. (D). A 26-mm Edwards Sapien valve is implanted (double dagger).

Table 1
Comparative results for each alternative access

	Antegrade	Transaortic	Transapical	Surgical Axillary	Percutaneous Axillary	Transcarotid	Transcaval
In-hospital mortality, %	0	8.1	7.4	4.3	3.4	2.5	4
Longer-term mortality	22% 6 mo	19% 1 y	9% 30 d	2.9% 30 d 20% 1-y	5.4% 30 d	4.3% 30 d	8% 30 d
Major bleeding, %	44.4	5.0	7.2	NA	0.5	0.1	12
Acute kidney injury, %	22.2	39.6		NA			12
Stroke, %	0	2.5	2.8	3	6.1	4.2	5
Vascular complications, %	33.3	0.5	3.8	2	2.5	1.5	13

Abbreviation: N/A, not applicable.

metallic frame (Aegis Surgical, Dublin, Ireland). Using a 3-cm transverse incision superior to the sternal notch, blunt dissection is performed to expose the plane between the brachiocephalic artery and innominate vein. The Aegis device optimized exposure and illumination to facilitate insertion of purse-string sutures by way of thoracic port instruments. Once prepared, the brachiocephalic artery is accessed with a pericardiocentesis needle to enable eventual exchange for a delivery sheath. Postvalve implantation, a long knot-tying instrument achieves hemostasis. The published data consist of 11 patients with earlier ambulation and shorter hospitalizations that propensity matched TA or TAo. Further studies are needed on this access route to determine generalizability of suprasternal access.

TRANSAXILLARY ACCESS

TAx access has long been used as an alternative access for TAVR, beginning with surgical exposure for sheath insertion, and it has now evolved to complete percutaneous access and hemostasis. Initially disseminated as an alternative access for Medtronic Corevalve implantation,[22] it has become the dominant alternative access in the United States.[20] Advantages of axillary access is the relative lack of atherosclerosis compared with femoral vessels, accessibility, and extrathoracic location. The medial section of the subclavian artery is thinner with a higher proportion of elastic fibers compared with the femoral artery, causing concern that the artery may be fragile. Another caveat is the proximity of the brachial plexus to the vessel and potential for

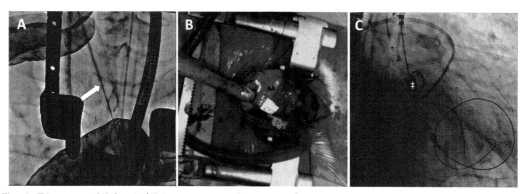

Fig. 4. TAo access. (*A*) Surgical TAo exposure and insertion of an 8F sheath (*arrow*) in the ascending aorta. (*B*) Insertion of a 20F sheath (*asterisk*) in the ascending aorta (AA). (*C*) A 29-mm Sapien XT valve is implanted (*double dagger*). RA, right atrium.

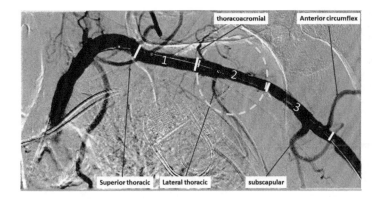

Fig. 5. Axillary artery anatomy relevant to transcatheter access. Angiogram of the axillary artery, its 3 divisions and side branches.

compromising the upper extremity via peripheral nerve injury or distal embolism.[23]

The axillary artery is divided into 3 segments (**Fig. 5**), with the most proximal section between the lateral margin of the first rib and medial border of the pectoralis minor muscle. The second segment is deep to the pectoralis minor muscle, whereas the third segment is between the lateral border of the pectoralis minor and inferior border of the teres major muscle. Computed tomographic analysis shows that the axillary artery is usually on average 1.5 mm smaller than the corresponding lower-extremity vessels.[24] Occasionally, a pacemaker or implantable cardioverter defibrillator encroaches on the deltopectoral groove, crowding the access point. In addition, large-bore axillary access should be avoided in the presence of an ipsilateral patent mammary graft to prevent ischemia during cannulation.

Operators should aim to access the distal end of the first segment or proximal second segment

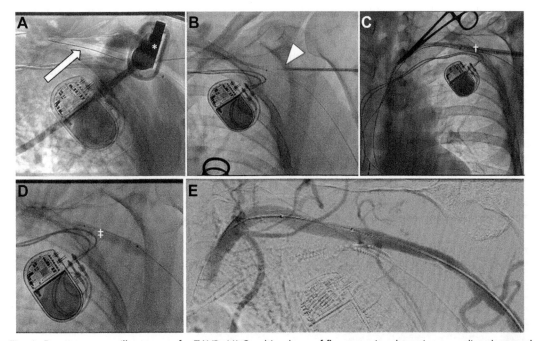

Fig. 6. Percutaneous axillary access for TAVR. (*A*) Combined use of fluoroscopic subtraction to outline the vessel and ultrasound (*asterisk*) to access the axillary artery using a 21-gauge needle and 0.018″ wire (*arrow*). (*B*) "Preclose" of the axillary artery using a Proglide Perclose (*triangle*) (Abbott Vascular, Santa Clara, CA). (*C*) Exchange for a 14F E-Sheath (*dagger*) (Edwards Lifesciences, Irvine, CA) over a stiff wire. (*D*) Balloon tamponade (*double dagger*) of the vessel postsheath removal and tightening of the Perclose sutures. (*E*) Completion angiogram showing no evidence of dissection or extravasation.

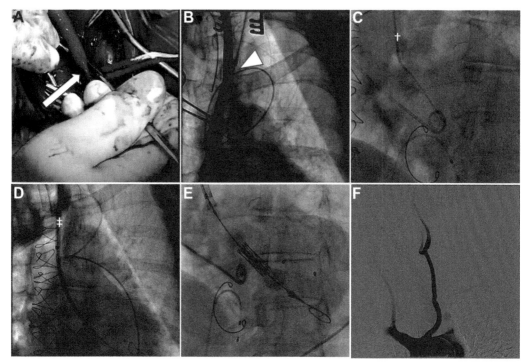

Fig. 7. TC TAVR. (A) Surgical exposure of the carotid artery (arrow). (B) Insertion of a 9F sheath in the carotid artery using the Seldinger technique (triangle). (C) Crossing the aortic valve using a JR4 catheter (dagger). (D) Exchanging for a 14F E-sheath (double dagger). (E) Delivery of a 26-mm Edwards Sapien 3 Ultra valve. (F) Completion angiography of the left carotid access site demonstrating no dissection or extravasation.

at a shallow angle to avoid sheath kinking (Fig. 6). The left axillary artery is more commonly used. Take care to avoid damaging the subclavian artery, as surgical rescue of this vessel requires a sternotomy. In preparation for large-bore TAVR access, the authors' center routinely prepares the ipsilateral radial artery with a 7F sheath and a 0.014 to 0.018″ wire for endovascular management and rescue. Using a combination of fluoroscopy and ultrasound, the axillary artery is punctured and dilated, and Proglide sutures are implanted in typical fashion before large-sheath insertion (see Fig. 6). Balloon tamponade between sheath exchanges minimizes blood loss, and the large-bore sheath should be inserted over a stiff wire. External compression against the second rib is feasible to maintain hemostasis in the case an ipsilateral peripheral arterial access is unavailable.[25] Following THV implantation, balloon tamponade prevents bleeding and facilitates hemostasis. Tightening of the Perclose sutures accompanied by short duration balloon tamponade should be sufficient for hemostasis. Given the torsion encountered by the axillary artery, flexible self-expanding or balloon expandable covered stents (VBX; Gore Medical, Flagstaff, AZ, USA) should be used for rescue; the latter in particular is advantageous because of its large range and ability to fit through a 7F sheath.

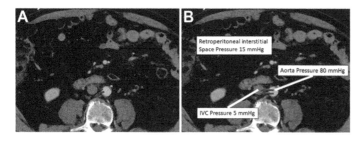

Fig. 8. Pathophysiology of an iatrogenic aortic-caval fistula. (A) Intuitively, most would believe that patients should exsanguinate (red arrows) from a rent in the aorta. (B) Because a breach is present in both the aorta and vena cava and the interstitial pressure of the retroperitoneal space exceeds the venous pressure, blood preferentially shunts from the aorta to the vena cava (straight red arrows). Permission received from Springer Publishing.[42]

Box 1
Computed tomography for planning transcaval access rationale and caveats

Objective: Identify a calcium-free crossing target

Rationale: A heavily calcified aorta cannot be traversed, and a window must be large enough to accommodate the intended sheath. The window should be larger than the outer diameter of the sheath in at least 1 dimension.

Example: 18F sheath for Medtronic Evolut R ≥7 mm

14 to 16F e-sheath for Edwards Sapien 3 ≥7.6 to 8.6 mm

Objective: Identify high-risk anatomy for caval-aortic traversal and large sheath insertion

Rationale: Several extravascular and intravascular anatomic variations have been identified that jeopardize safe traversal

Interposed structures: Arterial branches, interposed bowel, and major veins (eg, renal) cannot be traversed for obvious reasons

Pedunculated atheroma: Pedunculated aortic atheroma may embolize during catheter or closure device manipulation

Abdominal aneurysms: Ectasia and aneurysms are not contraindications, but the large size of the aorta may makes endovascular bailout challenging

Dissections: Chronic dissections can extend with large-bore sheath insertion and should be avoided

Leftward aorta: Aortas with a cephalad leftward trajectory may result in a tangential trajectory if a sheath is inserted and in leftward translation of the abdominal aorta while crossing. 20° leftward aortas should be avoided

Prior device implants: IVC filters, polyester aortic grafts, and even pacemakers have impeded TCav access. Although crossing an aortic graft is possible, it should be performed in experienced centers.

Objective: Identify vascular structures at risk during closure of possible endograft rescue

Rationale: The crossing site should be at least 15 mm away from the aortoiliac bifurcation and renal arteries. Important vessels, including accessory renal arteries and lumbar collaterals, in patients with important iliac disease should be noted, as endograft implantation will compromise these branches

Objective: Select preferred iliofemoral access for possible endograft insertion

Rationale: Endograft implantation at minimum requires a vessel that accepts a 12F access.

Should femoral arterial access be inadequate, then the patient will require appropriate risk:benefit counseling if operators decide to proceed

Objective: Perform measurements for equipment selection and corresponding bony landmarks for crossing plan

Rationale: Once a safe traversal point has been determined, measurements for selecting a snare, guide, and bail-out equipment

Key findings include the following:

- Crossing site(s) and correlating lumbar spinous level for crossing
- Distance from femoral vein puncture site to crossing site
- Distance from aortoiliac bifurcation
- Distance from renal arteries
- Abdominal aorta size at the crossing, 30 mm cephalad and 30 mm caudad

Aortocaval distance does not appear to be important

Permission received from Springer.

TAx access has catapulted to the most frequently used alternative access in the United States due to high rates of technical success and its extrathoracic nature. Retrospective studies have shown similar procedural outcomes between TF and TAx routes,[22,26] but most of these data originate from self-expanding valves and include the surgical cutdown technique. A single-center study reporting balloon-expandable platforms using TAx access reported 100 cases of complete percutaneous access with favorable outcomes.[27] Analysis of the US TVT showed that TAx access has been used in 2% of Sapien TAVR cases.[20] The device success rate was 97.3% and was accompanied by a major vascular complication rate of 2.5%. Propensity-matched analysis demonstrated that TAx access has lower 30-day mortality, shorter intensive care unit and hospital length of stay, but a higher stroke rate (6.1% TAx vs 3.1% transthoracic) compared with transthoracic alternative access (see Table 1). More recently, a 75-patient prospective registry using ACURATE-Neo valves (Boston Scientific, Natick, MA, USA) observed a high rate of complete percutaneous access (90.5%) and conscious sedation (95.2%).[28] Need for bail-out stenting and surgical vascular repair were 9.3% and 4%, respectively, and only 1 (1.3%) cerebral vascular event was reported.

Right axillary access is feasible, and additional technical challenges are encountered. No data exist for whether the right or left axillary artery is better for access, but the left more closely resembles the haptics of transfemoral access, and achieving coaxial alignment is easier.[29] Medtronic recommends against using Evolut (Medtronic, St. Paul, MN, USA) valves via the right axillary artery in root angles greater than 30°, whereas Sapien valves can be delivered but with some technical modifications.[29] Notably, inserting the sheath tip beyond the aortic valve to predilate, passively exposing the valve/delivery system in the ascending aorta and flexing the Commander delivery system (Edwards Lifesciences) away from the aortic valve will improve coaxial alignment.

TRANSCAROTID ACCESS

Superficial location, sturdy constitution, and deep surgical experience with the carotid artery increased its profile as a safe access for TAVR (Fig. 7). Achieved through surgical carotid exposure and establishing proximal and distal control of the vessel with tourniquets, the vessel is usually accessed near the level of the thyroid cartilage. After small sheath insertion, the stenotic aortic valve is crossed and exchanged for a stiff wire, allowing large-bore sheath exchange (see Fig. 7). Following THV implantation, the sheath is withdrawn, and hemostatic control is maintained by tightening the tourniquets. Meanwhile, surgical repair of the arteriotomy can be performed in standard fashion. Initial series of TC access used a vascular shunt to maintain

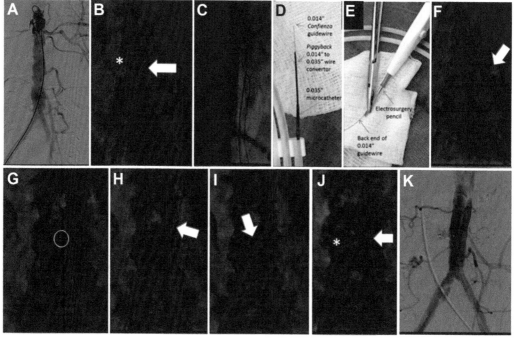

Fig. 9. Stereotypical case of TCav access and closure. (A) Scout angiogram using DSA of the abdominal aorta in the coplanar view. (B) A 6F IM (asterisk) guide is oriented in the IVC pointed toward the abdominal aorta. A 6F JR4 guide with a 25-mm Gooseneck snare (arrow) oriented orthogonally to the coplanar angle in preparation for wire crossing. (C) The image intensifier is rotated 90° to the coplanar angle and the IM catheter trajectory into the open snare in the abdominal aorta. (D) Assembly of a coaxial, serial telescoping system composed of a 0.014″ Confianza Pro 12 within a 0.014″ Piggyback, all nested inside a 0.035″ NAVICROSS. (E) The end of the of Confianza Pro 12 wire is clamped to an electrosurgical pencil with a hemostat. (F) With the application of 50 W of "cut" electrosurgical energy, the 0.014″ wire (arrow) traverses the IVC and abdominal aortic wall to the level of the snare. (G) The 0.014″ wire is captured and towed to the thoracic aorta. A 0.014″ Piggyback catheter (circle) crosses into the abdominal aorta. (H) Using the Piggyback 0.014″ → 0.035″ wire converter enables passage of a 0.035″ NAVICROSS (arrow) to facilitate delivery of a 0.035″ wire from the IVC into the abdominal aorta. (I) With the support a 0.035″ Lunderquist wire, a 14F Edwards Lifesciences E-sheath (arrow) is delivered to the abdominal aorta. (J) Using a small curl Agilis catheter (asterisk), an Amplatz Duct Occluder 10/8 (arrow) is deployed with the retention disc against the abdominal aortic wall. (K) Final DSA aortogram demonstrating minimal flow (type 0) across the TCav fistula. Permission received from Springer Publishing.[42]

antegrade flow but has largely been aban-doned.[30] Current practice at the authors' institu-tion is contralateral carotid and circle of Willis screening for advanced atherosclerosis, but this is not a universal practice. Although traditionally TC access has been under general anesthesia, data from France[31] suggest feasibility of TC TAVR using local and conscious sedation and noted that it was associated with lower stroke rates and less days in the hospital without compromising clinical outcomes.

Retrospective French registry data[32,33] show that TC access is associated with better out-comes compared with thoracic access; lower incidence of atrial fibrillation, less bleeding, acute kidney injury, and shorter hospital length of stay. US TVT data corroborated these out-comes and observed 0.4% rate of utilization in Sapien TAVR cases (see Table 1).[20] Compared with TAx TAVR,[34] TC TAVR has similar mortal-ities, less fluoroscopy and procedure time, and numerically lower stroke rates (nonstatistically significant), making it a favorable alternative ac-cess (see Table 1).

TRANSCAVAL ACCESS

A translational to catheterization laboratory innovation, TCav is the least conventional alter-native access. First validated in an animal model, the technique of harnessing electrosurgical po-wer to traverse the inferior vena cava (IVC) wall, retroperitoneal space, and abdominal aortic wall seems counterintuitive. At first glance, creating a vascular breach into the retro-peritoneal space results in exsanguination, but because the interstitial hydrostatic pressure of the abdomen exceeds IVC pressure, arterial blood preferentially shunts into the IVC. Suc-cessful use of TCav hinges on this concept, and the IVC must serve as a sink for arterial blood (Fig. 8).

TCav access planning requires detailed anal-ysis of the IVC/aorta to determine the crossing level, calcification, aortic size, distance from renal arteries (accessory renal arteries), distance to the iliacs, coplanar crossing angle, presence of interposed structures, and distance from the femoral vein (Box 1).[35,36]

Performing Transcaval Access
First, proper patient consent for alternative ac-cess and all necessary equipment for crossing, closure, and bailout should be assembled (Fig. 9). Attach the electrosurgical pad with care not to be close to any metallic implants (eg, hip replacement). Choose the largest

femoral artery for access in case of the need for endovascular bailout. After vascular access, anticoagulate with a goal of activated clotting time of greater than 250 seconds. Perform a scout abdominal aortogram under digital sub-traction angiography (DSA) at ~32 cm

---

Box 2
Equipment for transcaval access, closure, and bleeding management

Transcaval access

- Electrosurgical unit and pen (Bovie)
- 6F Judkins right guide
- Amplatz Gooseneck snares (~5 mm larger abdominal aortic diameter; Medtronic) (example: 20 mm diameter, use a 25-mm snare) (Medtronic, St Paul, MN)
- 6 to 7F Renal Double Curve-1 guide catheter or 6 to 7F IM guide catheter (renal length)
- 0.014″ microcatheters:

    0.014″ Finecross 135 cm (Terumo, Ann Arbor, MI, USA)

    0.014″ Piggyback 120 or 150 cm (Teleflex Medical, Morrisville, NC, USA)

    0.014″ Advance Microballoon 150 cm (Cook Medical, Bloomington, IN, USA)

- 0.035″ catheters:

    0.035″ CXI catheter 90 cm (Cook Medical)

    0.035″ NAVICROSS catheter 90 cm (Terumo, Ann Arbor, MI, USA)

    0.035″ Lunderquist Wire (Cook Medical, Bloomington, IN)

- 0.014″ crossing wires

    0.014″ Astato XS 20 wire 300 cm (Asahi Intecc, Tustin, CA, USA)

    0.014″ Confianza Pro 12 300 cm (Asahi Intecc)

Transcaval closure:

- Small curl Agilis (Abbott Structural, Santa Clara, CA)
- Amplatz Duct Occluder I 8/6 mm or 10/8 mm (Abbott Structural)
- 0.014″ Balance Middle Weight 300 cm

Bleeding complication rescue:

- Reliant Aortic Occlusion Balloon (Medtronic)
- Coda Aortic Occlusion Balloon (Cook Medical)
- 14 to 28 × 45 mm Endologix Ovation iX Iliac Limb Extender stents (Endologix, Irvine, CA)

Permission received from Springer Publishing.[42]

magnification using the coplanar angle preidentified. Afterward, exchange the pigtail catheter for a 6F JR4 guiding catheter and position a single-loop snare (Amplatz Gooseneck; Medtronic) in the abdominal aorta at the proposed crossing point, oriented toward the IVC. Next, the crossing catheter, usually a 6 to 7F Renal Double Curve or renal length internal mammary (IM) catheter is aimed at the snare at the corresponding lumbar spinous level in the IVC. Prepare a 0.014″ Astato 20 wire, 0.014″ microcatheter, and 0.035″ braided catheter as a serial telescoping crossing system. After crossing the system assembly, clamp the 0.014″ wire to the electrosurgical pencil and confirm coaxial trajectory of the wire to the snare center using orthogonal projections (see Fig. 8). Once confirmed, advance the wire while applying a short burst of 50 W of electrosurgical cutting, halting when the wire approximates the snare location. Close the snare around the wire and drag the 0.014″ wire cephalad to the thoracic descending aorta. Using the countertraction of the captured wire, advance the 0.014″ catheter and 0.035″ catheter in a telescoping fashion. Release the snared 0.014″ wire to exchange for the 0.035″ Lunderquist wire. Finally, exchange the small venous sheath for the large-bore sheath under high-resolution radiography to ensure smooth passage and scrutinize for sheath splaying.

Difficulty crossing should trigger caution and prompt troubleshooting steps. First, avoid wire buckling, as spring release of a buckled wire may create a slitlike orifice that is unmatched on the caval side and increase risk for bleeding.

Unexplained hemodynamic changes in the context of multiple crossing failures should prompt aorta angiography. Review that electrosurgical monopolar cutting of at least 50 W is being activated and the contact point between the coronary wire and electrosurgical pencil is clean. Several failed traversal attempts will char the wire, necessitating replacement. If a different crossing location is selected, knowledge of lumen size, interposing structures, proximity to vessels, and coplanar angles must be reassessed. The aortic wall may sometimes be resistant to catheter crossing despite wire traversal, in which case use a 2.5- to 3.0-mm noncompliant coronary balloon to facilitate traversal.

Transcaval Access Closure

Once the THV is implanted, reaffirm all access emergency bailout equipment is assembled (Box 2). Infuse protamine to normalize the activated clotting time and leave a 0.014″ 300-cm safety wire across the tract. Advance a small curl deflectable catheter through the delivery sheath, prepare a nitinol closure device, preferably an Amplatz Duct Occluder I (ADO I; Abbott Vascular, Santa Clara, CA, USA). Withdraw the large-bore TCav sheath close to the crossing site and passively expose the ADO I, forming a "ball." Retract the TCav sheath to the IVC and ensure the venous side is not obstructed to allow venous decompression. Finally, form a retention disc completely and deflect the catheter 90° and retract the system with sufficient tension to appose the aortic wall but avoid pulling through. Once apposed, passively expose the remainder of the device. Immediate angiography is important to recognize any bleeding early. Generally,

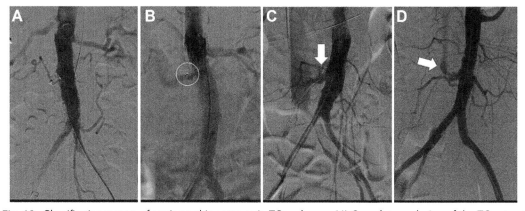

Fig. 10. Classification system of angiographic patterns in TCav closure. (*A*) Complete occlusion of the TCav tract after closure (type 0). (*B*) Patent, funnel-shaped fistula (*circle*) flowing into the IVC (type 1). (*C*) Patent fistula with a "cruciform" pattern of contrast flow (*arrow*) at the occluder (type 2). (*D*) Extravasation (*arrow*). Note that there is superimposed flow into the vena cava but the contrast staining pattern without clearance should be interpreted as retroperitoneal bleeding. Permission received from Springer Publishing.[42]

there are 4 patterns of closure (Fig. 10): Occluded (type 0), funneled (type I), cruciform (type II), and extravasation (type III).[37] Types 0 to 2 can be observed without intervention, and extravasation requires intervention. Transient blood pressure drops of 10 to 15 mm Hg are typical with shunting. If hypotension persists, consider oblique views to exclude extravasation.

In the event of extravasation, rapidly exchange for an aortic occlusion balloon and tamponade the TCav tract. Occlusion of the tract for 3- to 5-minute cycles can be done several times, but if there is no improvement, then proceed with covered stent implantation. In rare occasions, patients with right ventricular cardiomyopathy can experience hemodynamic embarrassment from the inability to accommodate aortic-caval shunting. To manage extravasation or arterial-venous shunting, occlusion of the tract using a covered stent is sometimes necessary. A self-expanding covered stent 10% to 20% larger than the aortic lumen is recommended, and the stent of choice is an Ovation iX aortic limb extender stent (Endologix, Irvine, CA, USA); however, a balloon expandable stent (VBX; Gore Medical) has been successfully used as well.

The feasibility of this access was demonstrated in preclinical work on animals[38] and subsequently performed in a series of 25 patients without femoral or another alternative access options.[39] A larger prospective study[40] was done and reported data on 100 patients at 17 centers with 99% successful TCav access (1 failure to cross), and 98% device success (no death or surgery bailout). The 1-year data on TCav tract closure were reported in 2019 and showed that 93% of patients had complete closure of the cavoaortic tract at 1 year.[41]

SUMMARY

Vascular access complications continue to negatively impact patients, and alternative access remains essential to treating complex cases of valvular heart disease. The infrequent use of alternative access requires that operators concentrate their focus on developing expertise with 1 to 2 techniques or refer patients to experienced tertiary centers. Although THV evolution may eventually further reduce the need for alternative access, high prevalence of advanced age, morbid obesity, peripheral vascular disease, and earlier onset diabetes will likely preserve the need for nonfemoral access. Furthermore, the authors' center promotes the philosophy that the best access be pursued in each individual case and not simply the most convenient. To this end, alternative access remains central to building a high-quality tertiary center for TAVR.

REFERENCES

1. Leon MB, Smith CR, Mack M, et al. Transcatheter aortic-valve implantation for aortic stenosis in patients who cannot undergo surgery. N Engl J Med 2010;363:1597–607.
2. Leon MB, Smith CR, Mack MJ, et al. Transcatheter or surgical aortic-valve replacement in intermediate-risk patients. N Engl J Med 2016; 374:1609–20.
3. Mack MJ, Leon MB, Thourani VH, et al. Transcatheter aortic-valve replacement with a balloon-expandable valve in low-risk patients. N Engl J Med 2019;380:1695–705.
4. Rogers T, Gai J, Torguson R, et al. Predicted magnitude of alternate access in the contemporary transcatheter aortic valve replacement era. Catheter Cardiovasc Interv 2018;92:964–71.
5. Genereux P, Webb JG, Svensson LG, et al. Vascular complications after transcatheter aortic valve replacement: insights from the PARTNER (Placement of AoRTic TraNscathetER Valve) trial. J Am Coll Cardiol 2012;60:1043–52.
6. Kadakia MB, Herrmann HC, Desai ND, et al. Factors associated with vascular complications in patients undergoing balloon-expandable transfemoral transcatheter aortic valve replacement via open versus percutaneous approaches. Circ Cardiovasc Interv 2014;7:570–6.
7. Vemulapalli S, Carroll JD, Mack MJ, et al. Procedural volume and outcomes for transcatheter aortic-valve replacement. N Engl J Med 2019;380: 2541–50.
8. Cribier A, Eltchaninoff H, Tron C, et al. Early experience with percutaneous transcatheter implantation of heart valve prosthesis for the treatment of end-stage inoperable patients with calcific aortic stenosis. J Am Coll Cardiol 2004;43:698–703.
9. Cribier A, Eltchaninoff H, Bash A, et al. Percutaneous transcatheter implantation of an aortic valve prosthesis for calcific aortic stenosis: first human case description. Circulation 2002;106:3006–8.
10. Hanzel GS, Harrity PJ, Schreiber TL, et al. Retrograde percutaneous aortic valve implantation for critical aortic stenosis. Catheter Cardiovasc Interv 2005;64:322–6.
11. Webb JG, Chandavimol M, Thompson CR, et al. Percutaneous aortic valve implantation retrograde from the femoral artery. Circulation 2006;113: 842–50.
12. Blackstone EH, Suri RM, Rajeswaran J, et al. Propensity-matched comparisons of clinical outcomes after transapical or transfemoral transcatheter

aortic valve replacement: a placement of aortic transcatheter valves (PARTNER)-I trial substudy. Circulation 2015;131:1989–2000.

13. Lichtenstein SV, Cheung A, Ye J, et al. Transapical transcatheter aortic valve implantation in humans: initial clinical experience. Circulation 2006;114:591–6.

14. Ribeiro HB, Nombela-Franco L, Munoz-Garcia AJ, et al. Predictors and impact of myocardial injury after transcatheter aortic valve replacement: a multicenter registry. J Am Coll Cardiol 2015;66:2075–88.

15. Mach M, Koschutnik M, Wilbring M, et al. Impact of COPD on outcome in patients undergoing transfemoral versus transapical TAVI. Thorac Cardiovasc Surg 2019;67:251–6.

16. Bapat V, Frank D, Cocchieri R, et al. Transcatheter aortic valve replacement using transaortic access: experience from the multicenter, multinational, prospective ROUTE registry. JACC Cardiovasc Interv 2016;9:1815–22.

17. Thomas T, Poulose AK, Harris KM. Transient aortic intramural hematoma complicating transaortic valve replacement. Aorta (Stamford) 2016;4:232–4.

18. Tsuyoshi Kaneko FY, Hirji S, Pelletier M, et al. Peripheral versus central access for alternative access transcatheter aortic valve replacement (TAVR): results from the TVT registry. J Am Coll Cardiol 2020;75:1177.

19. Tanawuttiwat T, O'Neill BP, Cohen MG, et al. New-onset atrial fibrillation after aortic valve replacement: comparison of transfemoral, transapical, transaortic, and surgical approaches. J Am Coll Cardiol 2014;63:1510–9.

20. Dahle TG, Kaneko T, McCabe JM. Outcomes following subclavian and axillary artery access for transcatheter aortic valve replacement: Society of the Thoracic Surgeons/American College of Cardiology TVT Registry Report. JACC Cardiovasc Interv 2019;12:662–9.

21. Codner P, Pugliese D, Kouz R, et al. Transcatheter aortic valve replacement by a novel suprasternal approach. Ann Thorac Surg 2018;105:1215–22.

22. Petronio AS, De Carlo M, Bedogni F, et al. Safety and efficacy of the subclavian approach for transcatheter aortic valve implantation with the CoreValve revalving system. Circ Cardiovasc Interv 2010;3:359–66.

23. McCabe JM, Kaki AA, Pinto DS, et al. Percutaneous axillary access for placement of microaxial ventricular support devices. Circ Cardiovasc Interv 2021;14:e009657.

24. Tayal R, Iftikhar H, LeSar B, et al. CT angiography analysis of axillary artery diameter versus common femoral artery diameter: implications for axillary approach for transcatheter aortic valve replacement in patients with hostile aortoiliac segment and advanced lung disease. Int J Vasc Med 2016;2016:3610705.

25. Cheney AE, McCabe JM. Alternative percutaneous access for large bore devices. Circ Cardiovasc Interv 2019;12:e007707.

26. Frohlich GM, Baxter PD, Malkin CJ, et al. Comparative survival after transapical, direct aortic, and subclavian transcatheter aortic valve implantation (data from the UK TAVI registry). Am J Cardiol 2015;116:1555–9.

27. Schafer U, Deuschl F, Schofer N, et al. Safety and efficacy of the percutaneous transaxillary access for transcatheter aortic valve implantation using various transcatheter heart valves in 100 consecutive patients. Int J Cardiol 2017;232:247–54.

28. Amat-Santos IJ, Santos-Martínez S, Conradi L, et al. Transaxillary transcatheter ACURATE neo aortic valve implantation – The TRANSAX multicenter study. Catheter Cardiovasc Interv 2020. https://doi.org/10.1002/ccd.29423.

29. Rajkumar CA, Cook C, Shalhoub J, et al. Facilitating right-sided axillary artery access for transcatheter aortic valve replacement using the Edwards Sapien 3 and ultra valves: technical considerations. Catheter Cardiovasc Interv 2020;96:E747–54.

30. Guyton RA, Block PC, Thourani VH, et al. Carotid artery access for transcatheter aortic valve replacement. Catheter Cardiovasc Interv 2013;82:E583–6.

31. Debry N, Delhaye C, Azmoun A, et al. Transcarotid transcatheter aortic valve replacement: general or local anesthesia. JACC Cardiovasc Interv 2016;9:2113–20.

32. Chamandi C, Abi-Akar R, Rodes-Cabau J, et al. Transcarotid compared with other alternative access routes for transcatheter aortic valve replacement. Circ Cardiovasc Interv 2018;11:e006388.

33. Allen KB, Chhatriwalla AK, Cohen D, et al. Transcarotid versus transapical and transaortic access for transcatheter aortic valve replacement. Ann Thorac Surg 2019;108:715–22.

34. James Hermiller DH, Moainie S, Kirker E, et al. Transcarotid versus subclavian/axillary access for transcatheter aortic valve replacement: real-world comparative outcomes utilizing the TVT registry. J Am Coll Cardiol 2019;74:B77.

35. Lederman RJ, Chen MY, Rogers T, et al. Planning transcaval access using CT for large transcatheter implants. JACC Cardiovasc Imaging 2014;7:1167–71.

36. Lederman RJ, Greenbaum AB, Rogers T, et al. Anatomic suitability for transcaval access based on computed tomography. JACC Cardiovasc Interv 2017;10:1–10.

37. Lederman RJ, Babaliaros VC, Greenbaum AB. How to perform transcaval access and closure for transcatheter aortic valve implantation. Catheter Cardiovasc Interv 2015;86:1242–54.

38. Halabi M, Ratnayaka K, Faranesh AZ, et al. Aortic access from the vena cava for large caliber

transcatheter cardiovascular interventions: pre-clinical validation. J Am Coll Cardiol 2013;61: 1745–6.

39. Greenbaum AB, O'Neill WW, Paone G, et al. Caval-aortic access to allow transcatheter aortic valve replacement in otherwise ineligible patients: initial human experience. J Am Coll Cardiol 2014;63: 2795–804.

40. Greenbaum AB, Babaliaros VC, Chen MY, et al. Transcaval access and closure for transcatheter

aortic valve replacement: a prospective investiga-tion. J Am Coll Cardiol 2017;69:511–21.

41. Lederman RJ, Babaliaros VC, Rogers T, et al. The fate of transcaval access tracts: 12-month results of the prospective NHLBI transcaval transcatheter aortic valve replacement study. JACC Cardiovasc Interv 2019;12:448–56.

42. Eng MH, Villablanca P, Frisoli T, et al. Transcaval ac-cess for large bore devices. Curr Cardiol Rep 2019; 21:134.

Neurologic Complications in Transcatheter Aortic Valve Replacement

Abel Ignatius, MD[a], Marvin H. Eng, MD[a],
Tiberio M. Frisoli, MD[b,c,*]

KEYWORDS

• Stroke • TAVR • Cerebral embolic protection • Atrial fibrillation

KEY POINTS

- Stroke remains a source of significant mortality, morbidity, and disability in the transcatheter aortic valve replacement (TAVR) population.
- Acute periprocedural and remote strokes have differing mechanisms, hence mitigation strategies.
- Although the use of cerebral embolic protection devices did not meet statistical significance for preventing stroke, larger analyses suggest they have value in preventing stroke.
- Post-TAVR stroke prevention is controversial and limited by the bleeding profile of patients as routine use of Factor Xa inhibitors and even dual antiplatelet therapy were a source of significant morbidity in prospective studies.

INTRODUCTION

Transcatheter aortic valve replacement (TAVR) has become the most commonly performed treatment for symptomatic severe aortic stenosis (AS) in patients across all surgical risk profiles.[1] TAVR provides a life-saving and lifestyle-improving treatment for patients across all surgical risk profiles.[2–5] Advancements in technology and operator experience have resulted in diminishing rates of mortality, paravalvular aortic insufficiency, postprocedure pacemaker implantation, and vascular complications.[6]

However, despite those advancements, the rate of postprocedural stroke has remained relatively stable over time, with multiple studies demonstrating a stroke rate in the 2% to 3% range at 30 days post-TAVR in procedures performed between 2007 and 2018.[7–10] These TAVR stroke rates are lower than the comparator surgical aortic valve replacement.[2,11]

Stroke is one of the most feared, debilitating, and costly complications of TAVR. Further reducing stroke remains a central objective in the treatment of aortic valve stenosis. In later discussion, the authors synthesize the state-of-the-art and future of post-TAVR stroke and its prevention.

DEFINITIONS AND DISTINCTIONS

Standardized criteria for the definition of stroke endpoints for TAVR clinical trials have been published by the Valve Academic Research Consortium. Diagnostic criteria involve "rapid onset of a focal or global neurological deficit with at least 1 of the following: change in level of consciousness, hemiplegia, hemiparesis, numbness or sensory loss affecting one side of the body, dysphagia or aphasia, hemianopia, amaurosis fugax, or other neurological signs or symptoms consistent with stroke."[6] In addition, there should be no readily identifiable nonstroke cause for the

[a] Center for Structural Heart Disease, Henry Ford Hospital, 2799 W Grand Boulevard, Detroit, MI 48202, USA; [b] Interventional Structural Cardiology, Center for Structural Heart Disease, Heart and Vascular Institute, Henry Ford Hospital, 2799 W Grand Boulevard, Detroit, MI 48202, USA; [c] Henry Ford Allegiance Hospital, 205 N East Avenue, Jackson, MI 49201, USA
* Corresponding author. Center for Structural Heart Disease, Henry Ford Hospital, 2799 W Grand Boulevard, Detroit, MI 48202.
E-mail address: tfrisol1@hfhs.org

Intervent Cardiol Clin 10 (2021) 519–529
https://doi.org/10.1016/j.iccl.2021.06.006
2211-7458/21/© 2021 Elsevier Inc. All rights reserved.

clinical presentation. Minor stroke is characterized by a modified Rankin score less than 2, whereas major stroke is characterized by a score ≥2.

Although the definition of stroke is relatively clear, how stroke has been defined and studied in TAVR is quite more complex.

True Incidence of Stroke Depends on the Definition and Adjudication

Different TAVR trials have adjudicated the stroke endpoint differently: some as disabling, others inclusive of those detected after careful examination, often by a neurologist, of subtle signs and symptoms and that may yield no lifestyle-limiting disabilities, and others detected with imaging, such as MRI, sometimes in asymptomatic patients.

Analysis of the transcatheter valve therapy (TVT) registry of about 100,000 TAVR procedures through the middle of 2017 shows stable stroke rates (TVT registry represents site-reported stroke rates) despite improvements in operator experience and device technology, of about 2% to 2.5%.[9] In comparison, trials (ie, SENTINEL, DEFLECT III) whereby stroke is adjudicated based on careful neurologic assessment (eg, National Institutes of Health Stroke Scale before and after TAVR), the rates are in the range of 9% to 15%; in trials for which new brain MRI lesions are a principal endpoint (ie, MISTRAL-C, CLEAN TAVI, SENTINEL), the rates are much higher.[10,12–14] Stroke rates in contemporary TAVR trials are shown in Fig. 1.

Importantly, nondisabling strokes should not necessarily be considered benign or truly asymptomatic, as these may be associated with steeper cognitive decline over time, an issue

that is of particular importance for the large and growing number of younger low-risk patients that are undergoing TAVR.[14]

Relationship of Stroke to the Transcatheter Aortic Valve Replacement Procedure Itself

Some strokes occur in the periprocedural period, whereas other strokes occur remotely from the procedure. It is critically important to make these distinctions, as they have implications for mitigating the risk of these events. An intraprocedural stroke has a different pathophysiological mechanism, incidence, and potential prevention strategy than a stroke remote from the TAVR.

TIMING, MECHANISM, AND PREDICTORS OF STROKE IN TRANSCATHETER AORTIC VALVE REPLACEMENT PATIENTS

Timing

Post-TAVR strokes have been classified as acute if occurring withing 24 hours, subacute if occurring from 1 day to 30 days post-TAVR, and late if occurring after 30 days. Acute strokes occurring during or shortly after TAVR represent most post-TAVR strokes. In cohort B of the landmark PARTNER trial, nearly two-thirds of the strokes related to TAVR at 1 year occurred within 30 days post-TAVR. In PARTNER, 85% of the 30-day strokes occurred within the first week, with the peak rate by day 2.[15] Several other studies have shown that stroke incidence following TAVR has a peak in the immediate period after the procedure (24–48 hours), with some studies reporting half of the total events occurring within 1 month.[16,17] Among 3191

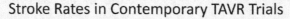

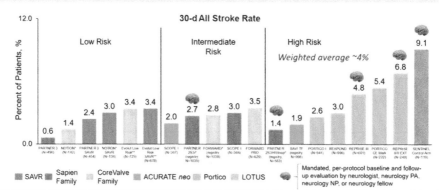

Fig. 1. Stroke rates vary across various contemporary TAVR trials, in part related to the definition of stroke used in the trial protocol. *, refers to Kaplan Meier estimates.

patients from the FRANCE-2 registry, strokes were reported in 4%, with 48.5% of these events occurring within the first 48 hours.[17]

Mechanism

Acute strokes are thought to be due to embolism of thrombus or fibrocalcific debris from the valve site or because of atherothrombotic emboli originating from ulcerative plaques in the aortic arch or great cerebral vessels. Such particles can be dislodged during wire/catheter/device manipulation across the aortic arch, during attempts to traverse the aortic annulus with wire and device, during balloon valvuloplasty, or valve deployment. Other potential causes of stroke caused by TAVR include hypotension associated with rapid ventricular pacing or hemodynamic instability during the procedure, especially in someone with preexisting cerebrovascular disease.[6] Less than 5% of acute strokes after TAVR are reported as hemorrhagic.[18]

Stroke that occurs after many days to weeks or months after TAVR is presumably less related to the TAVR procedure and more so to the patient's underlying stroke risk factors. Many patients who have AS also have other comorbidities that predispose them to ischemic stroke, such as advanced age, hypertension, diabetes, atherosclerotic and calcific arterial disease of the aorta and cerebral vessels, and atrial fibrillation.

Predictors/Risk Factors

It is important to establish reliable predictors of stroke after TAVR so that periprocedural and postprocedural care can be tailored on an individual basis. There are patient risk factors and procedural risk factors. Table 1 summarizes some of the reported risk factors, with more detailed discussion later.

In a meta-analysis, female sex and underlying chronic kidney disease (CKD) were baseline characteristics that were associated with higher risk of stroke post-TAVR.[19] Female sex is associated with smaller aortic annuli and left ventricular outflow tract dimensions, and therefore, higher mechanical interaction between the native and aortic valve prosthesis. This finding is supported by the PARTNER trial, which demonstrated a higher rate of strokes (6.3% vs 2.8%) in patients with smaller aortic annuli and valve area.[15] CKD was also identified as a patient-related risk factor (relative risk [RR]: 1.29; P = .03), thought to be related to its inherent role in atherogenesis and/or the absence of established guidelines regarding

Table 1	
Reported stroke risk factors in TAVR, categorized as patient- or procedure-related	
Patient-Related	**Procedure-Related**
Female Gender	Valve dislodgement/
Older Age	embolization
Atrial fibrillation	Non-transfemoral
Chronic kidney	TAVR Access
disease	
Smaller aortic	
annular area	
Degree of	
aortic valve	
calcification	
Bicuspid aortic	
valve	
Carotid artery	
disease	
Peripheral arterial	
disease	
Prior Stroke	

anticoagulation therapy for stroke prevention in these patients.[19]

There was a nonstatistically significant signal that balloon postdilation was associated with higher risk of stroke. The strongest procedure-related predictor of stroke occurring 1 to 30 days post-TAVR was new-onset atrial fibrillation (RR: 1.85; P = .005).

In a real-world sample of commercial TAVRs performed in 2017, for which the ischemic stroke rate was 2.4%, factors independently associated with post-TAVR ischemic stroke included a history of carotid artery disease, peripheral artery disease, atrial fibrillation or flutter, older age, bicuspid aortic valve, and female sex.[20,21]

Atrial fibrillation has been consistently reported in studies investigating risk factors for postprocedural stroke. New-onset atrial fibrillation has been identified as an independent predictor for 30-day stroke (odds ratio [OR] 2.27, P = .018) and chronic atrial fibrillation as a major contributor to late (>30 days) strokes occurring in 3.3% of patients after a median follow-up of 12 months.[16]

Other potential risk factors for stroke after TAVR include implantation of 2 valves, prior stroke, coronary artery disease, valve dislodgement/embolization, degree of aortic valve calcification, and small index aortic valve area (cutoff value of 0.4 cm^2/m^2).[16,17,22,23]

Presently, the balloon-expandable Sapien valve (Edwards Life Sciences, Inc, Irvine, CA, USA) and the self-expandable CoreValve Evolut system (Medtronic, Inc, Minneapolis, MN, USA) are the 2 devices primarily used for the TAVR procedure, with no strong evidence to suggest statistically significant differences in stroke rates between valve types.[17,19,24] A meta-analysis of transfemoral versus nontransfemoral (in this analysis, transcarotid and transsubclavian approaches) TAVR revealed an increased risk of stroke for the nontransfemoral route (OR 1.53; confidence interval 1.05–2.22) when adjusting for confounding factors.[21] It is possible that the risk adjustment does not fully account for the higher stroke predisposition of patients that require nontransfemoral TAVR. These nontransfemoral arterial alternative accesses were not associated with an increased risk of adjusted 30-day death, bleeding, or vascular complication. Current data suggest no difference in stroke rate with regard to transfemoral versus transapical approach.[19,24,25,26]

IMPLICATIONS OF STROKE TO THE PATIENT AND HEALTH CARE SYSTEM

Stroke has been shown to increase mortality in TAVR patients, with a 30-day mortality of 16.7% compared with 3.7% in patients without stroke.[8] One meta-analysis revealed periprocedural stroke associated with a more than 6 times greater risk of 30-day mortality.[27,28]

Silent or asymptomatic infarctions, as assessed by brain MRI, have been associated with steeper decline in cognitive function, including impairments in memory performance, psychomotor speed, and global cognitive function resulting in increased risk of dementia and depression.[29,30] Furthermore, stroke patients who survive to hospital discharge are significantly less likely to go home following TAVR (36.1% vs 78.9% in those without strokes, $P<.001$).[8]

In an analysis of younger patients (age <65), stroke was associated with significant financial strains in 33%, an inability to return to work in 56%, and a decrease in participation in social activities in 79%.[31] After a stroke, the additional annual change in disability increases at a faster rate than in those age-matched who did not have stroke.[32] Given the steep growth in TAVR volume, the impact is further amplified with wide-reaching consequences.

The financial burden of TAVR-related stroke also cannot be understated, with an estimated incremental cost of approximately $16,272 per patient and an added length of stay of about 2.5 days for major stroke.[33] In another analysis, stroke is associated with a 33% increase in average TAVR hospitalization cost (+$19,658),

a 6-day average increase in length of index hospitalization stay, and a 121% increase in nursing home and intermediate care facility discharge.[34]

STROKE PREVENTION

As discussed, post-TAVR strokes can be acute and often related to the procedure itself, or subacute-late and more related to the inherent stroke-predisposing milieu of the patient and the transcatheter heart valve.

Efforts to reduce rates of acute stroke have centered on meticulous intraprocedural technique, improved device technology, and intraprocedural cerebral embolic prevention device use. Prevention of subacute and late stroke revolves around pharmacologic antiplatelet or anticoagulant therapy as it relates to the transcatheter prosthesis and to the patient's inherent stroke risk factors, such as atrial fibrillation and atherosclerotic vascular disease. Device therapy with, for example, left atrial appendage closure is also under investigation for the prevention of subacute and late stroke after TAVR.

Intraprocedural Device Therapy

Cerebral embolic protection devices (CEPDs) were developed to reduce the risk of strokes and silent emboli by preventing procedural debris from reaching cerebral vasculature. Currently, the SENTINEL Cerebral Protection System (Boston Scientific, Natick, MA, USA) is the only Food and Drug Administration (FDA)-approved device available for use in the United States. It consists of 2 filters within a single 6F delivery catheter percutaneously placed from the right radial or brachial artery over a 0.014-in guidewire.[14] The filters are positioned in the brachiocephalic and the left common carotid arteries before TAVR (Fig. 2), covering about 90% of cerebral vascular circulation. The filters are then withdrawn into the catheter and removed after TAVR. The Sentinel device has been shown to capture debris, including thrombus, valve tissue, calcified debris, artery wall, myocardium, and foreign material, in 99% of TAVR patients, which weighed heavily in the decision by the FDA to approve the device. Fig. 3 shows debris as captured during TAVR, and Fig. 4 shows fluoroscopic examples of in vivo Sentinel deployment during TAVR and illustrates some techniques used to overcome more challenging anatomies.

The SENTINEL trial randomized 363 patients undergoing TAVR at 17 centers in the United States and 2 centers in Germany to CEPD versus no protection. The device, although

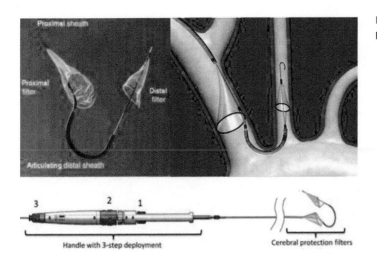

Fig. 2. The Sentinel cerebral embolic protection filter device.

manipulated and positioned in the great cerebral vessels, was shown to be safe: Sentinel-related complications were 0.4%. The rate of major adverse cardiac and cerebrovascular events at 30 days was 7.3% and not statistically different than that of the control group (9.9%).[14] Strokes at 30 days were 9.1% in control subjects and 5.6% in patients with devices, also statistically not significant (P = .25), in what was an underpowered study for this endpoint.

Despite not achieving statistical significance, the 72-hour data demonstrate 63% relative risk reduction and 5.2% absolute risk reduction in stroke.

The primary efficacy endpoint for this trial, importantly, not stroke but rather new lesion volume on diffusion-weighted MRI in protected territories, was lower in the device arm (178.0 mm^3) as compared with the control arm (102.8 mm^3) but did not meet statistical significance

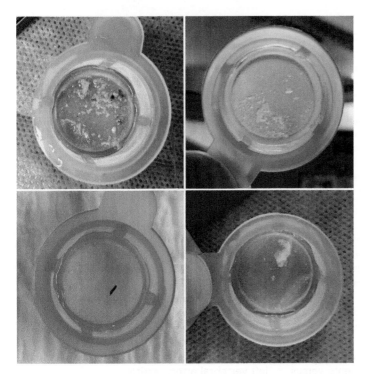

Fig. 3. Examples of debris retrieved from the Sentinel device during TAVR. (Courtesy of Tiberio Frisoli MD.)

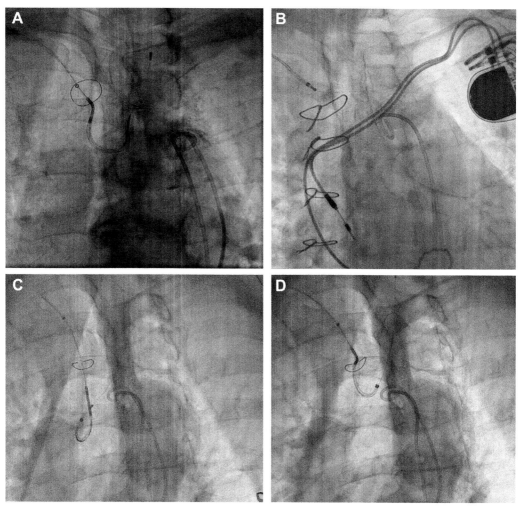

Fig. 4. Fluoroscopic images during TAVR that serve as examples of Sentinel deployment. (*A*) Typical appearance of Sentinel after deployment, with distal filter in left common carotid artery and proximal filter in brachiocephalic artery. (*B*) Example of how, in a bovine arch anatomy, the guidewire can be passed directly into the left carotid rather than into the ascending aorta, for delivery of the Sentinel. (*C*) Example of how, in bovine arch anatomy, when one is unable or prefers not to pass the guidewire directly into the left common carotid artery, the device can be flexed and turned around on itself in the distal ascending aorta to become coaxial with the left common carotid to allow wiring. (*D*) After the operator does what is shown in panel (*C*), the rotation that was applied to the device can be undone as it is pulled up into the left common carotid, after which the distal filter is pushed forward.

(P = .33). Thus, the SENTINEL trial was a negative trial. However, after adjusting for valve type and baseline T2/FLAIR lesion volume in a post hoc analysis, there were significant differences in new lesion volumes favoring embolic protection. There was also a correlation between lesion volume and neurocognitive decline at 30 days.

In the MISTRAL-C randomized controlled study, the Sentinel device had fewer new lesions and a smaller total lesion volume (95 mm^3 vs 197 mm^3). Neurocognitive deterioration was present in 4% of Sentinel CPS patients versus 27% without embolic protection.[10] In the randomized controlled CLEAN-TAVI trial, the number of new lesions was lower in the filter group compared with controls (4.00 vs 10.00), as was the new lesion volume (242 mm^3 vs 527 mm^3).[12] Meta-analysis data from the SENTINEL, MISTRAL-C, and CLEAN-TAVI trials showed a statistically significant reduction (P = .017) in new brain lesions favoring Sentinel, ultimately leading to FDA approval. Of note, the Sentinel device does not provide complete cerebrovascular protection, as there is no filter in the left vertebral artery territory.

Real-world registry data have been favorable for the Sentinel device. Stroke rates (disabling and nondisabling) at 7 days after TAVR were reduced by 70% (1.4% vs 4.6%; $P = .03$) at the University of Ulm and by 78% (1.4% vs 6.3%; $P<.01$) at Cedars-Sinai.[35,36] When patients from the SENTINEL trial were combined with the CLEAN-TAVI and SENTINEL-Ulm studies in a patient level pooled analysis of 1306 patients with propensity score matching, all stroke was significantly lower (1.88% vs 5.44%; $P = .003$; relative risk reduction (RRR) 65%).[37] A recently published retrospective analysis of the Nationwide Inpatient Sample database from 2017, of 525 patients who underwent TAVR with CEPD and 1050 propensity score-matched patients who underwent TAVR without CEPD, revealed a lower ischemic stroke risk (1% vs 3.8%; $P = .003$) and a higher cost of index hospitalization ($47,783 vs $44,578; $P = .002$), without an increased risk of procedural complications.[20]

A major barrier to widespread Sentinel use has been cost, as the Centers for Medicare and Medicaid Services did not reimburse for its use. As of October 2018, an add-on payment went into effect for Sentinel use during TAVR. Maximum new technology add-on payment for a case involving Sentinel was $1400 for fiscal year 2019. Cost is still a commonly cited barrier for use of this device.

The TriGuard (Keystone) Embolic Deflection Device is another form of cerebral embolic protection for use during TAVR. It is a nitinol mesh filter positioned in the aortic arch across the right brachiocephalic, left common carotid, and left subclavian arteries and is designed to deflect emboli away from cerebral circulation during TAVR. The DEFLECT III trial randomized 85 subjects undergoing TAVR at 13 centers in Europe and Israel from February 2014 to 2015 to TriGuard protection versus no protection. Results from this prospective study showed that the device was safe to use, and patients who underwent TAVR with TriGuard protection had fewer ischemic brain lesions, fewer neurologic deficits, and improved cognitive function at discharge and at 30 days compared with controls.[13] However, results from the late-breaking REFLECT II trial reported at the Transcatheter Cardiovascular Therapeutics Connect 2020 virtual conference showed that the TriGuard 3 failed to demonstrate a statistically significant difference in in-hospital and 30-day stroke compared with controls.[38]

Only about 20% of all TAVR procedures in the United States is performed with cerebral embolic protection; in Germany over the past 3 years, only 3.8% of all TAVR cases were done with cerebral protection.[39]

Many who do not use cerebral embolic protection regularly argue: it is a device that has never been proven in a randomized trial to reduce stroke; it does not protect all cerebral vessels; cost is significant if not prohibitive.

Many who do use cerebral embolic protection regularly tend to argue: the SENTINEL study was underpowered; although it did not meet its primary endpoint, the findings from registries and meta-analyses such as those discussed above are compelling; for such a devastating complication as stroke, the use of a device that is proven safe and effective at least at catching debris simply makes too much sense to be dismissed. A common rhetorical question cited by proponents is: "If your mother were to undergo TAVR, would you want cerebral embolic protection for her?"

At this time, a paucity of prospective randomized data showing a clinical stroke benefit, coupled with a significant cost has led to a lack of universal adoption of cerebral embolic protection in TAVR. The multicenter PROTECTED-TAVR trial aims to address this controversial issue. It is an ongoing randomized controlled trial scheduled for completion in 2022; the primary endpoint is clinically adjudicated stroke at 72 hours or discharge.

Post–Transcatheter Aortic Valve Replacement Medical Therapy for the Mitigation of Stroke Risk

Subclinical leaflet thrombosis, defined as hypoattenuated leaflet thickening (HALT) as detected by high-resolution computed tomography (CT) has been investigated as a potential risk factor for post-TAVR stroke. The prevalence of HALT among TAVR patients in PARTNER 3 was 10% and 24% at 30 days and 1 year after TAVR, respectively; spontaneous resolution of 30-day HALT occurred in 54% of patients at 1 year.[40] Although the individual endpoint of stroke was not different between HALT and no HALT groups, the pooled rates of stroke, transient ischemic attack (TIA), and thromboembolic complications were higher in HALT than no HALT groups (8.6 vs 1.6%; RRR 5.3). An analysis of the RESOLVE and SAVORY registries revealed no statistically significant difference in stroke rates between those with (4.12 strokes per 100 person-years) or without (1.92 strokes per 100 person-years) CT-adjudicated reduced leaflet motion.[41] However, they did note that subclinical leaflet thrombosis was associated with increased rates of TIAs (4.18 TIAs per 100 person-years vs 0.60 TIAs per 100 person-years). An analysis of the OCEAN-TAVI registry with CT data out to 3 years after TAVR showed that early HALT was present in 45 patients (9.3%) at a median time of 3 days.[42] The investigators found that the presence of early leaflet thrombosis was not associated with in-hospital stroke. Furthermore, the rates of ischemic and hemorrhagic stroke were similar between patients with and without early leaflet thrombosis at a mean follow-up of 1.8 years post-TAVR (0% vs 0.6%, P = .57; 0% vs 0.7%, P = .52, respectively). Overall, the association between HALT and stroke is still unclear.

Atrial fibrillation is common in patients undergoing TAVR and represents a major risk factor for acute, subacute, and late post-TAVR stroke.[43,44] Reported incidences of stroke among atrial fibrillation patients after TAVR range from 3% to 12% in the first year after TAVR, with a quarter of the strokes occurring within the first 24 hours and half within 30 days.[45,46] Guidelines recommend vitamin K antagonist with or without antiplatelet therapy for 3 to 6 months after TAVR in patients with indication for anticoagulation, with the antiplatelet intended to prevent thromboembolism before valve endothelialization.

In the POPular TAVI trial, cohort B, which looked at patients with an already-established indication for long-term anticoagulation, the addition of 3 months of clopidogrel to oral anticoagulation (either vitamin K antagonist or direct-acting oral anticoagulant) increased bleeding (34.6% vs 21.7% for all bleeding; 16.7% vs 8.9% for major, life-threatening, or disabling bleeding) without reducing stroke (5.8% vs 5.1% for ischemic stroke).[47] The Kaplan-Meier curves for bleeding separate almost immediately after TAVR and continue to separate out to 90 days when clopidogrel was discontinued, with most of the bleeding occurring within 1 week of TAVR.

The GALILEO trial, involving patients without an established indication for oral anticoagulation after TAVR, showed that rivaroxaban 10 mg daily with aspirin was associated with more bleeding and more death or thromboembolic complications than aspirin with clopidogrel.[48] Another analysis found that for patients with hemorrhagic late strokes (>30 days postprocedure), the use of anticoagulation was more common than antiplatelet therapy (48.3% vs 27.2%).[49]

The aforementioned studies raise an important question: how do we adequately mitigate the potential of late strokes in patients who have undergone TAVR without putting them at increased risk for bleeding? The ongoing prospective WATCH-TAVR randomized controlled trial aims to address this dilemma by investigating the safety and effectiveness of left atrial appendage occlusion with the WATCHMAN device in prevention of stroke and bleeding in patients with atrial fibrillation undergoing TAVR. It is tentatively scheduled for completion in November 2022.

In patients *without* an indication for long-term anticoagulation, practice guidelines recommend clopidogrel in addition to aspirin for the first 3 to 6 months after TAVR, for the purpose of mitigating the stent-mediated risk of thromboembolization before the valve has endothelialized. This intensified dual antiplatelet regimen has been shown in several series to result in major or life-threatening bleeding in up to 15% of patients 1 year after TAVR.[2,3,11] TAVR patients are particularly prone to bleeding, as they tend to be older with comorbidities that predispose to bleeding, such as gastrointestinal angiodysplasia, and with postprocedure conditions, such as transient thrombocytopenia, that further augment this risk. Balancing stroke prevention related to the transcatheter prosthesis and the patient's inherent stroke risk factors, with the bleeding tendencies that many TAVR patients possess, is a prominent focus of research.

Prospective studies, such as the ARTE trial, showed a lower incidence of bleeding with aspirin than with aspirin plus clopidogrel at 3 months.[50] In cohort A of POPular, a comparison of aspirin with clopidogrel to aspirin alone, for 3 months after TAVR, revealed that bleeding was significantly higher (26.6% vs 15.1% for all bleeding; 10.8% vs 5.1% for major, life-threatening, or disabling bleeding), without a benefit in ischemic outcomes (5.4 vs 5.1% for ischemic stroke; 9.9 vs 9.7% for composite of cardiovascular death, ischemic stroke, or myocardial infarction), for the patients with a dual antiplatelet regimen.[51] The quality of these pieces of data may call for a revision of post-TAVR guideline recommendations.

SUMMARY

Stroke remains an issue for the TAVR procedure. TAVR-related strokes are devastating to patients and their families, and very costly for health care systems. With the growth of TAVR volumes and the expansion of TAVR indications to lower-risk, younger, and often less symptomatic patients, the mission to bring TAVR stroke rates down is even more important. The predictors of stroke in TAVR are not yet well defined, although older age and female gender, carotid and peripheral arterial disease, bicuspid aortic valve anatomy, and atrial fibrillation are emerging as risk factors across studies; the detection and appropriate and prompt treatment of preexisting or newly diagnosed atrial fibrillation represent a central objective in the mitigation of stroke risk. For acute stroke, there is an evolving body of evidence suggesting cerebral embolic protection may mitigate the risk; more randomized controlled data are forthcoming. For subacute and late stroke, treating the intrinsic stroke-predisposing milieu of patient and transcatheter prosthesis requires careful individualized pharmacologic and nonpharmacologic therapy, balancing risk of stroke with that of bleeding.

CLINICS CARE POINTS

- When counseling patients on risks and benefits of TAVR, it is important to explain that TAVR has a proven excellent safety and efficacy profile, but that there is still a roughly 2% risk of clinically significant stroke.

- Patients should know that improving stroke rates is a priority among those performing and developing TAVR. Stroke prevention strategies currently being utilized and studied include devices placed during the TAVR procedure into or near the arteries that supply the brain, blood thinning medications, early diagnosis and treatment of atrial fibrillation, and further improved operator experience and TAVR device technology.

DISCLOSURE

Dr T.M. Frisoli is a physician proctor for Edwards Lifescience, Boston Scientific, and Medtronic.

REFERENCES

1. Carroll JD, Mack MJ, Vemulapalli S, et al. STS-ACC TVT registry of transcatheter aortic valve replacement. J Am Coll Cardiol 2020;76:2492–516.
2. Mack MJ, Leon MB, Thourani VH, et al, PARTNER 3 Investigators. Transcatheter aortic-valve replacement with a balloon-expandable valve in low-risk patients. N Engl J Med 2019;380(18):1695–705.
3. Leon MB, Smith CR, Mack MJ, et al, PARTNER 2 Investigators. Transcatheter or surgical aortic-valve replacement in intermediate-risk patients. N Engl J Med 2016;374(17):1609–20.
4. Mack MJ, Leon MB, Smith CR, et al. 5-year outcomes of transcatheter aortic valve replacement or surgical aortic valve replacement for high surgical risk patients with aortic stenosis (PARTNER 1): a randomised controlled trial. The Lancet 2015;385:2477–84.
5. Leon MB, Smith CR, Mack M, et al. Transcatheter aortic-valve implantation for aortic stenosis in patients who cannot undergo surgery. N Engl J Med 2010;363:1597–607.
6. Holmes DR Jr, Mack MJ, Kaul S, et al. 2012 ACCF/AATS/SCAI/STS expert consensus document on transcatheter aortic valve replacement. J Am Coll Cardiol 2012;59(13):1200–54.
7. Vlastra W, Jimenez-Quevedo P, Tchétché D, et al. Predictors, incidence, and outcomes of patients undergoing transfemoral transcatheter aortic valve implantation complicated by stroke. Circ Cardiovasc Interv 2019;12(3):e007546.
8. Huded CP, Tuzcu EM, Krishnaswamy A, et al. Association between transcatheter aortic valve replacement and early postprocedural stroke. JAMA 2019;321(23):2306–15.
9. Carroll JD, Vemulapalli S, Dai D, et al. Procedural experience for transcatheter aortic valve replacement and relation to outcomes: the STS/ACC TVT registry. J Am Coll Cardiol 2017;70(1):29–41.
10. Van Mieghem NM, van Gils L, Ahmad H, et al. Filter-based cerebral embolic protection with transcatheter aortic valve implantation: the randomised MISTRAL-C trial. EuroIntervention 2016;12(4):499–507.
11. Popma JJ, Deeb GM, Yakubov SJ, et al, Evolut Low Risk Trial Investigators. Transcatheter aortic-valve replacement with a self-expanding valve in low-risk patients. N Engl J Med 2019;380(18):1706–15.
12. Haussig S, Mangner N, Dwyer MG, et al. Effect of a cerebral protection device on brain lesions following transcatheter aortic valve implantation in patients with severe aortic stenosis: the CLEAN-TAVI randomized clinical trial. JAMA 2016;316(6):592–601.
13. Lansky AJ, Schofer J, Tchetche D, et al. A prospective randomized evaluation of the TriGuard™ HDH embolic DEFLECTion device during transcatheter aortic valve implantation: results from the DEFLECT III trial. Eur Heart J 2015;36(31):2070–8.
14. Kapadia SR, Kodali S, Makkar R, et al, SENTINEL Trial Investigators. Protection against cerebral embolism during transcatheter aortic valve replacement. J Am Coll Cardiol 2017;69(4):367–77.
15. Kapadia S, Agarwal S, Miller DC, et al. Insights into timing, risk factors, and outcomes of stroke and transient ischemic attack after transcatheter aortic valve replacement in the PARTNER trial (Placement

of Aortic Transcatheter Valves). Circ Cardiovasc Interv 2016;9(9):e002981.

16. Nombela-Franco L, Webb JG, de Jaegere PP, et al. Timing, predictive factors, and prognostic value of cerebrovascular events in a large cohort of patients undergoing transcatheter aortic valve implantation. Circulation 2012;126(25):3041–53.

17. Tchetche D, Farah B, Misuraca L, et al. Cerebrovascular events post-transcatheter aortic valve replacement in a large cohort of patients: a FRANCE-2 registry substudy. JACC Cardiovasc Interv 2014; 7(10):1138–45.

18. Miller DC, Blackstone EH, Mack MJ, et al, PARTNER Trial Investigators and Patients; PARTNER Stroke Substudy Writing Group and Executive Committee. Transcatheter (TAVR) versus surgical (AVR) aortic valve replacement: occurrence, hazard, risk factors, and consequences of neurologic events in the PARTNER trial. J Thorac Cardiovasc Surg 2012;143(4):832–43.e13.

19. Auffret V, Regueiro A, Del Trigo M, et al. Predictors of early cerebrovascular events in patients with aortic stenosis undergoing transcatheter aortic valve replacement. J Am Coll Cardiol 2016;68(7): 673–84.

20. Megaly M, Sorajja P, Cavalcante J, et al. Ischemic stroke with cerebral protection system during transcatheter aortic valve replacement. JACC Cardiovasc Interv 2020;13(18):2149–55.

21. Faroux L, Junquera L, Mohammadi S, et al. Femoral vs nonfemoral subclavian/carotid arterial access route for transcatheter aortic valve replacement: a systematic review and meta-analysis. J Am Heart Assoc 2020;9:e017460.

22. Takagi K, Naganuma T, Tada N, et al. The predictors of peri-procedural and sub-acute cerebrovascular events following TAVR from OCEAN-TAVI registry. Cardiovasc Revasc Med 2020;21(6):732–8.

23. Doerner J, Kupczyk PA, Wilsing M, et al. Cerebral white matter lesion burden is associated with the degree of aortic valve calcification and predicts peri-procedural cerebrovascular events in patients undergoing transcatheter aortic valve implantation (TAVI). Catheter Cardiovasc Interv 2018;91(4):774–82.

24. Athappan G, Gajulapalli RD, Sengodan P, et al. Influence of transcatheter aortic valve replacement strategy and valve design on stroke after transcatheter aortic valve replacement: a meta-analysis and systematic review of literature. J Am Coll Cardiol 2014;63(20):2101–10.

25. Thomas M, Schymik G, Walther T, et al. Thirty-day results of the SAPIEN aortic Bioprosthesis European Outcome (SOURCE) Registry: a European registry of transcatheter aortic valve implantation using the Edwards SAPIEN valve. Circulation 2010;122(1):62–9.

26. Rodés-Cabau J, Dumont E, Boone RH, et al. Cerebral embolism following transcatheter aortic valve implantation: comparison of transfemoral and transapical approaches. J Am Coll Cardiol 2011; 57(1):18–28.

27. Muralidharan A, Thiagarajan K, Van Ham R, et al. Meta-analysis of perioperative stroke and mortality in transcatheter aortic valve implantation. Am J Cardiol 2016;118(7):1031–45.

28. Vlastra W, Chandrasekhar J, Vendrik J, et al. Transfemoral TAVR in nonagenarians: from the CENTER collaboration. JACC Cardiovasc Interv 2019;12(10): 911–20.

29. Hassell ME, Nijveldt R, Roos YB, et al. Silent cerebral infarcts associated with cardiac disease and procedures. Nat Rev Cardiol 2013;10(12):696–706.

30. Vermeer SE, Prins ND, den Heijer T, et al. Silent brain infarcts and the risk of dementia and cognitive decline. N Engl J Med 2003;348(13):1215–22.

31. Daniel K, Wolfe CD, Busch MA, et al. What are the social consequences of stroke for working-aged adults? A systematic review. Stroke 2009;40(6):e431–40.

32. Dhamoon MS, Longstreth WT, Bartz TM, et al. Disability trajectories before and after stroke and myocardial infarction. JAMA Neurol 2017;74(12): 1439–45.

33. Arnold SV, Lei Y, Reynolds MR, et al. Costs of peri-procedural complications in patients treated with transcatheter aortic valve replacement: results from the Placement of Aortic Transcatheter Valve trial. Circ Cardiovasc Interv 2014;7(6):829–36.

34. Alqahtani F, Sengupta PP, Badhwar V, et al. Clinical and economic burden of acute ischemic stroke following transcatheter aortic valve replacement. Struct Heart 2018;3(1):72–3.

35. Seeger J, Gonska B, Otto M, et al. Cerebral embolic protection during transcatheter aortic valve replacement significantly reduces death and stroke compared with unprotected procedures. JACC Cardiovasc Interv 2017;10(22):2297–303.

36. Makkar RR, Thourani VH, Mack MJ, et al, PARTNER 2 Investigators. Five-year outcomes of transcatheter or surgical aortic-valve replacement. N Engl J Med 2020;382(9):799–809.

37. Seeger J, Kapadia SR, Kodali S, et al. Rate of peri-procedural stroke observed with cerebral embolic protection during transcatheter aortic valve replacement: a patient-level propensity-matched analysis. Eur Heart J 2019;40(17):1334–40.

38. Presented by Dr. Jeffrey W. Moses at the Transcatheter Cardiovascular Therapeutics Virtual Meeting (TCT Connect), October 14-18, 2020.

39. Stachon P, Kaier K, Heidt T, et al. The use and outcomes of cerebral protection devices for patients undergoing transfemoral transcatheter aortic valve replacement in clinical practice. JACC Cardiovasc Interv 2021;14(2):161–8.

40. Makkar RR, Blanke P, Leipsic J, et al. Subclinical leaflet thrombosis in transcatheter and surgical bioprosthetic valves: PARTNER 3 cardiac computed tomography substudy. J Am Coll Cardiol 2020; 75(24):3003–15.

41. Chakravarty T, Søndergaard L, Friedman J, et al, RESOLVE, SAVORY Investigators. Subclinical leaflet thrombosis in surgical and transcatheter bioprosthetic aortic valves: an observational study. Lancet 2017;389(10087):2383–92.

42. Yanagisawa R, Tanaka M, Yashima F, et al. Early and late leaflet thrombosis after transcatheter aortic valve replacement. Circ Cardiovasc Interv 2019;12(2):e007349.

43. Kirchhof P, Benussi S, Kotecha D, et al, ESC Scientific Document Group. 2016 ESC guidelines for the management of atrial fibrillation developed in collaboration with EACTS. Eur Heart J 2016; 37(38):2893–962.

44. January CT, Wann LS, Calkins H, et al. 2019 AHA/ACC/HRS Focused Update of the 2014 AHA/ACC/HRS guideline for the management of patients with atrial fibrillation: a report of the American College of Cardiology/American Heart Association Task Force on Clinical Practice Guidelines and the Heart Rhythm Society in collaboration with the Society of Thoracic Surgeons. Circulation 2019;140(2):e125–51.

45. Abdul-Jawad Altisent O, Durand E, Muñoz-García AJ, et al. Warfarin and antiplatelet therapy versus warfarin alone for treating patients with atrial fibrillation undergoing transcatheter aortic valve replacement. JACC Cardiovasc Interv 2016;9(16): 1706–17.

46. Jochheim D, Zadrozny M, Ricard I, et al. Predictors of cerebrovascular events at mid-term after transcatheter aortic valve implantation - results from EVERY-TAVI registry. Int J Cardiol 2017;244: 106–11.

47. Nijenhuis VJ, Brouwer J, Delewi R, et al. Anticoagulation with or without clopidogrel after transcatheter aortic-valve implantation. N Engl J Med 2020;382(18):1696–707.

48. Dangas GD, Tijssen JGP, Wöhrle J, et al, GALILEO Investigators. A controlled trial of rivaroxaban after transcatheter aortic-valve replacement. N Engl J Med 2020;382(2):120–9.

49. Muntané-Carol G, Urena M, Munoz-Garcia A, et al. Late cerebrovascular events following transcatheter aortic valve replacement. JACC Cardiovasc Interv 2020;13(7):872–81.

50. Rodés-Cabau J, Masson JB, Welsh RC, et al. Aspirin versus aspirin plus clopidogrel as antithrombotic treatment following transcatheter aortic valve replacement with a balloon-expandable valve: the ARTE (Aspirin Versus Aspirin + Clopidogrel Following Transcatheter Aortic Valve Implantation) randomized clinical trial. JACC Cardiovasc Interv 2017;10(13):1357–65.

51. Brouwer J, Nijenhuis VJ, Delewi R, et al. Aspirin with or without clopidogrel after transcatheter aortic-valve implantation. N Engl J Med 2020; 383(15):1447–57.

Early Leaflet Thickening, Durability and Bioprosthetic Valve Failure in TAVR

Brian C. Case, MD[a], Jaffar M. Khan, BM BCh, PhD[b,*],
Toby Rogers, MD, PhD[a,b]

KEYWORDS

- Transcatheter aortic valve replacement • Leaflet thickening • Durability
- Bioprosthetic valve failure • Structural valve degeneration

---

KEY POINTS

- Heterogeneity in definitions, and follow-up, of studies evaluating the durability of SAVR.
- Leaflet thickening present in THV; however, further studies are needed to determine whether THV leaflet thickening affects hemodynamic status, durability, and rate of clinical thromboembolic events.
- New standardized definitions of structural valve deterioration allow for future studies to adequately evaluate TAVR durability.
- Coronary access, valve-in-valve procedures, and lifetime management strategy for younger patients still need to be determined.

INTRODUCTION

Historically, surgical aortic valve replacement (SAVR) was the standard of care for the treatment of symptomatic patients with severe aortic stenosis (AS). However, over the last decade, transcatheter aortic valve replacement (TAVR) has become the established alternative to surgery for the treatment of patients with symptomatic, severe AS. Large, multicenter trials have shown the noninferiority, and even superiority, of TAVR to SAVR in high-risk surgical patients[1,2] and intermediate-risk surgical patients.[3,4]

In 2019, the Food and Drug Administration (FDA) approved TAVR for patients with a low surgical risk after multiple large multicenter trials established the role of TAVR for the treatment of low-risk patients with severe AS.[5–7] As younger patients, with a typical life expectancy of more than 10 years, receive TAVR they will most likely outlive their bioprosthetic valve. Indeed, all bioprosthetic valves, both surgical and transcatheter, have a finite lifespan before their leaflets inevitably degenerate, leading to stenosis or regurgitation. The unresolved question of TAVR valves is the long-term valve durability. The paucity of data regarding the durability of transcatheter heart valves (THVs) is often underscored as a weakness of TAVR, but the data for surgical bioprosthesis durability are also poor in

---

Funding: None.

Relationships with Industry: J.M. Khan and T. Rogers—proctor for Edwards and Medtronic. J.M. Khan and T. Rogers—inventors on patents, assigned to the NIH, on devices for transcatheter leaflet laceration. T. Rogers—advisory board: Medtronic. Equity interest: Transmural Systems. All other authors—None.
[a] Section of Interventional Cardiology, MedStar Washington Hospital Center, 110 Irving Street NW, Washington, DC 20010, USA; [b] Cardiovascular Branch, Division of Intramural Research, National Heart, Lung and Blood Institute, National Institutes of Health, 9000 Rockville Pike, Bethesda, MD 20892, USA
* Corresponding author.
E-mail address: Jaffar.Khan@nih.gov

2211-7458/21/© 2021 Elsevier Inc. All rights reserved.

quality. This review will discuss early leaflet thickening, valve durability, and bioprosthetic valve failure (BVF) in TAVR patients.

SURGICAL VALVE DURABILITY

Historically, surgery has been the standard of care for the treatment of severe AS. Given the fact that they have been around for longer, there is a larger number of studies reporting data on surgical aortic valve durability. However, there is a lot of variability in the study methodologies and definitions as well as inadequate follow-up. The heterogeneity of these studies makes the interpretation of the data challenging.

Largely, structural valve degeneration (SVD) in SAVR studies has been defined as valve reintervention with redo surgery, with SVD rates of 2% to 10% at 10 years and 10% to 20% at 15 years. However, this only accounts for valve failure that proceeds to redo surgery and does not account for patients who die or suffer from SVD treated medically. This leads to a substantial underestimate of the incidence of valve deterioration, hemodynamic compromise, and overall valve failure. This underestimation has been validated by studies in which SVD definitions include hemodynamics assessed by echocardiography, and which reported significantly higher SVD rates of 10% at 5 years and 30% at 10 years post-SAVR.[8]

A recent systematic review of preexisting literature on the actuarial freedom from SVD in SAVR patients and outcomes of SVD, yielding 167 studies and 12 FDA reports.[9] Authors found that 11 different definitions of SVD were used and only 11 studies used a core laboratory to collect data. Furthermore, mean follow-up ranged from less than 1 year all the way to 14 years with only 0% to 37% of patients remaining at risk at maximum follow-up. Thus, there is substantial variability in reporting SVD for surgical valves, with different definitions and inadequate long-term systematically collected core laboratory data. Rigorously collected long-term data with standardized definitions for surgical valves are needed to provide a benchmark for the durability of rapidly evolving transcatheter valves.

LEAFLET THICKENING

Leaflet thrombosis has been observed with both surgical and transcatheter bioprostheses. Symptomatic obstructive valve thrombosis results in an increase in the transvalvular gradient and reduction in the effective orifice area of the valve. However, overall, this event is rare in TAVR patients, with a rate of about 0.5%. Furthermore, there is a signal for a slightly higher rate of leaflet thrombosis in annular valves as compared with supra-annular valves. However, this needs to be further validated in larger, prospective studies.[10]

In contrast, subclinical thrombosis—meaning asymptomatic—causes thickening and reduced leaflet motion of the bioprosthetic valve. This finding could be missed on echocardiography as the transvalvular gradients often remain within the normal range. Commonly, this finding is only detected on computed tomography (CT) scan, which is not routinely performed outside of clinical trials. Early leaflet thickening (30 days) is found to be more frequent in THVs, as compared with surgical valves, with an estimated incidence rate of 5% to 40% of patients.[11] It is thought to be more frequent in THVs given the incomplete expansion of the THV in an oval aortic annulus and also the metallic nature of the struts.[12] That being said, there is no clear signal yet that leaflet thickening is associated with excess cerebrovascular accidents or premature structural valve deterioration. Recently, several clinical trials have attempted to address these questions further.

The LRT (Low-Risk TAVR) trial was an investigator-initiated, prospective, multicenter study, and was the first FDA-approved Investigational Device Exemption trial to evaluate the feasibility of TAVR in low-risk patients. In the LRT trial, leaflet thickening was a secondary endpoint. Subjects in the LRT trial underwent follow-up time-resolved contrast-enhanced cardiac CT at 30 days. Hypoattenuated leaflet thickening (HALT) was observed in 14.0% of subjects (n = 27 or 193) with an evaluable CT or transesophageal echocardiography at 30 days. This rate is similar to other studies in low-risk TAVR patients, for example, the PARTNER 3 trial (13%)[6] and the Evolut Low-Risk Trial (17.3%).[7] Additional, larger trials including the SAVORY (Subclinical Aortic Valve Bioprosthesis Thrombosis Assessed With Four-Dimensional Computed Tomography) and RESOLVE (Assessment of Transcatheter and Surgical Aortic Bioprosthetic Valve Thrombosis and Its Treatment With Anticoagulation) observational registries (13%)[13] showed similar rates in all surgical risk cohorts.

Further analysis in the LRT trial demonstrated that reduced leaflet motion was observed in 11.2% of subjects. Interestingly, in this analysis, HALT was observed in subjects who received balloon-expandable valves only, and not self-expanding valves. Furthermore, at 30 days, mean valve area and dimensionless index were lower in subjects with HALT, with a trend toward higher mean gradients. However, at 1 year, these differences appeared to resolve. Finally, clinically at 1 year, there was a numerically higher rate of stroke in subjects with HALT (3.8% vs 1.9%; P = .53), although the absolute number of events was small in both groups (1 of 27 with HALT vs 4 of 166 with no HALT).[14]

Next, a follow-up LRT Trial was performed, which was an investigator-initiated, prospective, multicenter study, and was the first and only U.S. FDA–approved investigational device exemption trial to evaluate the feasibility of TAVR with either balloon-expandable or self-expanding valves in low-risk patients with bicuspid AS. Baseline and follow-up echocardiography and CT to detect leaflet thickening were analyzed in an independent core laboratory.

At 30 days, 60 of 61 subjects underwent contrast-enhanced CT scans, which were analyzed for subclinical leaflet thrombosis. HALT was present in 6 patients (1 with a self-expanding THV and 5 with balloon-expandable THVs). HALT was observed in 10% of bicuspid TAVR patients at 30 days, which is similar to the previously published tricuspid LRT cohort (14%),[14] the PARTNER 3 trial (13%),[6] and the larger SAVORY (Subclinical Aortic Valve Bioprosthesis Thrombosis Assessed With Four-Dimensional Computed Tomography) and RESOLVE (Assessment of Transcatheter and Surgical Aortic Bioprosthetic Valve Thrombosis and Its Treatment With Anticoagulation) observational registries (13%).[13] Furthermore, the stroke rate in the bicuspid arm of the LRT trial was extremely low (only 1 nondisabling stroke at 30 days), so it was not possible to correlate THV leaflet thrombosis with clinical events.

At the current time, there is no evidence that leaflet thickening results in worsening valve durability. In the tricuspid arm of the LRT trial, patients with HALT had inferior THV hemodynamic status compared with those without HALT at 30 days. Patients with HALT had smaller aortic valve areas and Doppler velocity index (0.4 ± 0.1 vs 0.5 ± 0.1; P = .003) than those without HALT at 30 days. However, hemodynamic differences disappeared at 1 year and clinical outcomes were similar at the 1-year mark.[15] Longer follow-up of larger cohorts with serial echocardiography will be needed to determine whether THV leaflet thrombosis/thickening affects long-term THV hemodynamic status, durability, and rate of late thromboembolic events.

Further information was provided by the pivotal industry-sponsored low-risk TAVR trials

with the balloon-expandable and a self-expanding THVs. First, a substudy of the PARTNER 3 (The Safety and Effectiveness of the SAPEIN 3 Transcatheter Heart Valve in Low-Risk Patients With Aortic Stenosis)[16] enrolled 435 patients with low-surgical-risk AS who received either TAVR (n = 221) or surgery (n = 214) and who underwent serial 4-dimensional CT at 30 days and 1 year. They found that the incidence of HALT increased from 10% at 30 days to 24% at 1 year. Spontaneous resolution of 30-day HALT occurred in 54% of patients at 1 year, whereas new HALT appeared in 21% of patients at 1 year. HALT was more frequent in transcatheter versus surgical valves at 30 days (13% vs 5%; P = .03), but not at 1 year (28% vs 20%; P = .19). The presence of HALT did not significantly affect aortic valve mean gradients at 30 days or 1 year. Furthermore, patients with HALT at both 30 days and 1 year, compared with those with no HALT at 30 days and 1 year, had significantly increased aortic valve gradients at 1 year.

Second, a similar substudy was conducted evaluating patients who received a self-expanding THV in the Evolut Low-Risk trial. In this substudy patients from the Evolut Low-Risk trial who were not on oral anticoagulation underwent computed tomographic imaging at 30 days and 1 year after TAVR (n = 179) or SAVR (n = 139). At 30 days, the frequency of HALT was 17.3% for TAVR and 16.5% for surgery; and at 1 year, the frequency of HALT was 30.9% for TAVR and 28.4% for surgery. Aortic valve hemodynamic status was not influenced by the presence or severity of HALT. They concluded that the presence of computed tomographic imaging abnormalities on aortic bioprostheses was frequent but dynamic in the first year after self-expanding transcatheter and SAVR, but these findings did not correlate with aortic valve hemodynamics after aortic valve replacement in patients at low risk for surgery. Clearly, based on these studies, the impact of HALT on thromboembolic complications and SVD needs further assessment.

Naturally, it would be of interest to identify anatomic features that would place a THV at an increased risk for HALT and subsequent leaflet degeneration. A recent subanalysis of the LRT trial tried to determine anatomic characteristics associated with HALT, which may contribute to early THV degeneration.[17] The authors found that in patients who developed HALT, THV implantation depth was shallower than in patients who did not develop HALT. In addition, there were more patients in the HALT group with commissural malalignment, but this did not reach statistical significance. Furthermore, in a univariable regression model, no predetermined variables were shown to independently predict the development of HALT. Future, larger, prospective trials are needed to potentially identify anatomic risks associated with HALT.[17]

LEAFLET DEGENERATION

Just as with native aortic valve, bioprosthetic leaflet degeneration occurs when leaflet calcification develops and results in either valve stenosis, regurgitation, or both.[12] There are three components specific to a THV, as compared to a SAVR, which may impact early leaflet degeneration. First, when loading/crimping the THV into the delivery catheter, there is potential for trauma to the bioprosthetic leaflets. Second, after the THV is deployed, noncircular expansion could affect normal valvular functioning. Noncircularity may occur due to excessive native aortic leaflet calcification, ellipticity of the left ventricular outflow tract, and prosthetic valve oversizing. This is more commonly seen with self-expanding THVs, although the supra-annular position of the leaflets in the Evolut valve may mitigate the impact of noncircularity at the annulus. Finally, the presence of turbulence in the aortic root due to the combined presence of bulky calcium nodules in the sinuses of Valsalva and presence of the THV, which could potentially affect blood flow patterns, resulting in chronic mechanical stresses on the bioprosthetic leaflets, and in turn leading to early degeneration. A recent systematic review and meta-analysis identified younger age, patient-prosthesis mismatch, body surface area, and smoking as risk factors for SVD.[18]

VALVE DURABILITY

Failure modes of bioprosthetic aortic valves may be different for TAVR versus SAVR. When an SAVR valve fails, the etiology is usually due to a leaflet tear (leading to valve incompetence), calcification (leading to valve restenosis), or pannus formation. When a TAVR valve fails, the etiology could be from leaflet tear or calcification, but it could also be due to valve dislocation (albeit very rare) or worsening paravalvular leak.[19] Historically, the lack of standard definitions of SVD has made it difficult to analyze studies on the durability of both surgical and transcatheter bioprostheses.

However, since 2017, the European Association of Percutaneous Cardiovascular Interventions (EAPCI), endorsed by the European Society of Cardiology (ESC) and the European Association for Cardio-Thoracic Surgery (EACTS), proposed a consensus definition, applicable to both transcatheter and surgically implanted bioprosthetic valves. When describing the mechanism of valve failure, the etiology can be separated into 2 broad categories—(1) structural valve deterioration and (2) non-structural valve deterioration.[20]

SVD is the most common type of bioprosthetic valve dysfunction.[21] It is characterized by permanent intrinsic changes to the valve. Examples of structural valve deterioration include leaflet calcification, leaflet tear, valve seam disruption, and stent fracture. These abnormalities result from both patient-related factors and prothesis-related factors. The patient-related factors include dyslipidemia, diabetes, hypertension, metabolic syndrome, phosphocalcic dysregulation, and/or a component of an immune reaction. The prosthesis-related factors include absence of antimineralization treatment, flaws in the bioprosthesis design, severe prosthesis-patient mismatch, and/or small prosthesis size. These two factors lead to a spectrum of increased leaflet mechanical stress all the way to abnormal valvular flow leading to SVD.

Examples of nonstructural valve deterioration include leaflet thrombosis, endocarditis, and paravalvular leakage. These abnormalities tend to happen from TAVR specific factors including leaflet injury (due to crimping, loading, dilatation), abnormal trans-and/or-paravalvular flow patterns, and/or noncircular, irregular, incomplete stent deployment[8,22] (Fig. 1).

Once either SVD or nonstructural valve dysfunction is present, the next step in the cascade is hemodynamic valve deterioration. The ESC/EACTS created standardized definitions for this as well. Morphologic SVD needs at least multidetector CT to be diagnosed, whereas the diagnosis of hemodynamics is based on echocardiography or invasive hemodynamics. They define moderate hemodynamic valve deterioration is defined as a mean transprosthetic gradient ≥ 20 to < 40 mm Hg or ≥ 10 to 20 mm Hg change from baseline. Alternatively, moderate intraprosthetic aortic regurgitation, new or worsening ($> 1+/4+$) from baseline.[20] After this, the patient then develops severe hemodynamic valve deterioration and BVF. Severe hemodynamic valve deterioration is defined as a mean transprosthetic gradient ≥ 40 mm Hg or ≥ 20 mm Hg change from baseline or severe intraprosthetic aortic regurgitation. Alternatively, it can be defined by autopsy with findings likely related to the case of death,

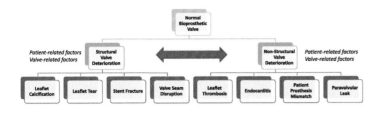

Fig. 1. Mechanisms of bio-prosthetic valve dysfunction.

valve-related death, or repeat intervention.[20] BVF is used when there are clinical symptoms and signs of bioprosthetic valve deterioration. Furthermore, ESC/EACTS define BVF as a patient-oriented composite outcome of death (confirmed by autopsy or by clinical diagnosis of bioprosthetic valve dysfunction before death), repeated intervention (including valve-in-valve TAVR, paravalvular leak closure or surgery), or severe hemodynamic structural valve deterioration (Fig. 2). In addition, it can be defined as early (≤30 days) or late (>30 days) after valve replacement.

Using the ESC/EACTS definitions, studies have demonstrated that the durability of THV is up to 7 and 8 years.[23–25] Previous analysis looked at clinical trials to try to assess long-term durability of TAVR. They concluded that the weighted incidence of SVD at 5 to 8 years was 1.3% (95% CI 0.7–1.9) and the weighted incidence of BVF at 6 to 8 years was 3.7% (95% CI 2.7–4.6).[26] An additional study looked at the 8-year durability of 990 patients treated with a self-expanding TAVR between 2007 and 2011 in Italy.[27] In this analysis, 78% of patients were alive at 8 years and the rate of moderate SVD was 3.0%, severe SVD was 1.6%, and BVF was seen in 2.5% of patients.[27] An additional trial, the UK TAVI Trial showed excellent long-term THV function. Between 5 and 10 years after implantation, 91% remained free of SVD with only 0.4% cases of severe SVD at 5.3 years after implantation and 8.7% cases of moderate SVD.[28] Finally, 2.4% patients demonstrated moderate to severe valve durability and 4.51% with BVF at 8 years in the local Italian REPLACE registry.[29] However, the main limitation of these earlier

trials is that most of the studies to date have had a high rate of mortality at 5 years in the high and extreme risk patients treated with TAVR. This is due to the consequence of the advanced age and comorbidities of the high-risk population being treated, and not necessarily valve failure itself.

The NOTION trial provides data on bioprosthetic valve durability from a randomized clinical trial in patients at low surgical risk of mortality. At 6 years, all-comers (TAVR and surgical) showed that the rate of SVD was higher with SAVR than TAVR (24.0% vs 4.8%; P<.001), with similar rates of all-cause mortality (42.5% for TAVR vs 37.7% for SAVR, P = .58) and no differences in terms of non-SVD (57.8% vs 54.0%, P = .52) and endocarditis (5.9% vs 5.8%, P = .95). Furthermore, TAVR and SAVR patients experienced a similar degree of BVF through 6 years (7.5% vs 6.7%; P = .89).[30] A summary of these trials is outlined in Figs. 3–5.

Lastly, in 2020, a PARTNER 2A substudy trial sought out to determine and compare the 5-year incidence of SVD, using the standardized definitions, in intermediate-risk patients with severe AS given annular TAVR (Second Generation SAPIEN-XT or Third Generation SAPIEN 3) or SAVR. The investigators found that compared with SAVR, the SAPIEN-XT TAVR cohort had a significantly higher 5-year exposure adjusted incidence rates (per 100 patient-years) of SVD (1.61 ± 0.24% vs 0.63 ± 0.16%), SVD-related BVF (0.58 ± 0.14% vs 0.12 ± 0.07%), and all-cause (structural or nonstructural) BVF (0.81 ± 0.16% vs 0.27 ± 0.10%) (P≤.01 for all). Alternatively, the 5-year rates of SVD (0.68 ± 0.18% vs 0.60 ± 0.17%; P = .71), SVD-related BVF (0.29 ± 0.12% vs

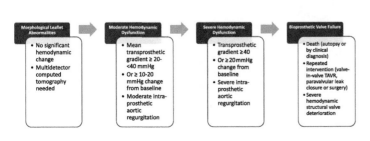

Fig. 2. European Society of Cardiology/European Association for Cardio-Thoracic Surgery Definition of Hemodynamic Valve Deterioration.

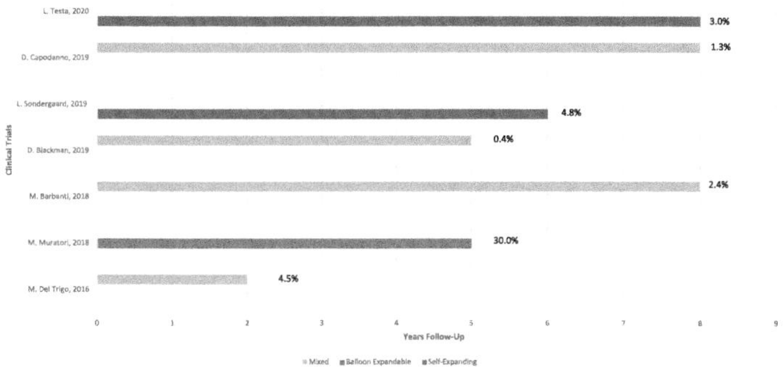

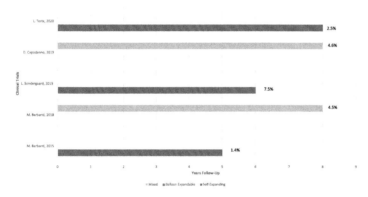

Fig. 3. Incidence of structural valve deterioration.

Fig. 4. Incidence of bioprosthetic valve failure.

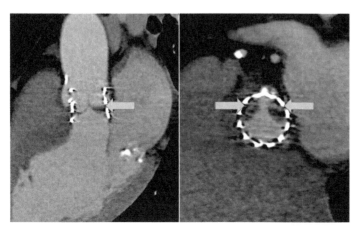

Fig. 5. Computed tomography imaging of bioprosthetic valve thickening.

0.14 ± 0.08%; *P* = .25), and all-cause BVF (0.60 ± 0.15% vs 0.32 ± 0.11%; *P* = .32) in SAPIEN 3 TAVR were not significantly different to a propensity score-matched SAVR cohort. Finally, when comparing the 5-year rates of SVD and SVD-related BVF were significantly lower in SAPIEN 3 (third generation) versus SAPIEN XT (second generation) TAVR matched cohorts. Their finding highlights that SVD rates may be higher in TAVR patients, but advancements in valve design have decreased the overall risk.[31]

CORONARY ACCESS

When discussing valve durability, and eventual valve failure, the issue of coronary access after the deployment of the valve is important. The incidence of coronary artery disease, and associated acute coronary syndrome, is common with patients receiving TAVR for AS, given the fact that these patients share common comorbidities. Given the structure of the THV, coronary access with a guide catheter to perform a percutaneous coronary intervention can be more challenging. For example, in low-risk patients who received a balloon-expandable THVs, the most challenging anatomy for coronary access (THV frame above and commissural suture post in front of a coronary ostium) was observed in 9% to 13% of subjects.[32] Furthermore, in low-risk patients who received a self-expanding THVs, CT simulation predicted sinus of Valsalva sequestration and resultant coronary obstruction during future TAVR-in-TAVR in up to 23% of patients. In addition, CT simulation predicted that the position of the pinned THV leaflets would hinder future coronary access in up to 78% of patients after TAVR-in-TAVR.[33]

VALVE-IN-VALVE

When bioprosthetic valve degeneration does occur, repeat intervention is needed. The patients' two options are SAVR or valve-in-valve (ViV) TAVR procedure. ViV procedures have demonstrated encouraging results in both patients with degenerated surgical aortic bioprostheses[34] and TAVR.[35] However, when TAV-in-TAV procedure is performed, the issue of coronary access becomes more problematic. In ViV TAVR procedures where a self-expanding THV is used, a recent study using CT simulation predicted that the position of the pinned THV leaflets would hinder future coronary access in up to 78% of patients.[33]

YOUNGER PATIENTS

Among patients in whom a bioprosthesis is appropriate, there are certain scenarios when SAVR is preferred over TAVR. The recent 2020 ACC/AHA Guidelines for the Management of Patients with Valvular Heart Disease: A Report of the American College of Cardiology/American Heart Association Joint Committee on Clinical Practice guidelines provides guidance on these patients.[36] They still recommend SAVR as the preferred treatment among patients younger than 65 years or with a life expectancy more than 20 years. SAVR or TAVR is recommended after shared decision-making among symptomatic patients ages 65 to 80 years with no other contraindications. These recommendations appear to be based on studies comparing the long-term mortality benefit of patients who underwent aortic valve replacement or mitral valve replacement with a mechanical or biologic prosthesis (surgical or transcatheter). They found that there was a long-term mortality benefit that was associated with a mechanical prosthesis, as compared with a biologic prosthesis, and this persisted until 70 years of age among patients undergoing mitral valve replacement and until 55 years of age among those undergoing aortic valve replacement. In addition, the incidence of reoperation was significantly higher among recipients of a biologic prosthesis than among recipients of a mechanical prosthesis. Alternatively, patients who received mechanical valves had a higher cumulative incidence of bleeding and, in some age groups, stroke than did recipients of a biologic prosthesis.[37]

It is important to note as well, anecdotally, that many patients do not want a mechanical valve, and commitment to anticoagulation, even if they are younger. It is important to have a shared decision with your patient to determine the management that is best for them. In addition, it is always a class I indication for all cases to be reviewed by a Heart Team to determine the aortic intervention. These age recommendations may change if we can better define the durability of both SAVR and TAVR in the future.

SUMMARY

Moving forward, establishing valve durability in larger cohorts and determining the relative freedom from structural valve deterioration of different valve designs is needed as TAVR is increasingly offered to and requested by younger patients with longer life expectancy. Ensuring adequate coronary access, especially following TAV-in-TAV, is imperative as more younger patients receive TAVR.

CLINICS CARE POINTS

- Large, multicenter trials have shown the non-inferiority, and even superiority, of TAVR to SAVR in high-risk, intermediate and low surgical risk patients.
- Structural valve degeneration in SAVR studies has been defined as valve re-intervention with redo surgery, with rates of 2-10% at 10 years and 10-20% at 15 years. Heterogeneity and underestimation.
- Leaflet thickening, and leaflet degeneration, is seen in both SAVR and TAVR valves.
- Consensus definitions of Structural Valve Deterioration by societies provides standardization and framework for future clinical trials.
- Ensuring adequate coronary access, especially following TAV-in-TAV, is imperative as more younger patients receive TAVR.

REFERENCES

1. Adams DH, Popma JJ, Reardon MJ, et al. Transcatheter aortic-valve replacement with a self-expanding prosthesis. N Engl J Med 2014;370: 1790–8.
2. Smith CR, Leon MB, Mack MJ, et al. Transcatheter versus surgical aortic-valve replacement in high-risk patients. N Engl J Med 2011;364:2187–98.
3. Leon MB, Smith CR, Mack MJ, et al. Transcatheter or surgical aortic-valve replacement in intermediate-risk patients. N Engl J Med 2016;374:1609–20.
4. Reardon MJ, Van Mieghem NM, Popma JJ, et al. Surgical or transcatheter aortic-valve replacement in intermediate-risk patients. N Engl J Med 2017; 376:1321–31.
5. Waksman R, Rogers T, Torguson R, et al. Transcatheter aortic valve replacement in low-risk patients with symptomatic severe aortic stenosis. J Am Coll Cardiol 2018;72:2095–105.
6. Mack MJ, Leon MB, Thourani VH, et al. Transcatheter aortic-valve replacement with a balloon-expandable valve in low-risk patients. N Engl J Med 2019;380:1695–705.
7. Popma JJ, Deeb GM, Yakubov SJ, et al. Transcatheter aortic-valve replacement with a self-expanding valve in low-risk patients. N Engl J Med 2019;380:1706–15.
8. Salaun E, Clavel MA, Rodes-Cabau J, et al. Bioprosthetic aortic valve durability in the era of transcatheter aortic valve implantation. Heart 2018;104: 1323–32.
9. Fatima B, Mohananey D, Khan FW, et al. Durability data for bioprosthetic surgical aortic valve: a systematic review. JAMA Cardiol 2019;4:71–80.
10. Latib A, Naganuma T, Abdel-Wahab M, et al. Treatment and clinical outcomes of transcatheter heart valve thrombosis. Circ Cardiovasc Interv 2015;8(4):e001779.
11. Kanjanauthai S, Pirelli L, Nalluri N, et al. Subclinical leaflet thrombosis following transcatheter aortic valve replacement. J Interv Cardiol 2018; 31:640–7.
12. Mylotte D, Andalib A, Theriault-Lauzier P, et al. Transcatheter heart valve failure: a systematic review. Eur Heart J 2015;36:1306–27.
13. Chakravarty T, Sondergaard L, Friedman J, et al. Subclinical leaflet thrombosis in surgical and transcatheter bioprosthetic aortic valves: an observational study. Lancet 2017;389:2383–92.
14. Waksman R, Corso PJ, Torguson R, et al. TAVR in low-risk patients: 1-year results from the LRT trial. JACC Cardiovasc Interv 2019;12:901–7.
15. Khan JM, Rogers T, Waksman R, et al. Hemodynamics and subclinical leaflet thrombosis in low-risk patients undergoing transcatheter aortic valve replacement. Circ Cardiovasc Imaging 2019;12: e009608.
16. Makkar RR, Blanke P, Leipsic J, et al. Subclinical leaflet thrombosis in transcatheter and surgical bioprosthetic valves: PARTNER 3 cardiac computed tomography substudy. J Am Coll Cardiol 2020;75: 3003–15.
17. Khan JM, Rogers T, Weissman G, et al. Anatomical characteristics associated with hypoattenuated leaflet thickening in low-risk patients undergoing transcatheter aortic valve replacement. Cardiovasc Revasc Med 2021;27:1–6.
18. Ochi A, Cheng K, Zhao B, et al. Patient risk factors for bioprosthetic aortic valve degeneration: a systematic review and meta-analysis. Heart Lung Circ 2020;29:668–78.
19. Arsalan M, Walther T. Durability of prostheses for transcatheter aortic valve implantation. Nat Rev Cardiol 2016;13:360–7.
20. Capodanno D, Petronio AS, Prendergast B, et al. Standardized definitions of structural deterioration and valve failure in assessing long-term durability of transcatheter and surgical aortic bioprosthetic valves: a consensus statement from the European Association of Percutaneous Cardiovascular Interventions (EAPCI) endorsed by the European Society of Cardiology (ESC) and the European Association for Cardio-Thoracic Surgery (EACTS). Eur Heart J 2017;38:3382–90.
21. Johnston DR, Soltesz EG, Vakil N, et al. Long-term durability of bioprosthetic aortic valves: implications from 12,569 implants. Ann Thorac Surg 2015;99:1239–47.

22. Bagur R, Pibarot P, Otto CM. Importance of the valve durability-life expectancy ratio in selection of a prosthetic aortic valve. Heart 2017;103:1756–9.

23. Barbanti M, Petronio AS, Ettori F, et al. 5-year outcomes after transcatheter aortic valve implantation with core valve prosthesis. JACC Cardiovasc Interv 2015;8:1084–91.

24. Muratori M, Fusini L, Tamborini G, et al. Five-year echocardiographic follow-up after TAVI: structural and functional changes of a balloon-expandable prosthetic aortic valve. Eur Heart J Cardiovasc Imaging 2018;19:389–97.

25. Del Trigo M, Munoz-Garcia AJ, Wijeysundera HC, et al. Incidence, timing, and predictors of valve hemodynamic deterioration after transcatheter aortic valve replacement: multicenter registry. J Am Coll Cardiol 2016;67:644–55.

26. Capodanno D, Sondergaard L, Tamburino C. Durability of transcatheter bioprosthetic aortic valves: the story so far. EuroIntervention 2019;15:846–9.

27. Testa L, Latib A, Brambilla N, et al. Long-term clinical outcome and performance of transcatheter aortic valve replacement with a self-expandable bioprosthesis. Eur Heart J 2020;41:1876–86.

28. Blackman DJ, Saraf S, MacCarthy PA, et al. Long-term durability of transcatheter aortic valve prostheses. J Am Coll Cardiol 2019;73:537–45.

29. Barbanti M, Costa G, Zappulla P, et al. Incidence of long-term structural valve dysfunction and bioprosthetic valve failure after transcatheter aortic valve replacement. J Am Heart Assoc 2018;7:e008440.

30. Sondergaard L, Ihlemann N, Capodanno D, et al. Durability of transcatheter and surgical bioprosthetic aortic valves in patients at lower surgical risk. J Am Coll Cardiol 2019;73:546–53.

31. Pibarot P, Ternacle J, Jaber WA, et al. Structural deterioration of transcatheter versus surgical aortic valve bioprostheses in the PARTNER-2 trial. J Am Coll Cardiol 2020;76:1830–43.

32. Rogers T, Greenspun BC, Weissman G, et al. Feasibility of coronary access and aortic valve reintervention in low-risk TAVR patients. JACC Cardiovasc Interv 2020;13:726–35.

33. Forrestal BJ, Case BC, Yerasi C, et al. Risk of coronary obstruction and feasibility of coronary access after repeat transcatheter aortic valve replacement with the self-expanding Evolut valve: a computed tomography simulation study. Circ Cardiovasc Interv 2020;13:e009496.

34. Dvir D, Webb JG, Bleiziffer S, et al. Transcatheter aortic valve implantation in failed bioprosthetic surgical valves. JAMA 2014;312:162–70.

35. Landes U, Webb JG, De Backer O, et al. Repeat transcatheter aortic valve replacement for transcatheter prosthesis dysfunction. J Am Coll Cardiol 2020;75:1882–93.

36. Writing Committee M, Otto CM, Nishimura RA, et al. 2020 ACC/AHA guideline for the management of patients with valvular heart disease: executive summary: a report of the American College of Cardiology/American Heart Association Joint Committee on Clinical Practice Guidelines. J Am Coll Cardiol 2021;77:450–500.

37. Goldstone AB, Chiu P, Baiocchi M, et al. Mechanical or biologic prostheses for aortic-valve and mitral-valve replacement. N Engl J Med 2017;377:1847–57.

Treatment of Bicuspid Aortic Valve Stenosis Using Transcatheter Heart Valves

Pedro Engel Gonzalez, MD[1],
Dharam J. Kumbhani, MD, SM*

KEYWORDS

- Bicuspid aortic valve • Transcatheter aortic valve replacement • Aortic stenosis

---

KEY POINTS

- Bicuspid aortic valve (BAV) anatomy presents unique anatomic challenges for transcatheter aortic valve replacement given the noncircular annulus with asymmetric heavy calcification, as well as a concurrent aortopathy in up to half of these patients.
- The use of new-generation transcatheter heart valves (THV), and the routine use of multidetector row computed tomography, and increased clinical experience have led to better safety outcomes, excellent device success, and promising short-term outcomes in TAVR for BAV aortic stenosis.
- Further dedicated studies are needed to clarify the long-term outcomes and durability of THV in patients with BAV, the effect of concomitant aortopathy, and the role of cerebral embolic protection devices.

INTRODUCTION

The development of transcatheter aortic valve replacement (TAVR) has been a paradigm shift in the treatment of severe symptomatic aortic stenosis (AS). In the last decade, early studies showed a clear benefit with TAVR in prohibitive and high-surgical-risk patients.[1,2] More recently, TAVR use has expanded to patients with AS at lower surgical risks,[3,4] mainly due to advances in the TAVR technology, improvements in procedural technique, and enhanced methods of annular sizing.[5] With the publication of the Placement of Aortic Transcatheter Valves (PARTNER 3) and Evolut Low Risk trials in 2019[6,7] and the US Food and Drug Administration (FDA) approval of TAVR for low-risk patients, the number of low-risk patients with AS treated with TAVR is increasing, and, overall, the annual volume of TAVR has exceeded those of all forms of surgical aortic valve replacement (SAVR) for the first time in 2019.[8]

As we expand TAVR into low-risk patients, a larger proportion of potential TAVR candidates will have bicuspid aortic valve (BAV) anatomy. Approximately 1% to 2% of the general population has a BAV and is most frequently associated with AS.[9] Among the patients with BAV, 37% have moderate-to-severe AS at the time of their initial evaluation with echocardiography.[10] Before the TAVR era, patients with BAV represented approximately 49% of all patients undergoing SAVR and 62% among those aged 50 to 70 years.[11] Randomized controlled clinical trials comparing SAVR with TAVR have excluded patients with BAV; however, they have been included in prospective studies and registries,[12,13] and in 2019, the FDA approved

---

Division of Cardiology, Department of Internal Medicine, University of Texas Southwestern Medical Center, Dallas, TX, USA
[1]Present address: 2799 W Grand Boulevard K14, Detroit, MI 48202.
* Corresponding author. UT Southwestern Medical Center, 2001 Inwood Road, Suite WC05.852, Dallas, TX 75390-9254.
E-mail address: dharam.kumbhani@utsouthwestern.edu
Twitter: @engelpedro (P.E.G.)

Intervent Cardiol Clin 10 (2021) 541–552
https://doi.org/10.1016/j.iccl.2021.06.002
2211-7458/21/© 2021 Elsevier Inc. All rights reserved.

TAVR for low-surgical-risk patients with symptomatic severe AS regardless of aortic valve morphology. Given the progressive expansion of TAVR toward younger and lower-risk patients, heart teams are encountering patients with BAV more frequently at a time when evidence-based guidelines are evolving to incorporate recommendations on surgical-based or catheter-based therapies for this particular group of patients. This review delineates the important anatomic and clinical considerations in managing patients with BAV with TAVR, as well as systemically discusses the existing evidence in this space.

BICUSPID AORTIC VALVE MORPHOLOGY

BAV disease is the most common congenital heart defect, and it is not isolated to the aortic valve leaflets because it is a genetic disorder that also affects the aorta and/or cardiac development; therefore, nonvalvular coexisting findings occur in up to 50% of adults with BAV with the most common abnormality being dilation of the thoracic aorta.[14] Even when it pertains to the abnormal bileaflet valve, it is not a homogenous condition. The BAV is made of 2 unequal-sized leaflets with an eccentric closure line and doming of the leaflets (during diastole). The larger leaflet has a central raphe or ridge that results from the fusion of commissures, and these fused commissures are susceptible to disruption as occurs with balloon valvuloplasty. The distribution of tissue and calcification is usually different between the 2 cusps irrespective of whether or not a raphe is present, possibly because cusps differ in size from the

time of birth and the cusp with the largest surface area undergoes greater calcium deposition.[15]

Hence, the identification of the different morphologic types and phenotypes is essential for procedural success. Diagnosis is best made on a prospectively gated computed tomography (CT), as echocardiography can miss most of these cases.[16] There are several classification systems for the different BAV morphologies, but the most widely used classification is by Sievers and Schmidtke. Valve morphology is classified based on the number, position, and symmetry of the cusps and the presence of raphes. Type 0 has 2 symmetric leaflet/cusps and 1 commissure without a raphe. Type 1 has a single raphe due to fusion of the left coronary cusp with either the right or noncoronary cusps, and Type 2 arises when 2 raphes are present with fusion of both the right and noncoronary cusps (Fig. 1).[13] Of these, type 1 is the most common (90%), of which fusion of left and right cusps is seen in ~70% of patients, followed by right and noncoronary fusion in about 10% to 20%.[17] Other classification systems have been proposed like the one by Jilaihawi and colleagues,[18] which takes into account the interaction between the transcatheter heart valve (THV) frame and the aortic valve (AV) complex (which may have implications with regard to expansion and orientation of the valve). There are regional and racial differences with the incidence of BAV being more common in an Asian population when compared with Westerners, and with the former group presenting more often with Sievers type 0 and also with excess calcium burden.[19]

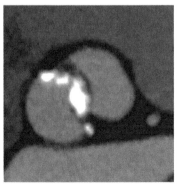 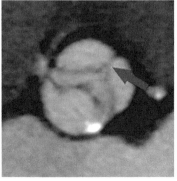 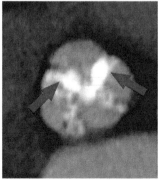

Sievers Type 0   **Sievers Type 1**   **Sievers Type 2**

Fig. 1. Bicuspid aortic valve Sievers classification. Red arrows indicate fused raphes in Sievers type 1 and 2 bicuspid morphologies. (*Adapted from* Waksman R, Craig PE, Torguson R, et al. Transcatheter Aortic Valve Replacement in Low-Risk Patients with Symptomatic Severe Bicuspid Aortic Valve Stenosis. *JACC Cardiovasc Interv.* 2020;13(9):1019-1027.[13])

OTHER ANATOMIC CONSIDERATIONS

Concern for poor clinical outcomes after implantation of THV in patients with BAV stems from the unique anatomic challenges like a noncircular annulus with asymmetric heavy calcification (**Fig. 2**),[20] which could lead to higher incidence of significant paravalvular leak (PVL) (which is defined as greater than mild), incomplete valve expansion, higher risk of annular rupture, periprocedural strokes, and need for a permanent pacemaker (PPM). Even if the annular shape itself is more circular, the supra-annular geometry, especially at the level of the sinus of Valsalva, is more frequently elliptical in patients with BAV.[21] The dimensions of the aortic annulus are also generally larger in BAV than in tricuspid aortic valves (TAVs), increasing the likelihood of having an annulus size outside of the range covered by currently available THVs.[22] Another concern is that conduction disturbances may be higher with certain morphologies—for instance, in patients with Right/Left fusion due to a raphe, there can be an increase in the compression forces applied on the contralateral stent frame toward the noncoronary cusp area, which is very close to the His bundle.[23] On the other hand, Left/Right fusion is much more likely to have progression of valve dysfunction at an earlier age with mixed aortic valve disease (AS and aortic regurgitation), which portends an aggressive disease course often requiring intervention earlier in life.[24,25]

Other considerations are the height and location of the coronary ostia, as well as the presence of a horizontal aorta defined as an angle of less than 30° between the plane perpendicular to the aortic annulus (**Fig. 3**) and the horizontal reference line on multidetector row computed tomography (MDCT).[26] A horizontal aorta may complicate accurate positioning of the prosthesis during TAVR, particularly when using a self-expanding valve. Need for a second valve and postdilation, longer fluoroscopy time and increased device embolization, and higher rates of significant PVL have been described.[27] Patients with BAV may have more frequent coronary artery anomalies when compared with patients with TAV.[26] However, the larger sinus of Valsalva in patients with BAV stenosis compared with TAV hypothetically should be protective from coronary obstruction during TAVR. The evidence has shown very low and similar incidence of coronary obstruction in both patients with BAV and TAV.[28]

In addition to the aforementioned conditions, aortic root dilation occurs in 50% to 60% of patients with a normally functioning bicuspid valve (due to both genetic and hemodynamic factors that affect the wall elasticity), increasing the risk of aortic dissection.[29] Most commonly, there is isolated tubular dilation of the ascending aorta itself, although the root may be involved as well. It is possible that progression of BAV aortopathy may be further accelerated by mechanical wall shear stress, in particular when associated with concomitant valvulopathy such as AS.[30] At present, guidelines recommend that aneurysms measuring 4.5 cm or larger be replaced at the same time as SAVR in patients with BAV, and that replacement should be considered at 5.5 cm (5.0–5.5 cm if there are additional risk factors) if the patient otherwise does not require AVR.[31] Hence, it is essential to assess the thoracic aorta preprocedurally in patients with

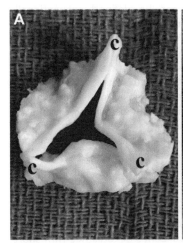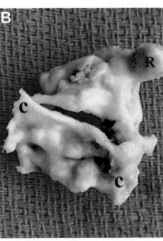

Fig. 2. Gross specimens of a calcific (*A*) tricuspid aortic valve and a (*B*) bicuspid aortic valve (Sievers type 1 left/right). (*Adapted from* Radermecker MA, Sprynger M, Hans G. TAVR for Stenotic Bicuspid Aortic Valve: Feasible, Continuously Improving Results With Another Red Flag. *J Am Coll Cardiol.* 2020;76(22):2591-2594.[20])

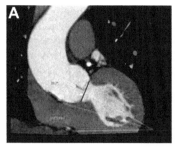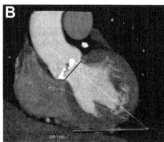

Fig. 3. Horizontal aorta in 2 patients with bicuspid aortic valve stenosis. Horizontal aorta is defined as an angle of <30° between the plane perpendicular to the aortic annulus plan and a horizontal reference line. (*Adapted from* Kong WKF, Delgado V, Bax JJ. Bicuspid Aortic Valve: What to Image in Patients Considered for Transcatheter Aortic Valve Replacement? *Circ Cardiovasc Imaging.* 2017;10(9).[26])

BAV. SAVR should still be the mainstay therapy for patients with a significant aortic aneurysm because it would be undesirable to leave a life-threatening aneurysm untreated with TAVR. On the other hand, the natural history of BAV aneurysm may be more benign than previously thought and, theoretically, abnormal wall shear stress from AS may be reduced after TAVR and decrease the future risk of aneurysm progression. At this moment, there are no data to support this latter hypothesis.

IMAGING FOR TRANSCATHETER AORTIC VALVE REPLACEMENT IN BICUSPID AORTIC VALVE

MDCT is key and the preferred imaging modality in the selection and planning of TAVR in patients with BAV.[32] MDCT allows for an excellent assessment of the aortic valve calcification, in particular, the amount and distribution, which may pose challenges during the THV deployment. MDCT also allows for conventional measurements (annulus size measurements with modifications when appropriate, sinus of Valsalva width, height of coronary ostia) and an assessment of the number of cusps, presence of raphe, and dimensions of the whole aortic valve complex, which can help plan the procedure, anticipate the THV expansion, and avoid potential complications.[33]

Identification of the exact annular plan can be challenging, and there is no established consensus methodology to define the aortic annulus plane in BAV. In addition, the AV complex shape (from annulus to the leaflet tips) is nontubular (flared or tapered) in two-thirds of patients with BAV, with the tapered configuration accounting for a minority of patients (14% to 40.1%) with the narrowest dimensions and point of resistance located above the annulus at the commissural level (Fig. 4).[22,34,35] A less circular deployment, THV oversizing, and subsequent risk of THV underexpansion or annulus

injury can occur if sized according to annulus dimension in a tapered configuration. However, THV sizing should still be primarily based on the annulus size, which has been shown to be reliable and safe in patients with BAV.[34,35] For the minority of patients with a tapered configuration, a supra-annular sizing strategy can be considered to select a smaller THV than suggested by annulus dimension,[22,36,37] but these supra-annular techniques of measurements are not standardized, have inferior reproducibility than annulus measurement, and would result in a beneficial modification of THV size in a minority of patients.[35]

When defining the aortic annulus in BAV, the 3 points (the most basal attachment points of the 3 cusps into the left ventricular outflow tract) that usually demark the annulus plane in TAV may be difficult to define, particularly in type 0 BAV. In this situation, Kong and colleagues[26] proposed using the 2 hinge points of the 2 existing cusps, and the third point to define the annular plane is derived from a plane perpendicular to the landing zone of the prosthesis (Fig. 5). Conversely, in type 1 BAV, the hinge points of the 3 cusps can be identified and the annulus plane can be defined conventionally (see Fig. 5).[26] It is likely that the interaction between the BAV anatomy and the prosthesis type is more important for the final TAVR result than just the size of the aortic annulus; therefore, for BAV sizing an integrative approach that takes into account the multilevel dimensions (from the annulus to aortic root) and multiple parameters (area, perimeter, supra-annular or intercommissural distance/area, and median/minimum/maximum diameter) is important.[33]

EARLY EXPERIENCE

Initially, our understanding of the safety and efficacy of TAVR for patients with BAV was based on limited clinical series or registries with short-term data because this procedure was

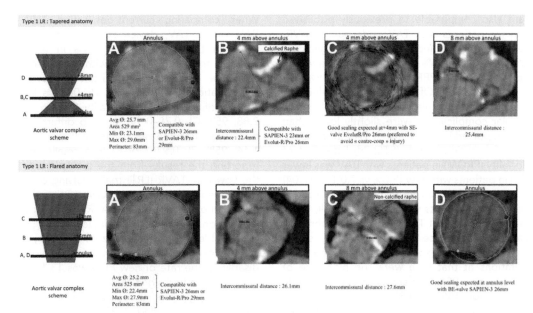

Fig. 4. Computed tomographic scan sizing strategy and transcatheter heart valve design choice in bicuspid aortic valve. (*Top*) Aortic valve sizing at different level of a tapered bicuspid aortic valve type 1 left/right bicuspid aortic valve. (*A*) Annulus level, (*B*) 4 mm above annulus, (*C*) 8 mm above annulus, (*D*) simulated Evolut-R/Pro 26 mm (*dashed blue and pink circle*). (*Bottom*) Aortic valve sizing at a different level of a flared bicuspid aortic valve type 1 left/right bicuspid aortic valve. (*A*) Annulus level, (*B*) 4 mm above annulus, (*C*) 8 mmx above annulus, (*D*) simulated SAPIEN 3 26 mm (*blue circle*). (*Adapted from* Vincent F, Ternacle J, Denimal T. Transcatheter Aortic Valve Replacement in Bicuspid Aortic Valve Stenosis. *Circulation.* 2021; 143(10):1043-1061.[33])

considered off label in the United States and because these patients were excluded from all randomized TAVR trials. The early experience suggested an adverse signal related to increased significant PVL,[38] valve malposition,[39] and higher PPM rates.[40] To overcome the issue of studies with small sample size and poor generalizability, Reddy and colleagues[41] performed a systematic review and meta-analysis to evaluate the outcomes of TAVR for patients with BAV, which involved studies with at least 1 month of outcome data. In this analysis (51% SAPIEN valve [Edwards Lifesciences, Irvine, CA, USA], 46% CoreValve "Classic" [Medtronic, Dublin, Ireland]), the device success rate was 95% (95% confidence interval [CI], 90.2%–98.5%), and the incidences of annular rupture, device malposition, and second valve implants

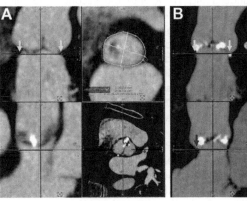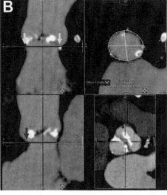

Fig. 5. Aortic annulus dimensions sizing with multidetector row computed tomography according to type of bicuspid aortic valve (BAV). (*A*) Type 0 BAV. Arrows indicate the hinge points of the 2 cusps into the left ventricular outflow tract. The third point will be derived from a plane perpendicular to the landing zone of the prosthesis (*red line* in lower, left panel). (*B*) Type 1 BAV. The hinge points of the right (*red point*), left (*green point*), and no-coronary (*yellow point*) cusps can be identified on cross-sectional plane, as well as in the orthogonal planes (*yellow arrows* in coronal plane and *red arrow* in sagittal plane). (*Adapted from* Kong WKF, Delgado V, Bax JJ. Bicuspid Aortic Valve: What to Image in Patients Considered for Transcatheter Aortic Valve Replacement? *Circ Cardiovasc Imaging.* 2017;10(9).[26])

were also comparable to previously published data for patients with TAV undergoing TAVR. However, the pooled incidence of significant PVL was 12.2% (95% CI, 3.1%–24.7%) and the requirement for PPM was 17.9% (95% CI, 14.1%– 21.9%).[42] Of note, rates of all-cause death, life-threatening bleeds, and major vascular complications were slightly lower than those reported in patients with TAV, but the society of thoracic surgeons (STS) Predicted Risk of Mortality (PROM) in patients with BAV was lower than in patients with TAV (5.0% vs 7.0%, $P = .04$) which may reflect a lower comorbidity burden in the younger patients with BAV.[41] Overall, these data suggested that TAVR for BAV is technically feasible, that device success and early safety event rates were excellent, and that the main limitations at that time were the high rate of PVL and new PPM implantation; this is notable because both PVL and PPM are associated with increased long-term morbidity and mortality despite otherwise successful TAVR in patients with TAV.[43]

CONTEMPORARY STUDIES

More recently, several studies have focused on contemporary TAVR devices (SAPIEN 3 [Edwards Lifesciences] and Evolut R and Evolut PRO [Medtronic]) in patients with BAV (Table 1). In a study by Yoon and colleagues[28] using the propensity scored-matched Bicuspid AS TAVR Registry, which included 226 patients with BAV receiving contemporary THV (both balloon-expandable and self-expandable) who were compared with patients with TAV, there were no significant differences in procedural complications (conversion to surgery, second valve implantation, significant PVL, absence of device success, new PPM) or 2-year all-cause mortality rates. In terms of outcomes across bicuspid phenotype, there was no significant difference in procedural and clinical outcomes between type 0 and type 1 BAV. Similarly, in a study using data from the American College of Cardiology (ACC) STS transcatheter valve therapy (TVT) Registry, Halim and colleagues[44] observed that 3.2% of 170,959 eligible TAVR procedures were performed in patients with BAV, of which 3705 were done with current-generation THV (both balloon-expandable and self-expandable devices). When current-generation devices were used to treat patients with BAV, device success increased (93.5% vs 96.3%, $P = .001$) and the incidence of significant aortic valve regurgitation declined (14.0% vs 2.7%, $P<.001$) when compared with older-generation devices.

When comparing current-generation THV in BAV versus TAV, device success was slightly lower in the BAV group (96.3% in BAV vs 97.4% in tricuspid, $P = .07$), with slightly higher incidence of residual significant aortic valve regurgitation (2.7% vs 2.1%, $P<.001$), a lower 1-year adjusted risk of mortality (hazard ratio, 0.88; 95% CI, 0.78–0.99), and no difference in the 1-year adjusted risk of stroke (hazard ratio, 1.14; 95% CI, 0.94–1.39).[44] In a smaller study reporting the results from the bicuspid arm of the Low Risk TAVR (LRT) trial involving 61 low-risk (based on their STS PROM) patients with BAV who underwent TAVR with third-generation balloon-expandable and self-expandable THV there was zero mortality and 1.6% strokes (none of which were considered disabling); the rate of new PPM was 13.1% and just 1 patient had significant PVL.[13]

In a more recent analysis based on the STS TVT Registry including 2691 propensity-score-matched pairs of patients undergoing TAVR with third-generation balloon-expandable devices for BAV versus TAV, there was no statistically significant difference in in-hospital mortality (1.7% vs 1.6%, $P = .75$) or 1-year mortality (10.5 vs 12.0%).[45] However, the risk of in-hospital stroke (2.1% vs 1.2, $P = .05$) was significantly greater among those with bicuspid AS, and this difference was sustained at 30 days. The rate of new PPM was also higher in patients with BAV versus those with TAV (7.3% vs 5.9%, $P = .05$). Valvular hemodynamics, including PVL, was not significantly different at 30 days, and both groups had significant and comparable improvement in functional and health status after TAVR.[45]

There are 2 recent studies that compare outcomes in patients with BAV with those with TAV undergoing TAVR with the second- and third-generation self-expandable THV (Evolut R or Evolut PRO). In an analysis from the ACC STS TVT Registry patients in which 932 patients with BAV were propensity matched with patients with TAV (STS PROM scores 5.3% ± 4.2%), the rates of all-cause mortality at 30 days (2.6% vs 1.7%, $P = .018$) and 1 year (10.4 vs 12.1%, $P = .63$), as well as the rate of stroke at 30 days (3.4% vs 2.7%, $P = .41$) and 1 year (3.9% vs 4.4%, $P = .93$), were comparable. There was no significant difference in the rate of new PPM in the patients with BAV versus those with tricuspid valve (15.4% vs 13.7%, $P = .3$). The rate of significant aortic regurgitation was much higher in the BAV group immediately post-procedure (5.6% vs 2.1%, $P≤.001$); however, at 1 year this difference had vanished (4.7% vs

Table 1
Contemporary studies of transcatheter aortic valve replacement in patients with bicuspid aortic valve

Study	Patients (n)	SAPIEN 3 (%)	Evolut R or Evolut PRO (%)	Mortality (%)	All Stroke (Disabling and Nondisabling)	Significant PVL (%)	New PPM (%)	Conversion to Surgery	Valve Embolization	Need for Second Valve
Yoon et al,[28] 2017[a]	226	70.7	10.2	2.7	3.4	2.7	16.4	1.3%	NR	1.3
Makkar et al,[45] 2019[b]	2691	100	0	2.6	2.5	2.0	7.3	0.9	0.1	0.4
Halim et al,[44] 2020[c]	3705	73.4	11.3	1.6	2.1	2.6	NR	0.7	NR	0.7
Waksman et al,[13] 2020[d]	61	74	26	0	1.6	1.6	13.1	NR	NR	0%
Forrest et al,[49] 2020[e]	932	0	100	1.7	3.4	5.6	14.3	NR	NR	NR
Forrest et al,[12] 2021[f]	150	0	100	0.7	4.0	0	15.1	0.7	1.3	3.1

30-day outcomes.

Abbreviations: NR, not reported; PVL, paravalvular leak; PPM, permanent pacemaker; STS PROM, STS Predicted Risk of Mortality.

[a] This study included 546 pair of patients who were propensity-score matched to a TAV cohort, but only data for patients receiving new-generation devices is being presented. STS PROM 4.6%.

[b] STS PROM 4.9%.

[c] In-hospital outcomes are being presented in this study. STS PROM 3.8%.

[d] STS PROM 1.5%.

[e] 30-day clinical outcomes and in-hospital postprocedure assessment of PVL being presented. STS PROM 5.3%.

[f] STS PROM 1.4%.

3.9%, $P = .6$); this could have been explained partially by the higher frequency of the aortic valve reintervention in patients with BAV observed in this study, albeit this rate was generally low (0.8% at 30 days and 1.7% at 1 year). In the prospective Low Risk Bicuspid Study, which included a single arm of 150 patients deemed to be low-risk (STS PROM <3%) patients, there was a low incidence of all-cause mortality at 30 days (0.7%) and there was no significant PVL reported; however, the rate of all strokes was 4.0% (disabling strokes comprised only 0.7%) and the incidence of new PPM was 15.1%.

PARAVALVULAR LEAK AND PERMANENT PACEMAKER

The exact mechanism underlying increased PVL is not well defined, but it is likely due to an interaction between factors such as a more heavily and heterogeneously calcified BAV (when compared with TAV), asymmetrical morphology of the aortic valve complex, and difficulty in sizing that can lead to malapposition or poor expansion of the THV leading to PVL. Of note, there is no clear correlation of the BAV phenotype with clinical outcomes after TAVR, regardless of whether the Sievers or the Jilahawi classification system is used.[18,28,46] Previously it was thought that PVL was mostly due to the presence of an elliptical annuli, which would not be expected to conform to a circular prosthesis. In the systematic review by Reddy and colleagues[41] the mean ellipticity index (the ratio of the maximum and minimum annulus diameters) was 1.24 in patients with BAV, which was similar to their TAV counterparts thus indicating this is likely not the driving mechanism. In addition, in experienced hands with the use of new-generation self-expandable and balloon-expandable valves, the PVLs could be reduced to very low levels. The rates of significant PVL in this analysis were much lower (3.4%) when new-generation THVs were used.[41] The SAPIEN 3 valve has an outer polyethylene terephthalate-sealing skirt at its lower portion and a more accurate positioning mechanism when compared with its prior iterations. The Evolut PRO valve has an outer pericardial wrap added to the inflow portion of the valve to decrease PVL. The LOTUS mechanical (Boston Scientific, Marlborough, MA, USA) expanding valve has an outer adaptive seal with the ability to be repositioned and retrieved; however, this valve has been recently withdrawn from the market.

The rates of PPM have continued to be elevated even in the studies with new-generation THV, and this continues to be one of the main limitations of TAVR in the BAV population, as well as in the low-risk population overall. The high pacemaker rates are likely due to the difficulty in valve positioning due to irregular leaflet shape and calcification, as well as the inability to achieve a coaxial position during valve deployment. These issues can lead to lower implantation depths, which are known to be associated with higher rates of new PPM implantation. Intraprocedural factors such as reducing the valve implant by only 3 mm could reduce the need for PPM implantation by 52%.[47] It is recommended to deploy the SAPIEN 3 in a 90% aortic/10% ventricular fashion and also aiming for higher deployment with the Evolut valves. It is important to note that the rate of new PPM is lower with patients with TAV undergoing TAVR with a balloon-expandable valve(6.6%),[6] and a recent observational study with patients with BAV receiving a SAPIEN 3 elicited a comparable rate (7.3%).[45] Patients with BAV disease tend to be younger and with less concomitant comorbidities; therefore, the high rate of PPM implantation could continue to hinder the expansion of TAVR for this population.

STROKES AND CEREBRAL EMBOLIC PROTECTION

The stroke rate after TAVR was initially at 5% to 10% in very-high-risk patients and is now as low as 0.5% to 0.9% in the latest randomized trials performed in low-risk patients with TAV.[6,7] BAV is associated with a significant higher risk of dislodging particles 1000 μm or larger after TAVR,[48] which is thought to be due to the greater calcium burden and usually may require more frequent balloon dilation before and after the THV deployment. In spite of these findings, it is unclear whether TAVR for BAV is associated with a higher rate of stroke when compared with TAVR for TAV. Among the studies that involved mostly newer-generation valves with significant power to assess for stroke, only the study by Makkar and colleagues[45] was associated with a higher rate of stroke in comparison to patients with TAV and the incidence rate was relatively low (2.5%). Otherwise, the incidence of stroke in BAV after TAVR ranged from 1.6% to 4.0% in these studies (patients had low to intermediate risk).[12,18,28,44,49] Cerebral embolic protection (CEP) captures debris (ie, foreign body material, endothelium, calcific debris, myocardial tissue) after TAVR, but thus far there has been no adequately powered randomized trials demonstrating efficacy of CEP devices in either TAV or BAV. The Sentinel device (Claret Medical, now Boston Scientific) was the first CEP device approved by the FDA based on the results from the Cerebral Protection in Transcatheter Aortic Valve Replacement (SENTINEL) Trial, and it is still the device being used predominantly in current practice. The exact number of patients with BAV in this study is unclear and likely very low, hence the utility of CEP during TAVR in BAV is still largely unknown and further studies are needed to clarify this question.

PROSTHESIS CHOICE

There are advantages and disadvantages of the new-generation balloon-expandable and self-expanding valves that are important for TAVR operators to understand so that the best valve design for a particular patient with BAV can be selected. The contemporary studies discussed in previous sections are revealing excellent device implantation success, low rate of safety outcomes, and promising short-term hemodynamic data and outcomes. A horizontal aorta is known to complicate accurate positioning of a self-expanding valve, and a balloon-expandable valve might be preferred if this anatomy is present. Balloon-expandable valves also exert greater radial force when compared with self-expanding devices and may potentially circularize the native annulus minimizing potential sites for PVLs. However, this might not be a decisive factor because as discussed in previous sections both valve designs now feature an external sealing skirt/wrap, which has significantly decreased the rates of significant PVL and the rates are comparable to those in patients with TAV. In addition, self-expanding valves might offer a slightly better hemodynamic profile regarding the rates of prosthesis-patient mismatch, which might be of particular importance in patients with smaller annuli. For the minority of patients with tapered or funnel anatomy, a supra-annular sizing has been suggested to be of incremental value to select a smaller THV than suggested by annulus dimensions and avoid the oversizing-related risks.[36] As an extension, in the TAV population, the incidence of prosthesis-patient mismatch in low-risk patients can be as high as 62.1%,[6] and the rate is significantly lower in the supra-annular self-expanding THV.[7,50] Dedicated prospective studies in patients with BAV comparing the 2 main THV designs are needed to confirm the hemodynamic performance differences, and more importantly, to determine if these differences have a clinically significant impact on the outcome or durability of the prosthesis.

Currently, both THV types offer a lower profile delivery system, which allows for more accurate position. Identification of an annular plane in BAV can be very challenging as described in earlier sections, and the self-expanding valves offer the ability to recapture the device before deployment that theoretically could be advantageous (when compared with balloon-expanding valves) for deploying the THV at the optimal landing zone.

Overall, operators should likely continue to use the THV valve they have more experience with because both valve systems have a learning curve that is known to be important and shared decision making and careful consideration of the patient's anatomy and preferences is also required.

BALLOON SIZING AND PREIMPLANT BALLOONING

Balloon sizing complements MDCT and is recommended based on the difficulty in assessing the geometry and size of the annulus using imagination alone. Balloon sizing is especially important in situations when there is ambiguity between valve sizing or when the measurements fall between 2 valve sizes. In addition, in the presence of heavily calcified cusps or long leaflets, balloon sizing can mimic valve implantation and also help identify patients at risk of coronary obstruction. This technique can help predict how severe, eccentric calcification may behave and the complications that can arise from it.[51] Preimplant balloon dilation may also help circularize BAVs to some extent, and many centers routinely predilate for BAVs even as the practice has been largely abandoned for routine implantations.

DURABILITY

Patients with BAV usually present at a younger age with significant AS meeting criteria for aortic valve replacement, which is why it is essential to better understand the long-term durability of THV in this population. Based on a study using event simulation models, the durability of the THV must be 70% shorter than that of a surgical bioprosthesis to have an impact on overall life expectancy in low-risk older patients; however, in younger patients life expectancy was reduced when the durability was 30% to 50% shorter than that of surgical valves.[52] Hence, in younger low-risk patients, valve durability must be carefully considered and weighed against other patient factors such as life expectancy. The durability of surgical and transcatheter bioprosthetic valves is not indefinite, thus for low-surgical-risk patients younger than 50 years, without a contraindication to anticoagulation, a mechanical valve is still recommended by the guidelines.[31] The long-term durability of THV for TAV beyond 5 to 8 years is poorly understood, but the short-term durability seems similar and adequate between balloon-expandable valves and self-expanding valves.[53] Numerous factors unique to TAVR (that tend to be more commonly present in patients with BAV) may affect long-term durability including THV crimping, postdilation, noncircular implantation, PVL, and leaflet thrombosis.[54] CT studies of patients with BAV undergoing TAVR have found suboptimal and asymmetrical expansion, which may result in suboptimal hemodynamic features that will likely impact long-term valve performance and the rate of valve degeneration.[22,55] Despite these theoretic concerns some of the largest studies to date in patients with BAV with new-generation THV showed that the valve hemodynamics (aortic valve area and mean gradient) was comparable with that of a cohort with TAV and sustained up to 1 year.[45,49] In one small study that assessed for subclinical hypoattenuated leaflet thickening (HALT), the incidence was 10% at 30 days, which is comparable to the 13% incidence rate observed in the PARTNER 3 trial.[6,13] Whether HALT affects long-term durability is also still unknown.

The choice of initial bioprosthesis, especially for younger patients who are expected to outlive the THV life span, should consider the relative safety and efficacy of potential subsequent interventions. In a recent observational propensity score-matched cohort of TAVR-in-TAVR valve versus TAVR-in-SAVR valve, the former group was associated with similar procedural success and safety but the rate of mild and moderate aortic regurgitation was higher after TAVR-in-TAVR procedures.[56,57]

SUMMARY

Prospective registries and clinical studies have elicited promising results suggesting that TAVR in BAV is safe, device success and procedural outcomes are excellent, and the short-term outcomes and hemodynamic data (30 days to 1 year) are encouraging. These contemporary studies with new-generation valves indicate that outcomes of TAVR in BAV are comparable to those in TAV; this is likely due to the increased experience with TAVR, improved THV technology, and the routine use of MDCT. However,

given the paucity of randomized controlled data regarding the use of TAVR in BAV due to exclusion from pivotal studies and the lack of long-term outcomes and valve performance studies, SAVR should continue to be the therapeutic modality of choice in this patient population in light of the well-established low rates of procedural complications and auspicious long-term outcomes data.[58] In TAVR for BAV, the issue of higher rates of significant PVL has mostly been resolved with the new iteration of THV and the current procedural techniques. The relative high rate of new implantation of PPM in a young population and the lack of durability data of the THV continue to be issues to address not only in the patients with BAV but also in the low-risk population in general. There are mixed results regarding the incidence of stroke when compared with patients with TAV anatomy, but the absolute rates are low in recent analyses and further studies assessing the utility of CEP in this population are needed. Future studies to evaluate the effect of concomitant aortopathy, as well as valve durability are a must. In sum, TAVR in selected patients with BAV in experienced TAVR centers is a reasonable option and the contemporary registry data may be able to guide clinical practice until randomized clinical trials are available studying the appropriate treatment of AS in patients with BAV.

DISCLOSURE

The authors have nothing to disclose.

REFERENCES

1. Adams DH, Popma JJ, Reardon MJ, et al. Transcatheter aortic-valve replacement with a self-expanding prosthesis. N Engl J Med 2014;370(19):1790–8.
2. Smith CR, Leon MB, Mack MJ, et al. Transcatheter versus surgical aortic-valve replacement in high-risk patients. N Engl J Med 2011;364(23):2187–98.
3. Leon MB, Smith CR, Mack MJ, et al. Transcatheter or Surgical Aortic-Valve Replacement in Intermediate-Risk Patients. N Engl J Med 2016; 374(17):1609–20.
4. Reardon MJ, Van Mieghem NM, Popma JJ, et al. Surgical or Transcatheter Aortic-Valve Replacement in Intermediate-Risk Patients. N Engl J Med 2017;376(14):1321–31.
5. Otto CM, Kumbhani DJ, Alexander KP, et al. 2017 ACC Expert Consensus Decision Pathway for Transcatheter Aortic Valve Replacement in the Management of Adults With Aortic Stenosis: A Report of the American College of Cardiology

Task Force on Clinical Expert Consensus Documents. J Am Coll Cardiol 2017;69(10):1313–46.

6. Mack MJ, Leon MB, Thourani VH, et al. Transcatheter Aortic-Valve Replacement with a Balloon-Expandable Valve in Low-Risk Patients. N Engl J Med 2019;380(18):1695–705.

7. Popma JJ, Deeb GM, Yakubov SJ, et al. Transcatheter Aortic-Valve Replacement with a Self-Expanding Valve in Low-Risk Patients. N Engl J Med 2019;380(18):1706–15.

8. Carroll JD, Mack MJ, Vemulapalli S, et al. STS-ACC TVT Registry of Transcatheter Aortic Valve Replacement. J Am Coll Cardiol 2020;76(21):2492–516.

9. Michelena HI, Prakash SK, Della Corte A, et al. Bicuspid aortic valve: identifying knowledge gaps and rising to the challenge from the International Bicuspid Aortic Valve Consortium (BAVCon). Circulation 2014;129(25):2691–704.

10. Kong WK, Regeer MV, Ng AC, et al. Sex Differences in Phenotypes of Bicuspid Aortic Valve and Aortopathy: Insights From a Large Multicenter, International Registry. Circ Cardiovasc Imaging 2017;10(3):e005155.

11. Roberts WC, Ko JM. Frequency by decades of unicuspid, bicuspid, and tricuspid aortic valves in adults having isolated aortic valve replacement for aortic stenosis, with or without associated aortic regurgitation. Circulation 2005;111(7):920–5.

12. Forrest JK, Ramlawi B, Deeb GM, et al. Transcatheter Aortic Valve Replacement in Low-risk Patients With Bicuspid Aortic Valve Stenosis. JAMA Cardiol 2021;6(1):50–7.

13. Waksman R, Craig PE, Torguson R, et al. Transcatheter Aortic Valve Replacement in Low-Risk Patients With Symptomatic Severe Bicuspid Aortic Valve Stenosis. JACC Cardiovasc Interv 2020;13(9):1019–27.

14. Siu SC, Silversides CK. Bicuspid aortic valve disease. J Am Coll Cardiol 2010;55(25):2789–800.

15. Roberts WC, Ko JM. Weights of individual cusps in operatively-excised congenitally bicuspid stenotic aortic valves. Am J Cardiol 2004;94(5):678–81.

16. Tanaka R, Yoshioka K, Niinuma H, et al. Diagnostic value of cardiac CT in the evaluation of bicuspid aortic stenosis: comparison with echocardiography and operative findings. AJR Am J Roentgenol 2010; 195(4):895–9.

17. Sievers HH, Schmidtke C. A classification system for the bicuspid aortic valve from 304 surgical specimens. J Thorac Cardiovasc Surg 2007;133(5):1226–33.

18. Jilaihawi H, Chen M, Webb J, et al. A Bicuspid Aortic Valve Imaging Classification for the TAVR Era. JACC Cardiovasc Imaging 2016;9(10):1145–58.

19. Jilaihawi H, Wu Y, Yang Y, et al. Morphological characteristics of severe aortic stenosis in China: imaging corelab observations from the first Chinese transcatheter aortic valve trial. Catheter Cardiovasc Interv 2015;85(Suppl 1):752–61.

20. Radermecker MA, Sprynger M, Hans G. TAVR for Stenotic Bicuspid Aortic Valve: Feasible, Continuously Improving Results With Another Red Flag. J Am Coll Cardiol 2020;76(22):2591–4.

21. Shibayama K, Harada K, Berdejo J, et al. Comparison of aortic root geometry with bicuspid versus tricuspid aortic valve: real-time three-dimensional transesophageal echocardiographic study. J Am Soc Echocardiogr 2014;27(11):1143–52.

22. Tchetche D, de Biase C, van Gils L, et al. Bicuspid Aortic Valve Anatomy and Relationship With Devices: The BAVARD Multicenter Registry. Circ Cardiovasc Interv 2019;12(1):e007107.

23. Fedak PW, Verma S, David TE, et al. Clinical and pathophysiological implications of a bicuspid aortic valve. Circulation 2002;106(8):900–4.

24. Egbe AC, Luis SA, Padang R, et al. Outcomes in Moderate Mixed Aortic Valve Disease: Is it Time for a Paradigm Shift? J Am Coll Cardiol 2016;67(20):2321–9.

25. Fernandes SM, Khairy P, Sanders SP, et al. Bicuspid aortic valve morphology and interventions in the young. J Am Coll Cardiol 2007;49(22):2211–4.

26. Kong WKF, Delgado V, Bax JJ. Bicuspid Aortic Valve: What to Image in Patients Considered for Transcatheter Aortic Valve Replacement? Circ Cardiovasc Imaging 2017;10(9):e005987.

27. Chan PH, Alegria-Barrero E, Di Mario C. Difficulties with horizontal aortic root in transcatheter aortic valve implantation. Catheter Cardiovasc Interv 2013;81(4):630–5.

28. Yoon SH, Bleiziffer S, De Backer O, et al. Outcomes in Transcatheter Aortic Valve Replacement for Bicuspid Versus Tricuspid Aortic Valve Stenosis. J Am Coll Cardiol 2017;69(21):2579–89.

29. Ward C. Clinical significance of the bicuspid aortic valve. Heart 2000;83(1):81–5.

30. Guzzardi DG, Barker AJ, van Ooij P, et al. Valve-Related Hemodynamics Mediate Human Bicuspid Aortopathy: Insights From Wall Shear Stress Mapping. J Am Coll Cardiol 2015;66(8):892–900.

31. Otto CM, Nishimura RA, Bonow RO, et al. 2020 ACC/AHA Guideline for the Management of Patients With Valvular Heart Disease: Executive Summary: A Report of the American College of Cardiology/American Heart Association Joint Committee on Clinical Practice Guidelines. Circulation 2020;143(5):e35–71.

32. Falk V, Baumgartner H, Bax JJ, et al. 2017 ESC/EACTS Guidelines for the management of valvular heart disease. Eur J Cardiothorac Surg 2017;52(4):616–64.

33. Vincent F, Ternacle J, Denimal T, et al. Transcatheter Aortic Valve Replacement in Bicuspid Aortic Valve Stenosis. Circulation 2021;143(10):1043–61.

34. Kim WK, Renker M, Rolf A, et al. Annular versus supra-annular sizing for TAVI in bicuspid aortic valve stenosis. EuroIntervention 2019;15(3):e231–8.

35. Weir-McCall JR, Attinger-Toller A, Blanke P, et al. Annular versus supra-annular sizing for transcatheter aortic valve replacement in bicuspid aortic valve disease. J Cardiovasc Comput Tomogr 2020;14(5):407–13.

36. Xiong TY, Feng Y, Li YJ, et al. Supra-Annular Sizing for Transcatheter Aortic Valve Replacement Candidates With Bicuspid Aortic Valve. JACC Cardiovasc Interv 2018;11(17):1789–90.

37. Xiong TY, Li YJ, Feng Y, et al. Understanding the Interaction Between Transcatheter Aortic Valve Prostheses and Supra-Annular Structures From Post-Implant Stent Geometry. JACC Cardiovasc Interv 2019;12(12):1164–71.

38. Mylotte D, Lefevre T, Sondergaard L, et al. Transcatheter aortic valve replacement in bicuspid aortic valve disease. J Am Coll Cardiol 2014;64(22):2330–9.

39. Yousef A, Simard T, Webb J, et al. Transcatheter aortic valve implantation in patients with bicuspid aortic valve: A patient level multi-center analysis. Int J Cardiol 2015;189:282–8.

40. Perlman GY, Blanke P, Dvir D, et al. Bicuspid Aortic Valve Stenosis: Favorable Early Outcomes With a Next-Generation Transcatheter Heart Valve in a Multicenter Study. JACC Cardiovasc Interv 2016;9(8):817–24.

41. Reddy G, Wang Z, Nishimura RA, et al. Transcatheter aortic valve replacement for stenotic bicuspid aortic valves: Systematic review and meta analyses of observational studies. Catheter Cardiovasc Interv 2018;91(5):975–83.

42. Mack MJ, Brennan JM, Brindis R, et al. Outcomes following transcatheter aortic valve replacement in the United States. JAMA 2013;310(19):2069–77.

43. Nazif TM, Dizon JM, Hahn RT, et al. Predictors and clinical outcomes of permanent pacemaker implantation after transcatheter aortic valve replacement: the PARTNER (Placement of AoRtic TraNscathetER Valves) trial and registry. JACC Cardiovasc Interv 2015;8(1 Pt A):60–9.

44. Halim SA, Edwards FH, Dai D, et al. Outcomes of Transcatheter Aortic Valve Replacement in Patients With Bicuspid Aortic Valve Disease: A Report From the Society of Thoracic Surgeons/American College of Cardiology Transcatheter Valve Therapy Registry. Circulation 2020;141(13):1071–9.

45. Makkar RR, Yoon SH, Leon MB, et al. Association Between Transcatheter Aortic Valve Replacement for Bicuspid vs Tricuspid Aortic Stenosis and Mortality or Stroke. JAMA 2019;321(22):2193–202.

46. Lei WH, Liao YB, Wang ZJ, et al. Transcatheter Aortic Valve Replacement in Patients with Aortic Stenosis Having Coronary Cusp Fusion versus Mixed Cusp Fusion Nonraphe Bicuspid Aortic Valve. J Interv Cardiol 2019;2019:7348964.

47. Urena M, Rodes-Cabau J. Conduction Abnormalities: The True Achilles' Heel of Transcatheter Aortic Valve Replacement? JACC Cardiovasc Interv 2016;9(21):2217–9.

48. Kroon H, von der Thusen JH, Ziviello F, et al. Heterogeneity of debris captured by cerebral embolic protection filters during TAVI. EuroIntervention 2020;16:1141–7.

49. Forrest JK, Kaple RK, Ramlawi B, et al. Transcatheter Aortic Valve Replacement in Bicuspid Versus Tricuspid Aortic Valves From the STS/ACC TVT Registry. JACC Cardiovasc Interv 2020;13(15):1749–59.

50. Hahn RT, Leipsic J, Douglas PS, et al. Comprehensive Echocardiographic Assessment of Normal Transcatheter Valve Function. JACC Cardiovasc Imaging 2019;12(1):25–34.

51. Das R, Puri R. Transcatheter Treatment of Bicuspid Aortic Valve Disease: Imaging and Interventional Considerations. Front Cardiovasc Med 2018;5:91.

52. Tam DY, Wijeysundera HC, Naimark D, et al. Impact of Transcatheter Aortic Valve Durability on Life Expectancy in Low-Risk Patients With Severe Aortic Stenosis. Circulation 2020;142(4):354–64.

53. Patel KV, Omar W, Gonzalez PE, et al. Expansion of TAVR into Low-Risk Patients and Who to Consider for SAVR. Cardiol Ther 2020;9(2):377–94.

54. Kataruka A, Otto CM. Valve durability after transcatheter aortic valve implantation. J Thorac Dis 2018;10(Suppl 30):S3629–36.

55. Guyton RA, Padala M. Transcatheter Aortic Valve Replacement in Bicuspid Aortic Stenosis: Early Success But Concerning Red Flags. JACC Cardiovasc Interv 2016;9(8):825–7.

56. Landes U, Sathananthan J, Witberg G, et al. Transcatheter Replacement of Transcatheter Versus Surgically Implanted Aortic Valve Bioprostheses. J Am Coll Cardiol 2021;77(1):1–14.

57. Bavry AA, Kumbhani DJ. As Patients Live Longer, Are We on the Cusp of a New Valve Epidemic? J Am Coll Cardiol 2021;77(1):15–7.

58. Goland S, Czer LS, De Robertis MA, et al. Risk factors associated with reoperation and mortality in 252 patients after aortic valve replacement for congenitally bicuspid aortic valve disease. Ann Thorac Surg 2007;83(3):931–7.

Revascularization in the Transcatheter Aortic Valve Replacement Population

Mohammad Alkhalil, MD, DPhil[a,b], Ahmad Jabri, MD[c],
Rishi Puri, MBBS, PhD[d], Ankur Kalra, MD[d,e,f,*]

KEYWORDS

- Coronary artery disease • Percutaneous coronary intervention
- Transcatheter aortic valve replacement • Aortic stenosis

KEY POINTS

- The role of asymptomatic coronary artery disease (CAD) in the context of patients undergoing transcatheter aortic valve replacement (TAVR) remains controversial because supporting evidence remains sparse. Data regarding the prognostic role of CAD are inconsistent, and a prospective trial randomizing patients to pre-TAVR revascularization and deferral of treatment is ongoing.
- Acute coronary syndromes post-TAVR are common, and prosthesis choice impacts the ease and feasibility of successful revascularization. Lower height profile balloon-expandable valves enable selective catheter engagement more as compared with taller self-expanding prostheses.
- Use of computed tomography, multiple trial-error engagements with catheters, and guide extensions may be required for successful coronary intervention.

INTRODUCTION

Transcatheter aortic valve replacement (TAVR) has become the most commonly performed procedure in valvular heart interventions.[1,2] Concomitant coronary artery disease (CAD) is frequently observed in patients with aortic stenosis, and early reports linked the 2 pathologic conditions based on the shared profile of conventional cardiovascular risk factors.[3,4] In the Cardiovascular Health Study, hypercholesterolemia, for example, was associated with the presence of aortic valve disease.[4] However, intensive low-density lipoprotein cholesterol reduction had neutral effect on clinical events related to aortic stenosis, challenging any causal relationship with aortic stenosis progression.[5]

Subsequently, cardiovascular risk factors were realized to act as confounding variables, yet underscoring the strong relationship between aortic stenosis and CAD.[6,7] In the German Aortic Valve Registry that included 15,964 patients who underwent TAVR between 2011 and 2013, CAD was identified in approximately 50% of the whole cohort.[8] The prevalence of CAD is strongly related to the mean Society of Thoracic Surgeons (STS) risk score and was reflected by the progressive reduction in the presence of CAD across randomized clinical trials over the last decade.[9] Up to 6 in 7 patients with extreme

[a] Department of Cardiothoracic Services, Freeman Hospital, Newcastle-upon-Tyne NE7 7DN, UK; [b] Vascular Biology, Newcastle University, Newcastle-upon-Tyne NE7 7DN, UK; [c] Case Western Reserve University/Metro-Health Medical Center, Cleveland, OH 44109, USA; [d] Department of Cardiovascular Medicine, Heart, Vascular, and Thoracic Institute, Cleveland Clinic, Cleveland, OH 44195, USA; [e] Section of Cardiovascular Research, Heart, Vascular, and Thoracic Department, Cleveland Clinic Akron General, Akron, OH, USA; [f] Department of Cardiovascular Medicine, Heart, Vascular, and Thoracic Institute, Cleveland Clinic, 224 West Exchange Street, Suite 225, Akron, OH 44302, USA
* Corresponding author. Department of Cardiovascular Medicine, Heart, Vascular, and Thoracic Institute, Cleveland Clinic, 224 West Exchange Street, Suite 225, Akron, OH 44302.
E-mail addresses: kalramd.ankur@gmail.com; kalraa@ccf.org

Intervent Cardiol Clin 10 (2021) 553–563
https://doi.org/10.1016/j.iccl.2021.06.003
2211-7458/21/© 2021 Elsevier Inc. All rights reserved.

or high surgical risk were reported to have CAD compared with 1 in 7 patients with low STS risk who underwent TAVR.[10–13]

The management of CAD in these patients remains controversial with 2 opposing approaches to either "prophylactically" or "expectedly" manage CAD in patients undergoing TAVR. This review article discusses the rationale and the prognostic role of CAD in patients undergoing TAVR and evaluates existing evidence related to revascularization strategies in this group.

RATIONALE OF CORONARY REVASCULARIZATION IN TRANSCATHETER AORTIC VALVE REPLACEMENT

In patients without aortic stenosis, coronary revascularization is indicated to relieve symptoms and improve quality of life.[14] Up to 40% of patients with aortic stenosis may present with angina pectoris, and coronary revascularization should be considered as part of patients' management plan. Importantly, aortic stenosis is associated with high systolic and diastolic wall stress, and a reduced coronary flow reserve.[15] Subsequently, patients with severe aortic stenosis may report anginal symptoms despite having normal coronary arteries.

The more challenging scenario is when interventional cardiologists are faced with patients undergoing TAVR and concomitant CAD but lack typical angina pectoris symptoms. Data from patients who underwent surgical aortic valve replacement showed that the presence of nonrevascularized CAD was linked to increased procedural and long-term mortality.[16] More importantly, coronary revascularization was associated with a reduction in procedural risk and long-term mortality.[17,18] Extrapolating these data to the TAVR population is a common practice, and current guidelines support revascularization of severe proximal CAD as part of the TAVR workup.[1,2] This approach has possible mechanistic and practical advantages. Coronary revascularization may minimize myocardial ischemia during rapid ventricular pacing. Previous reports highlighted the relationship between prolonged and repeated rapid pacing and adverse outcomes in TAVR patients.[19,20] However, the role of revascularized CAD was not specifically evaluated in these studies. It is plausible that myocardium at jeopardy, particularly if it is large and related to proximal coronary stenosis, may contribute to ventricular stunning, dysfunction, and prolong hypotension during rapid pacing.[21] Although these features have

been associated with worse clinical outcomes, coronary revascularization to mitigate the procedural and long-term risks in TAVR patients is yet to be determined.

The practical advantage is related to accessing coronary arteries following TAVR. The bioprosthetic valve may add challenges to selectively engaging the coronary arteries. Previous studies have reported the feasibility of performing coronary angiography and (PCI) post-TAVR.[22,23] Notably, the success rate was lower with self-expanding compared with balloon-expandable valves, requiring more catheters, and more frequently semiselective engagement of coronary ostia.[23] Moreover, these studies are of relatively small sample size, and with current paradigm shift toward using TAVR in low-risk patients, access to coronary arteries is likely to be a more common practice. Therefore, upfront coronary revascularization before TAVR may overcome these difficulties and provide operators with an opportunity to avoid future challenges.

PROGNOSTIC ROLE OF CORONARY ARTERY DISEASE IN TRANSCATHETER AORTIC VALVE REPLACEMENT PATIENTS

Historically, patients with aortic stenosis with concomitant CAD were more likely to be older with higher incidence of major comorbidities.[16–18] When adjusting for other prognostic variables, the impact of CAD on mortality in patients undergoing TAVR was not consistent, questioning whether CAD is a true independent risk factor in this population.[9] It may be argued that CAD is merely a marker of other comorbidities, particularly because it was closely associated with STS risk score in randomized clinical trials.[10–13] However, the significant heterogeneity in defining CAD poses considerable limitations in determining its prognostic role in patients undergoing TAVR. The binary classification of CAD when assessing procedural risk using STS score does not reflect the nature and severity of CAD, contributing to the current challenges in delineating the prognostic role of CAD in TAVR patients. CAD may be defined as residual narrowing $\geq$50% or $\geq$70% in the epicardial coronary arteries before TAVR procedure. In addition, previous myocardial infarction (MI) or coronary revascularization is also widely accepted as a reasonable definition of CAD. Although these definitions may serve as a surrogate of CAD, their impact on prognosis is unlikely to be identical, particularly when taking into consideration the timing of coronary events or ongoing myocardial ischemia related to residual coronary stenoses. Recent acute coronary syndrome may increase periprocedural risk, a phenomenon that is well established in patients undergoing cardiac surgery.[24] On the other hand, the influence of remote MI may predominantly be related to left ventricular systolic dysfunction.[25] Similarly, using different cutoffs to estimate the severity of coronary artery stenosis without factoring whether these lesions were revascularized may translate into various degrees of ischemic myocardium and plausibly clinical outcomes.[25] Notwithstanding the interobserver variability in estimating the degree of stenosis using angiography, quantitative coronary angiography was not used in defining CAD in most studies. Objective evaluation of CAD using functional or physiologic assessment may help delineate the role of obstructive CAD in patients undergoing TAVR. More recently, the role of computed tomography (CT) has been proposed as a tool to define CAD and was compared with invasive angiography in TAVR patients. A meta-analysis of 1275 patients conducted by van den Boogert and colleagues[26] showed an excellent sensitivity and negative predictive value (>90%) of CT in identifying CAD greater than 50% on invasive angiography. CT is a crucial tool to offer a safe TAVR procedure and also provides an opportunity to assess CAD. However, its specificity remains acceptable (60%–70%) and may be considered a drawback in evaluating CAD in TAVR patients.[26] Future studies, such as CT-CA (NCT03291925), will add further insight into the role of CT in patients undergoing TAVR.

Predictably, clinical outcomes data regarding the role of CAD in TAVR have not been consistent.[27,28] Sankaramangalam and colleagues[28] reported in a meta-analysis of 8013 patients that CAD was associated with 20% increased risk of death at 1 year following TAVR compared with patients without CAD. In contrast, a more recent meta-analysis by Lateef and colleagues[27] demonstrated that CAD was not associated with increased 1-year mortality post-TAVR. The lack of association between CAD and mortality risk remained evident even after including studies with 100% prevalence of CAD or those where PCIs were performed prior or during TAVR.[27] This finding was borne out in a retrospective analysis of 271 patients where significant CAD (defined as stenosis ≥70% or ≥50% in left main stem or vein graft) was not associated with increased mortality.[29] However, using the synergy between percutaneous coronary

intervention with taxus and cardiac surgery (SYNTAX) score, the investigators showed that patients with high SYNTAX score have the highest mortality compared with intermediate or low SYNTAX scores.[29] These findings were subsequently confirmed in a meta-analysis of 8334 patients demonstrating that CAD complexity, defined using SYNTAX score, was related to death following TAVR.[30] Furthermore, residual SYNTAX score (>8) was associated with 70% increased risk of death following TAVR.[30,31] Although considered indirect evidence, incomplete revascularization underscores the role of PCI in mitigating the risk of death following TAVR.

The relatively short duration of follow-up in TAVR studies did not permit a full evaluation of the role of CAD.[9] In addition, the risk of residual CAD is heterogeneous, and reported studies have mostly used mortality as a marker of risk, although other composite endpoints, such as MI and clinically urgent revascularization, should also be factored in when assessing CAD in future TAVR studies.

SELECTIVE VERSUS ROUTINE CORONARY REVASCULARIZATION

Routine revascularization for proximal CAD with a degree of stenosis ≥70% is supported by current guidelines.[1,2] The shared symptoms between CAD and aortic stenosis make it more difficult to assess the contribution of CAD to the patients' burden of anginal symptoms and support a role of routine coronary revascularization in patients undergoing TAVR. Angiography-guided revascularization appeared safe, although data were derived from small studies with a relatively short follow-up duration.[32,33] In addition, the interobserver variability in quantifying the degree of stenosis and identifying significant lesions may add further challenges to the use of angiogram-based approach.

The use of noninvasive stress tests to aid in decision making for coronary revascularization is not extensively studied.[25] Although these tests have been reported to be safe, their specificity in identifying CAD is considered acceptable at most.[25,34] Importantly, a positive ischemia testing is likely to be less specific in the presence of concomitant aortic stenosis.[35] Aortic stenosis contributes to subendocardial ischemia as a result of increased end-diastolic pressure and the demands of the afterload. When CAD and aortic stenosis coexist, it becomes challenging to interpret whether the subendocardial ischemia is secondary to CAD or aortic stenosis.

Moreover, once aortic stenosis is relieved, angiographically evident CAD may have sufficient flow to perfuse a less demanding myocardium. In a small study of 25 patients with severe aortic stenosis and normal coronary arteries, almost half of the patients had ischemic changes on electrocardiogram or echocardiography in response to dipyridamole infusion.[35] These changes disappeared after aortic valve replacement, highlighting the role of wall stress and afterload as ischemic components beyond epicardial coronary stenosis.[35] This finding should not be surprising because myocardial ischemia was not a discriminating factor in identifying suitable patients who may benefit from coronary revascularization.[36]

On the other hand, coronary ischemia assessment using fractional flow reserve (FFR) highlighted incremental benefits of coronary revascularization over medical treatment.[37] However, patients with severe aortic stenosis were excluded from these studies, and the effects of aortic stenosis and left ventricular hypertrophy in achieving maximal hyperemia should be considered when interpreting FFR results. Nonetheless, Pesarini and colleagues[38] showed no significant change in FFR value before and after TAVR, suggesting that FFR is a reliable measure of flow-limiting lesions in the context of severe aortic stenosis. Remarkably, patients with borderline FFR tend to have major variation in FFR post-TAVR, which is inflected on the management of only a small proportion of TAVR patients.[38] Another study investigated the role of instantaneous wave-free ratio (iFR) in evaluating the significance of CAD before and after TAVR. There was no change in the mean iFR value pre-TAVR and post-TAVR regardless of the degree of coronary stenosis.[39] However, individual iFR values varied widely and were more marked in patients with a large drop in transaortic gradient following valve implantation.[39] Therefore, the use of iFR to guide coronary revascularization requires further studies to determine its safety and reliability in this group.

Although the use of intravascular imaging is well established in patients undergoing PCI, data in patients undergoing TAVR are relatively sparse. Intravascular ultrasound-derived minimal luminal area (MLA) is potentially applicable in these patients.[40] Using the MLA cutoff greater than 6 mm^2 for left main coronary disease and greater than 4 mm^2 for non–left main disease may guide the decision to defer revascularization, although this needs to be determined in future prospective studies.[40]

TIMING OF CORONARY REVASCULARIZATION

The best timing of coronary revascularization in patients who are being evaluated for TAVR has not yet been established. Previously, PCI was not commonly performed in patients with severe aortic stenosis because it was thought to be associated with a high risk of procedural complications. This finding was supported by a meta-analysis by Kotronias and colleagues[41] where revascularization pre-TAVR did not show any benefit in relation to 30-day cardiovascular mortality, MI, acute kidney injury (AKI), stroke, or 1-year mortality (Table 1). However, there was an increased rate of major vascular complications and 30-day mortality.[41] It is important to highlight that this meta-analysis examined high-risk patients and did not include the lower-risk population with longer life expectancy.[41] Goel and colleagues[42] demonstrated that PCI can be safely performed in patients with severe aortic stenosis without a significant increase in mortality compared with patients without aortic disease. The feasibility and safety of PCI pre-TAVR have been also explored by Abdel-Wahab and colleagues,[32] whereby they compared 30-day and 6-month clinical outcomes in 2 groups: PCI plus TAVR and isolated TAVR. The 30-day mortality and periprocedural MI were not statistically significant between the 2 groups.[32] Moreover, the 30-day incidence of stroke, major bleeding, and major vascular complications did not differ in both groups.[32] Similarly, improvements in patients' symptoms were comparable between the 2 groups.[32] Another major concern when performing PCI before TAVR is the use of dual antiplatelet therapy (DAPT) and the increased bleeding risk associated with the use of DAPT post-TAVR.[43] Although there are no specific data evaluating bleeding risks with PCI before TAVR versus PCI after TAVR, the need for DAPT should be considered when making the decision of when to perform PCI in TAVR-eligible patients.

The option of concomitant PCI and femoral TAVR seems to be enticing, as it allows for treatment of both issues without increasing the number of arterial accesses. In a small study by Conradi and colleagues[44] of 28 patients, two-thirds of the patients underwent the staged approach involving PCI followed by TAVR, and one-third underwent the combined approach of PCI plus TAVR. There were no differences in periprocedural MI or stroke but longer fluoroscopy times and higher contrast medium usage in the latter group.[44] Ochiai and colleagues[45]

Table 1
Previous meta-analyses reporting outcomes of patients undergoing transcatheter aortic valve replacement according to the status of coronary artery disease

Meta-Analysis	Number of Studies	Number of Patients	Comparison	Endpoint	Outcome
D'Ascenzo et al,[58] 2013	7	2472	CAD vs no CAD	All-cause mortality	OR, 1.0; 95% CI, 0.67–1.50
Phan et al,[59] 2015	5	1634	TAVR vs TAVR plus PCI	30 d all-cause mortality	RR, 0.80; 95% CI, 0.35–1,83
Taha et al,[60] 2015	3	979	Residual SYNTAX of 0 vs residual SYNTAX ≤10	30 d all-cause mortality	OR, 1.08; 95% CI, 0.65–1.80
Bajaj et al,[61] 2017	7	1631	TAVR vs TAVR plus PCI	30 d all-cause mortality	OR, 0.91; 95% CI, 0.51–1.63
Kotronias et al,[41] 2017	9	3858	TAVR vs TAVR plus PCI	30 d all-cause mortality	OR, 1.42; 95% CI, 1.08–1.87
Sankaramangalam et al,[28] 2017	15	8013	CAD vs no CAD	30 d all-cause mortality	OR, 1.07; 95% CI, 0.82–1.40
Yang et al,[62] 2017	4	209	Concomitant PCI and TAVR vs staged PCI and TAVR	30 d all-cause mortality	OR, 1.47; 95% CI, 0.47–4.62
Witberg et al,[63] 2018	6	3107	ICR (using residual SYNTAX) vs no CAD or reasonable ICR	All-cause mortality	OR, 1.85; 95% CI, 1.42–2.40 (for no CAD) OR, 1.69; 95% CI, 1.26–2.28 (for reasonable ICR)
Bao et al,[64] 2018	5	1634	TAVR vs TAVR plus PCI	30 d all-cause mortality	OR, 1.25; 95% CI, 0.52–3.05
D'Ascenzo et al,[30] 2018	13	8334	The impact of CAD severity and PCI using SYNTAX and residual SYNTAX, respectively	One-year all-cause mortality	OR, 1.71; 95% CI, 1.24–2.36 (for SYNTAX >22) OR, 0.34; 95% CI, 0.012–0.93 for residual SYNTAX <8)
Lateef et al,[27] 2020	11	5580	TAVR vs TAVR plus PCI	30 d all-cause mortality	OR, 1.30; 95% CI, 0.85–1.98
Prasitlumkum et al,[65] 2020	11	7299	Previous CABG vs no CABG	All-cause mortality	RR, 0.96; 95% CI, 0.80–1.16

Abbreviations: CABG, coronary artery bypass graft; CI, confidence interval; ICR, incomplete revascularization; OR, odds ratio; RR, relative risk.
    Data from Refs.[27,28,30,58–65]

compared clinical outcomes according to timing of PCI in relation to TAVR procedure. The decision about PCI timing, pre-TAVR, concomitant, or post-TAVR was made by the heart team according to the patients' clinical status and location of the target lesion. PCI performed simultaneously with TAVR was not associated with an increased risk of AKI, major vascular complications, life-threatening bleeding, or adverse clinical events compared with the staged pre-TAVR or post-TAVR.[45] The study also suggested a potential advantage of post-TAVR PCI with reduced risk of ischemia and hemodynamic instability during PCI.[45]

CORONARY EVENTS FOLLOWING TRANSCATHETER AORTIC VALVE REPLACEMENT

Coronary events, including acute coronary syndrome (ACS), following TAVR are not uncommon, with 10% of patients presenting with at least 1 episode of ACS following TAVR.[46] The highest incidence of ACS has been recorded within 1 year from the procedure.[46] Male gender, preexisting CAD, and nonfemoral accesses are considered risk factors for ACS post-TAVR.[46] The most common presentation of ACS post-TAVR was non-ST segment elevation myocardial infarction (NSTEMI), and in a study by Vilalta and colleagues,[46] the rate of NSTEMI was 64.1%, followed by unstable angina at 34.6%, and STEMI at 1.3%. The low incidence of STEMI in this population has been attributed to the presence of collateral circulation in the elderly population undergoing TAVR, the use of systemic anticoagulation post-TAVR, and careful revascularization strategy before TAVR.[46] A recent study by Faroux and colleagues[47] recorded similar ACS presentations post-TAVR.[47] In this multicenter cohort study of 270 patients, the incidence of type 1 and type 2 NSTEMI was 31.9% and 31.5%, respectively, compared with 8.1% STEMI over median follow-up of 12 months post-TAVR. Revascularization was associated with a reduction in all-cause mortality by 46%, after multiple adjustments to known risk factors.

Post-TAVR ACS was associated with 4% to 10% in-hospital mortality and high mid-term mortality of 37% to 43% within 2 years of follow-up.[46,47] About one-quarter of patients develop congestive heart failure and another quarter develop AKI. STEMI presentation was associated with increased morality risk, whereas revascularization at the time of ACS was linked to a reduction in mortality risk.[47] Interestingly,

Faroux and colleagues[47] compared coronary catheterization images done before TAVR or during TAVR, and at the presentations of ACS and noticed that most coronary lesions were newly developed lesions that were nonexistent or not significant before TAVR.[47] Other mechanisms of ACS were proposed, such as coronary hypoperfusion related to the TAVR bioprosthesis, coronary embolism secondary to subclinical leaflet thrombosis, and impaired coronary flow dynamic.[9]

Notably, the proportion of patients who underwent coronary angiography for ACS presentation post-TAVR was relatively low.[46,47] Access to coronary arteries was challenging in 1 in 40 patients, and catheter techniques data in post-TAVR PCI patients are still evolving.[46,47] Boukantar and colleagues[48] reported higher fluoroscopic times, radiation dosage, and contrast medium use when compared with standard PCI without the presence of TAVR with selective engagement of both coronary ostia in 50% patients. Similarly, Allali and colleagues[49] showed similar challenges with up to 10 guiding catheters used to engage coronary ostia, and failure to engage the culprit artery during emergency PCI. Interestingly, both studies reported use of self-expanding valves, often times dictating different approaches to access the coronaries. Blumenstein and colleagues[23] reported that coronary angiography was easily performed with balloon-expandable valves (but not self-expanding valves). The investigators described more frequent use of different catheters or performing an aortogram in the self-expanding group. Importantly, careful planning and procedural experience may facilitate successful engagements of coronary ostia, particularly when choosing TAVR valve in low-risk patients.[50] In a study by Zivelonghi and colleagues,[22] patients with both balloon-expandable and self-expanding valves had satisfactory coronary ostia engagement. Extra assistance from guidewire was needed for selective engagement in 4% of the targeted vessels, and only 1 vessel access was not achieved in the study because of high implantation of the balloon-expandable valve. Importantly, rotational atherectomy as well as intravascular imaging was also successfully performed in patients after TAVR.[22,51] A recent study has proposed the use of guiding catheter extension for better engagement of coronary ostia (Fig. 1).[52]

These studies highlighted the need for special consideration when positioning a self-expanding valve to ensure easy access to coronary ostia in the future. These considerations are related to

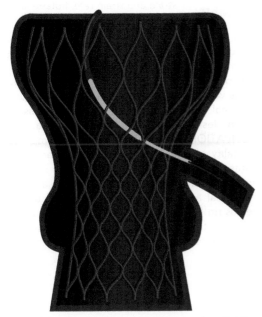

Fig. 1. The use of guiding catheter extension. Guiding catheter extensions can help in improving the engagement of coronary ostia.

valve depth and alignment of the TAVR commissures. Placing the self-expanding valve 4 mm below the annular plane will ensure that the valve skirt is not overlaying over the coronary ostia, unless patients have low coronary height.[53] The skirt height of current Evolut valves is 13-mm with the exception of the 34-mm Evolut R, where the skirt height is 14 mm. The implantation depth needs to be balanced to

allow future coronary access and minimize pacemaker rate.[53] Coaxial engagement is feasible in this position unless the native aortic leaflets interfere with accessing coronary ostia. Importantly, in the presence of sufficient sinus of Valsalva width, higher implantation may not lead to coronary obstruction because of the narrow waist of the self-expanding valve.[53] However, this may pose challenges to selective coronary angiography, as access will have to occur from a diamond above the coronary artery ostium. Recent data suggest some markers to help in alignment of the new commissure of the self-expanding valve.[54] Although the commissure is recommended to be introduced facing the anterior wall of the aorta, it is not possible to determine the final position until after the valve has been released.[53] Ensuring the Evolut "Hat" marker is facing the outer curve or central forward positions at deployment may render overlap of the coronary ostia with new valve commissures less likely, facilitating future coronary access (Fig. 2).[54,55]

Similar considerations are applicable to balloon-expandable valves. Because of the lack of the valve waist, the balloon-expandable valve is associated with a higher risk of coronary obstruction with partial overlay of coronary ostia reported in more than one-third of patients.[56,57] Importantly, however, access to coronary ostia has been less challenging in balloon-expandable valves.[50,57] Higher implantation may compromise coronary access, although this may remain feasible using the cells in the top row; the newer generation valve has 38%

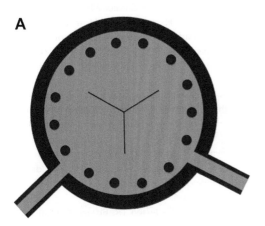

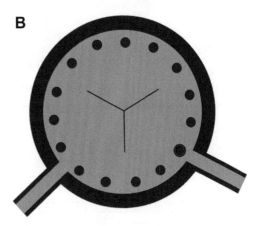

Fig. 2. (A) A cross-sectional view of the location of transcatheter heart valve in relation to the coronary ostia. The valve cells are aligned with the ostia allowing access. (B) A cross-sectional view of the location of transcatheter heart valve in relation to the coronary ostia. The valve cells are offset from the ostia, which can impede access.

larger area than Sapien XT.[53] Another consideration is related to a low sinotubular junction (STJ), whereby the balloon-expandable frame may extend beyond the STJ, making superior access (above the bioprosthetic valve) very challenging.[53] Unlike the self-expanding valve, crimped orientation had no impact on commissural alignment in the balloon-expanding valve.[55]

To aid in the visualization of anatomy and decision of reaccess post-TAVR, a multidetector CT can be used (Fig. 3). The 3-dimensional (3D) reconstruction allows the visualization of the stent frame in relation to the coronary ostia; however, the commissural posts are not well visualized.[53] The used contrast medium needs to be taken into consideration when using it in evaluation before elective coronary catheterization, specifically in renal insufficiency patients. Furthermore, motion artifact, image quality, and user interpretation of 3D structures can vary and affect the visualization of leaflet orientation of the TAVR to the coronary ostia.[53] Despite these restrictions, 3D CT still offers anatomic visualization of the valve in relation to the surrounding structures and aids in reducing challenges and longer times of PCI post-TAVR.

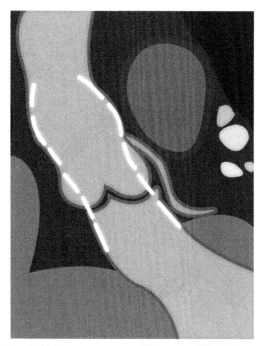

Fig. 3. Valve appearance on CT imaging. 3D CT imaging can offer visualization of the valve in relation to the surrounding anatomic structures and help reduce challenges and time to PCI post-TAVR.

SUMMARY

CAD commonly coexists with aortic stenosis, and decision regarding revascularization remains debatable. A selective approach has been proposed in which PCI may be considered in patients with large areas of ischemic myocardium, proximal lesions in major epicardial vessels, and/or lesions that contribute to angina. The ACTIVATION trial (ISRCTN75836930) compared mortality and rehospitalization at 1 year in patients with symptomatic, severe aortic stenosis and ≥1 proximal stenosis of ≥70% in a major epicardial artery who were randomized to PCI versus no PCI pre-TAVR. Future studies will aid in generating guidelines and more consistency when approaching CAD in patients undergoing TAVR.

DISCLOSURE

None.

REFERENCES

1. Patel MR, Calhoon JH, Dehmer GJ, et al. ACC/AATS/AHA/ASE/ASNC/SCAI/SCCT/STS 2017 Appropriate Use Criteria for Coronary Revascularization in Patients With Stable Ischemic Heart Disease: a rEPORT of the American College of Cardiology Appropriate Use Criteria Task Force, American Association for Thoracic Surgery, American Heart Association, American Society of Echocardiography, American Society of Nuclear Cardiology, Society for Cardiovascular Angiography and Interventions, Society of Cardiovascular Computed Tomography, and Society of Thoracic Surgeons. J Am Coll Cardiol 2017;69:2212–41.
2. Baumgartner H, Falk V, Bax JJ, et al. 2017 ESC/EACTS Guidelines for the management of valvular heart disease. Eur Heart J 2017;38:2739–91.
3. Aronow WS, Schwartz KS, Koenigsberg M. Correlation of serum lipids, calcium, and phosphorus, diabetes mellitus and history of systemic hypertension with presence or absence of calcified or thickened aortic cusps or root in elderly patients. Am J Cardiol 1987;59:998–9.
4. Stewart BF, Siscovick D, Lind BK, et al. Clinical factors associated with calcific aortic valve disease. Cardiovascular Health Study. J Am Coll Cardiol 1997;29:630–4.
5. Rossebo AB, Pedersen TR, Boman K, et al. Intensive lipid lowering with simvastatin and ezetimibe in aortic stenosis. N Engl J Med 2008;359:1343–56.
6. Otto CM, Lind BK, Kitzman DW, et al. Association of aortic-valve sclerosis with cardiovascular mortality and morbidity in the elderly. N Engl J Med 1999; 341:142–7.

7. Ortlepp JR, Schmitz F, Bozoglu T, et al. Cardiovascular risk factors in patients with aortic stenosis predict prevalence of coronary artery disease but not of aortic stenosis: an angiographic pair matched case-control study. Heart 2003;89:1019–22.

8. Walther T, Hamm CW, Schuler G, et al. Perioperative results and complications in 15,964 transcatheter aortic valve replacements: prospective data from the GARY Registry. J Am Coll Cardiol 2015;65:2173–80.

9. Faroux L, Guimaraes L, Wintzer-Wehekind J, et al. Coronary artery disease and transcatheter aortic valve replacement: JACC state-of-the-art review. J Am Coll Cardiol 2019;74:362–72.

10. Smith CR, Leon MB, Mack MJ, et al. Transcatheter versus surgical aortic-valve replacement in high-risk patients. N Engl J Med 2011;364:2187–98.

11. Popma JJ, Adams DH, Reardon MJ, et al. Transcatheter aortic valve replacement using a self-expanding bioprosthesis in patients with severe aortic stenosis at extreme risk for surgery. J Am Coll Cardiol 2014;63:1972–81.

12. Mack MJ, Leon MB, Thourani VH, et al. Transcatheter aortic-valve replacement with a balloon-expandable valve in low-risk patients. N Engl J Med 2019;380:1695–705.

13. Popma JJ, Deeb GM, Yakubov SJ, et al. Transcatheter aortic-valve replacement with a self-expanding valve in low-risk patients. N Engl J Med 2019;380:1706–15.

14. Knuuti J, Wijns W, Saraste A, et al. 2019 ESC Guidelines for the diagnosis and management of chronic coronary syndromes. Eur Heart J 2020;41:407–77.

15. Tansuphaswadikul S, Silaruks S, Lehmongkol R, et al. Frequency of angina pectoris and coronary artery disease in severe isolated valvular aortic stenosis. J Med Assoc Thai 1999;82:140–9.

16. Beach JM, Mihaljevic T, Svensson LG, et al. Coronary artery disease and outcomes of aortic valve replacement for severe aortic stenosis. J Am Coll Cardiol 2013;61:837–48.

17. Lund O, Nielsen TT, Pilegaard HK, et al. The influence of coronary artery disease and bypass grafting on early and late survival after valve replacement for aortic stenosis. J Thorac Cardiovasc Surg 1990;100:327–37.

18. Mullany CJ, Elveback LR, Frye RL, et al. Coronary artery disease and its management: influence on survival in patients undergoing aortic valve replacement. J Am Coll Cardiol 1987;10:66–72.

19. Fefer P, Bogdan A, Grossman Y, et al. Impact of rapid ventricular pacing on outcome after transcatheter aortic valve replacement. J Am Heart Assoc 2018;7:e009038.

20. Axell RG, White PA, Giblett JP, et al. Rapid pacing-induced right ventricular dysfunction is evident after balloon-expandable transfemoral aortic valve replacement. J Am Coll Cardiol 2017;69:903–4.

21. Axell RG, Giblett JP, White PA, et al. Stunning and right ventricular dysfunction is induced by coronary balloon occlusion and rapid pacing in humans: insights from right ventricular conductance catheter studies. J Am Heart Assoc 2017;6:e005820.

22. Zivelonghi C, Pesarini G, Scarsini R, et al. Coronary catheterization and percutaneous interventions after transcatheter aortic valve implantation. Am J Cardiol 2017;120:625–31.

23. Blumenstein J, Kim WK, Liebetrau C, et al. Challenges of coronary angiography and intervention in patients previously treated by TAVI. Clin Res Cardiol 2015;104:632–9.

24. Thielmann M, Massoudy P, Neuhauser M, et al. Prognostic value of preoperative cardiac troponin I in patients with non-ST-segment elevation acute coronary syndromes undergoing coronary artery bypass surgery. Chest 2005;128:3526–36.

25. Danson E, Hansen P, Sen S, et al. Assessment, treatment, and prognostic implications of CAD in patients undergoing TAVI. Nat Rev Cardiol 2016;13:276–85.

26. van den Boogert TPW, Vendrik J, Claessen B, et al. CTCA for detection of significant coronary artery disease in routine TAVI work-up: a systematic review and meta-analysis. Neth Heart J 2018;26:591–9.

27. Lateef N, Khan MS, Deo SV, et al. Meta-analysis comparing outcomes in patients undergoing transcatheter aortic valve implantation with versus without percutaneous coronary intervention. Am J Cardiol 2019;124:1757–64.

28. Sankaramangalam K, Banerjee K, Kandregula K, et al. Impact of coronary artery disease on 30-day and 1-year mortality in patients undergoing transcatheter aortic valve replacement: a meta-analysis. J Am Heart Assoc 2017;6:e006092.

29. Khawaja MZ, Asrress KN, Haran H, et al. The effect of coronary artery disease defined by quantitative coronary angiography and SYNTAX score upon outcome after transcatheter aortic valve implantation (TAVI) using the Edwards bioprosthesis. EuroIntervention 2015;11:450–5.

30. D'Ascenzo F, Verardi R, Visconti M, et al. Independent impact of extent of coronary artery disease and percutaneous revascularisation on 30-day and one-year mortality after TAVI: a meta-analysis of adjusted observational results. EuroIntervention 2018;14:e1169–77.

31. Witberg G, Regev E, Chen S, et al. The prognostic effects of coronary disease severity and completeness of revascularization on mortality in patients undergoing transcatheter aortic valve replacement. JACC Cardiovasc Interv 2017;10:1428–35.

32. Abdel-Wahab M, Mostafa AE, Geist V, et al. Comparison of outcomes in patients having isolated transcatheter aortic valve implantation versus

combined with preprocedural percutaneous coronary intervention. Am J Cardiol 2012;109:581–6.

33. Abramowitz Y, Banai S, Katz G, et al. Comparison of early and late outcomes of TAVI alone compared to TAVI plus PCI in aortic stenosis patients with and without coronary artery disease. Catheter Cardiovasc Interv 2014;83:649–54.

34. Cremer PC, Khalaf S, Lou J, et al. Stress positron emission tomography is safe and can guide coronary revascularization in high-risk patients being considered for transcatheter aortic valve replacement. J Nucl Cardiol 2014;21:1001–10.

35. Baroni M, Maffei S, Terrazzi M, et al. Mechanisms of regional ischaemic changes during dipyridamole echocardiography in patients with severe aortic valve stenosis and normal coronary arteries. Heart 1996;75:492–7.

36. Maron DJ, Hochman JS, Reynolds HR, et al. Initial invasive or conservative strategy for stable coronary disease. N Engl J Med 2020;382:1395–407.

37. De Bruyne B, Pijls NH, Kalesan B, et al. Fractional flow reserve-guided PCI versus medical therapy in stable coronary disease. N Engl J Med 2012;367:991–1001.

38. Pesarini G, Scarsini R, Zivelonghi C, et al. Functional assessment of coronary artery disease in patients undergoing transcatheter aortic valve implantation: influence of pressure overload on the evaluation of lesions severity. Circ Cardiovasc Interv 2016;9:e004088.

39. Scarsini R, Pesarini G, Zivelonghi C, et al. Physiologic evaluation of coronary lesions using instantaneous wave-free ratio (iFR) in patients with severe aortic stenosis undergoing transcatheter aortic valve implantation. EuroIntervention 2018;13:1512–9.

40. Patel JS, Kapadia SR. Coronary artery disease and transcatheter aortic valve replacement: when to intervene. Interv Cardiol Clin 2018;7:471–5.

41. Kotronias RA, Kwok CS, George S, et al. Transcatheter aortic valve implantation with or without percutaneous coronary artery revascularization strategy: a systematic review and meta-analysis. J Am Heart Assoc 2017;6:e005960.

42. Goel SS, Agarwal S, Tuzcu EM, et al. Percutaneous coronary intervention in patients with severe aortic stenosis: implications for transcatheter aortic valve replacement. Circulation 2012;125:1005–13.

43. Brouwer J, Nijenhuis VJ, Delewi R, et al. Aspirin with or without clopidogrel after transcatheter aortic-valve implantation. N Engl J Med 2020;383(15):1447–57.

44. Conradi L, Seiffert M, Franzen O, et al. First experience with transcatheter aortic valve implantation and concomitant percutaneous coronary intervention. Clin Res Cardiol 2011;100:311–6.

45. Ochiai T, Yoon SH, Flint N, et al. Timing and outcomes of percutaneous coronary intervention in patients who underwent transcatheter aortic valve implantation. Am J Cardiol 2020;125:1361–8.

46. Vilalta V, Asmarats L, Ferreira-Neto AN, et al. Incidence, clinical characteristics, and impact of acute coronary syndrome following transcatheter aortic valve replacement. JACC Cardiovasc Interv 2018;11:2523–33.

47. Faroux L, Munoz-Garcia E, Serra V, et al. Acute coronary syndrome following transcatheter aortic valve replacement. Circ Cardiovasc Interv 2020;13:e008620.

48. Boukantar M, Gallet R, Mouillet G, et al. Coronary procedures after TAVI with the self-expanding aortic bioprosthesis Medtronic CoreValve, not an easy matter. J Interv Cardiol 2017;30:56–62.

49. Allali A, El-Mawardy M, Schwarz B, et al. Incidence, feasibility and outcome of percutaneous coronary intervention after transcatheter aortic valve implantation with a self-expanding prosthesis. Results from a single center experience. Cardiovasc Revasc Med 2016;17:391–8.

50. Tarantini G, Nai Fovino L, Le Prince P, et al. Coronary access and percutaneous coronary intervention up to 3 years after transcatheter aortic valve implantation with a balloon-expandable valve. Circ Cardiovasc Interv 2020;13:e008972.

51. Htun WW, Grines C, Schreiber T. Feasibility of coronary angiography and percutaneous coronary intervention after transcatheter aortic valve replacement using a Medtronic self-expandable bioprosthetic valve. Catheter Cardiovasc Interv 2018;91:1339–44.

52. Bharadwaj AS, Bhatheja S, Sharma SK, et al. Utility of the guideliner catheter for percutaneous coronary interventions in patients with prior transcatheter aortic valve replacement. Catheter Cardiovasc Interv 2018;91:271–6.

53. Yudi MB, Sharma SK, Tang GHL, et al. Coronary angiography and percutaneous coronary intervention after transcatheter aortic valve replacement. J Am Coll Cardiol 2018;71:1360–78.

54. Tang GHL, Zaid S, Gupta E, et al. Impact of initial evolut transcatheter aortic valve replacement deployment orientation on final valve orientation and coronary reaccess. Circ Cardiovasc Interv 2019;12:e008044.

55. Tang GHL, Zaid S, Fuchs A, et al. Alignment of transcatheter aortic-valve neo-commissures (ALIGN TAVR): impact on final valve orientation and coronary artery overlap. JACC Cardiovasc Interv 2020;13:1030–42.

56. Ribeiro HB, Webb JG, Makkar RR, et al. Predictive factors, management, and clinical outcomes of coronary obstruction following transcatheter aortic valve implantation: insights from a large multicenter registry. J Am Coll Cardiol 2013;62:1552–62.

57. Katsanos S, Debonnaire P, van der Kley F, et al. Position of Edwards SAPIEN transcatheter valve in the

aortic root in relation with the coronary ostia: implications for percutaneous coronary interventions. Catheter Cardiovasc Interv 2015;85:480–7.

58. D'Ascenzo F, Conrotto F, Giordana F, et al. Mid-term prognostic value of coronary artery disease in patients undergoing transcatheter aortic valve implantation: a meta-analysis of adjusted observational results. Int J Cardiol 2013;168:2528–32.

59. Phan K, Wong S, Phan S, et al. Early outcomes of isolated transcatheter aortic valve implantation versus combined with percutaneous coronary intervention. Int J Cardiol 2015;179:258–61.

60. Taha S, Moretti C, D'Ascenzo F, et al. Impact of residual coronary artery disease on patients undergoing TAVI: a meta-analysis of adjusted observational studies. Int J Cardiol 2015;181:77–80.

61. Bajaj A, Pancholy S, Sethi A, et al. Safety and feasibility of PCI in patients undergoing TAVR: a systematic review and meta-analysis. Heart Lung 2017;46: 92–9.

62. Yang Y, Huang FY, Huang BT, et al. The safety of concomitant transcatheter aortic valve replacement and percutaneous coronary intervention: a systematic review and meta-analysis. Medicine (Baltimore) 2017;96:e8919.

63. Witberg G, Zusman O, Codner P, et al. Impact of coronary artery revascularization completeness on outcomes of patients with coronary artery disease undergoing transcatheter aortic valve replacement: a meta-analysis of studies using the residual SYNTAX Score (Synergy Between PCI With Taxus and Cardiac Surgery). Circ Cardiovasc Interv 2018;11: e006000.

64. Bao L, Gao Q, Chen S, et al. Feasibility and safety of combined percutaneous coronary intervention among high-risk patients with severe aortic stenosis undergoing transcatheter aortic valve implantation: a systematic review and meta-analysis. Eur J Cardiothorac Surg 2018;54:1052–9.

65. Prasitlumkum N, Kewcharoen J, Kanitsoraphan C, et al. Previous coronary artery bypass graft is not associated with higher mortality in transcatheter aortic valve replacement: systemic review and meta-analysis. Acta Cardiol 2020;75:26–34.

Transcatheter Aortic Valve Replacement
Advances in Procedural Technology and Approaches

John C. Lisko III, MD, MPH[a], Nikoloz Shekiladze, MD[a],
Pratik Sandesara, MD[a],
Chandan M. Devireddy, MD, MBA, FSCAI[b],*

KEYWORDS

- TAVR • Bicuspid aortic valve • Cerebral embolic protection • Innovation • Vascular closure

---

KEY POINTS

- Continued innovation will expand the indications of transcatheter aortic valve replacement (TAVR).
- New technologies will continue to make TAVR a safe a reproducible technique.
- Valve durability and the feasibility of routine redo TAVR remain uncertain.

CASE PRESENTATION
Case Presentation—Alternate Access Transcatheter Aortic Valve Replacement with Cusp-Overlap Technique

An 82-year-old woman with a past medical history significant for coronary artery disease status post prior 3-vessel coronary artery bypass grafting, mitral valve repair with a semirigid mitral ring and history of chronic kidney disease stage III, and peripheral artery disease presents to the Structural Heart and Valve Clinic with a chief complaint of progressively worsening shortness of breath and recent syncope. Echocardiography reveals severe aortic stenosis (mean gradient: 48 mm Hg; aortic valve area: 0.8 cm^2). The patient undergoes subsequent left-heart catheterization revealing patent bypass grafts. Her electrocardiogram is notable for a right bundle branch block. Gated cardiac computed tomography reveals an annular perimeter of 58 mm, an annular area of 285 mm^2, and stenosis in both femoral arteries (circumferential calcium, minimal diameter <5.5 cm). Given the patient's symptoms and high risk for pacemaker implantation, the heart team deems her a candidate for transcaval transcatheter aortic valve replacement using a self-expandable valve with the cusp overlap technique.

INTRODUCTION

Transcatheter aortic valve replacement (TAVR) is now the dominant form of aortic valve replacement (AVR).[1] Since the first implant in 2002, randomized controlled trials (RCT) have been completed in patients at all levels of surgical risk, showing superior or equal outcomes to surgical AVR.[2,3]

Advances in technology have made the technique simpler, safer, and reproducible; however, several important questions remain unanswered:

1. Can new valve platforms improve patient outcomes?
2. Is TAVR safe and feasible in patients with bicuspid aortic valves?

---

[a] Division of Cardiology, Emory University School of Medicine, Peachtree Street NE, 4th Floor Davis-Fischer Building, Atlanta, GA 30308, USA; [b] Division of Cardiology, Emory University School of Medicine, Emory University Hospital Midtown, Peachtree Street NE, 4th Floor Davis-Fischer Building, Atlanta, GA 30308, USA
* Corresponding author.
E-mail address: cdevire@emory.edu

Intervent Cardiol Clin 10 (2021) 565–578
https://doi.org/10.1016/j.iccl.2021.06.008
2211-7458/21/© 2021 Elsevier Inc. All rights reserved.

3. Can novel pacing and access strategies simplify TAVR?
4. Can vascular closure devices (VCDs) decrease access site complications?

Herein, the authors describe advances in transcatheter heart valves (THV) and adjunctive technologies, with an emphasis on Heart Team decision making and ongoing clinical trials.

NEW VALVE TECHNOLOGIES
SAPIEN 3 Ultra

The SAPIEN 3 Ultra THV System (Fig. 1) (Edwards Lifesciences, Irvine, California, USA) is a design iteration of the SAPIEN 3 THV System and was approved on December 28, 2018, obtaining an expanded indication to treat low-risk patients in 2019. The most important differences between Ultra and S3 pertain to the textured polyethylene terephthalate (PET) outer skirt, which has an approximately 40% increased height designed to allow up to 50% more surface contact area with native valve anatomy, aimed at improved annular sealing. In addition, the outer skirt was replaced by a textured sealing PET structure, which was designed to promote enhanced healing and endothelialization. The added external skirt design has been introduced in 20-mm, 23-mm, and 26-mm SAPIEN 3 Ultra valves, but not in the 29-mm valve, which remains the current S3 model. This new-iteration valve was initially introduced along with the SAPIEN 3 Ultra Delivery System (Edwards Lifesciences), which was designed to allow the THV to be crimped directly onto the deployment balloon, eliminating the need for valve alignment and reducing the number of procedural steps and the Axela Sheath (Edwards Lifesciences), which had a reduced profile of 14French across all valve sizes. However, reports of burst balloons during some implantation procedures using the new delivery system, which resulted in a few cases of vascular injury, bleeding, and the need for surgical intervention, led the Food and Drug Administration (FDA) to issue a class I recall for the SAPIEN 3 Ultra delivery system in August 2019. Following this recall, the new delivery system and the Axela Sheath were replaced by the previous-generation Edwards Commander (Edwards Lifesciences) and the eSheath (Edwards Lifesciences).[4]

In S3U registry, which is a physician-led, post-approval, multicenter registry of transfemoral transcatheter aortic valve replacement (TAVR) with SAPIEN 3 Ultra, the 30-day safety and efficacy outcomes were evaluated in 139 consecutive patients at 9 participating centers. In-hospital, there were no cases of death, stroke, or conversion to open heart surgery. Major vascular complications occurred in 3 patients (2.2%), as well as major or life-threatening bleeding in 3 patients (2.2%). There were 2 moderate (1.4%) and no moderate/severe paravalvular leaks. At 30 days, there were no deaths, myocardial infarction (MI), or strokes, and the incidence of new permanent pacemaker implantation was 4.4%. Overall, this registry study showed good in-hospital and 30-day clinical outcomes.[5]

In a recent retrospective single-center study from Germany, Rheude and colleagues[6] compared outcomes of SAPIEN 3 Ultra versus SAPIEN 3 in a one-to-one propensity score-matched cohort of patients (n = 310). All in-

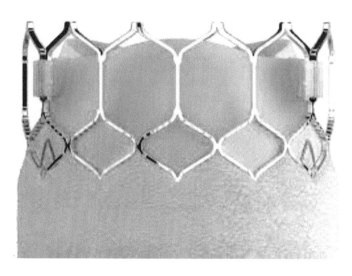

Fig. 1. Sapien 3 ultra valve. (© 2021 Edwards Lifesciences LLC, Irvine, CA [https://www.edwards.com/devices/heart-valves/transcatheter].)

hospital outcomes were comparable between S3 and S3 Ultra, including major vascular complications (12.3% vs 11.0%; $P = .723$), pacemaker implantation (5.8% vs 4.5%; $P = .608$), and rate of moderate or greater paravalvular leakage (PVL) (1.3% vs 2.7%; $P = .414$). There was a significantly lower rate of mild PVL with Ultra compared with S3 (18.7% vs 43.0%; $P<.001$). In conclusion, this propensity-matched comparison showed high device success rates with both valves, comparable rates of death and other clinical outcomes up to 30 days after TAVR, and overall significant reduction in mild PVL with S3 Ultra valve compared with S3.

Jena Valve

The self-expanding JenaValve (Fig. 2) (JenaValve Technology, Inc, Irvine, CA, USA) is made of a porcine pericardial root mounted on a low-profile nitinol stent frame. It relies on an active clip fixation of the native aortic valve leaflets.[7] This platform does not require significant radial force for deployment unlike other transcatheter aortic valve designs, thereby minimizing interactions with aortic structures. The unique clip fixation mechanism can provide secure anchoring to the native leaflets even in the absence of calcification and therefore may be used successfully for the treatment of noncalcified pure aortic regurgitation (AR). A sealing ring at the bottom of the valve is made of 24 diamond-shaped cells that provide annular conformability and sealing. The valve design with anatomic positioning of locators provides alignment with the native valve and limits interactions with the conduction system. Locators fixate on native leaflets, thereby preventing coronary obstruction. The valve is available in 3 different sizes (23 mm, 25 mm, and 27 mm) for implantation in native aortic annuli ranging from 21 to 27 mm in diameter. The device is deployed in a 3-step procedure using either a sheathless 32F delivery catheter via transapical approach or an 18F transfemoral delivery system comprising 3 coaxial catheters. Rapid pacing is not required during the procedure.[7,8]

In 2013, Seiffert and colleagues[9] presented initial clinical evidence that the JenaValve prosthesis might be a reasonable option in selected high-risk patients with severe noncalcified AR. Implantation was successful in all cases (n = 5) with no relevant remaining AR or signs of stenosis in any of the patients. No major device-related or procedure-related adverse events occurred, and all 5 patients were alive at 3-month follow-up. JenaValve received the CE mark approval for treatment of patients with

aortic stenosis (AS) in 2011 and for treatment of patients with noncalcified AR since 2013.[10]

A pivotal study for CE mark approval was a multicenter, prospective single-arm study conducted in Germany on 73 patients with severe aortic stenosis who were implanted with transapical JenaValve.[11] Sixty-seven elective implantations were attempted in these patients. TAVR was successful in 60 patients (89.6%) with perioperative stroke seen in 2 cases (3%). Most of the successfully treated patients revealed no or minimal PVL (86.4%). At 6 months, transvalvular gradients, systolic function, prevalence of PVL, and the effective orifice area (EOA) remained comparable to early postprocedural measurements. The overall mortality at 20 days was 7.6%.

One-year outcomes of transapical aortic valve implantation with second-generation JenaValve devices in AR were analyzed in the 30-patient Jupiter registry.[12] Procedural success was achieved in 96.7% (29/30). Mortality at 30 days was 10.0% (3/30). Combined safety endpoint at 30 days (all-cause mortality, major stroke, life-threatening or disabling bleeding, acute kidney injury stage III, periprocedural MI, major vascular complication, and repeated procedure for valve related dysfunction) in accordance with the Valve Academic Research Consortium Document (VARC-I) endpoint definitions was met in

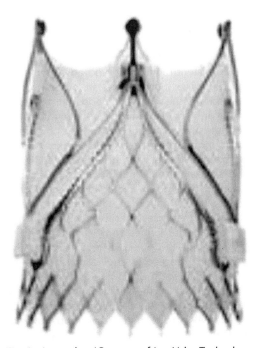

Fig. 2. Jena valve. (*Courtesy of* JenaValve Technology, Inc; with permission.)

13.3% of patients (4/30). Trivial or absence of PVL was seen in 84.6% (22/26), and mild PVL was seen in 15.4% (4/26). Rate of permanent pacemaker implantation was 3.8% (1/26). One-year Kaplan-Meier survival was 79.9%.

The first patient treated with a transfemoral delivery system was in 2014, with new generations of delivery systems developed since then. An 18F delivery catheter allows stepwise deployment using a rotator knob with a deflector allowing for accurate and precise placement of locators over cusps and a controller mechanism to maintain position. The ongoing ALIGN-AR pivotal trial (NCT04415047) will examine the use of JenaValve patients with symptomatic severe AR and high surgical risk.

In 2020, JenaValve received a "Breakthrough Device" designation from the FDA as the first transcatheter device to achieve this designation for severe AR and AR-dominant mixed aortic valve disease in patients at high risk for surgery.[13]

Evolut PRO+

The Evolut PRO+ TAVR System (Fig. 3) (Medtronic Plc, Dublin, Ireland) is the newest generation of the self-expanding valve within Evolut family, which received FDA approval September 2019. The advantage of this generation valve is that it can treat the broad annulus range and offers low delivery profile (the 23-, 26- and 29-mm valves with access vessel down to 5-mm and 34-mm valve with access vessel down to 6 mm). Consistent with the Evolut platform design, the PRO+ valve is designed with a self-expanding nitinol frame that conforms to the native annulus with consistent radial force and advanced sealing. The valve incorporates an outer porcine pericardial tissue wrap that adds surface area contact and tissue interaction between the valve and the native aortic annulus to help potentially reduce incidence of paravalvular leaks. Adding the external tissue wrap to the large 34-mm valve size, which was not previously available, is a major change in Evolut PRO+ compared with Evolut PRO, allowing utilization in patients with larger anatomies. The Evolut PRO+ valves can treat annulus ranges from 18 mm to 30 mm.

The Evolut PRO transcatheter aortic valve (Medtronic) represents the earlier-generation self-expanding valve within the CoreValve Evolut family. Building off the Evolut R valve platform, the Evolut PRO valve was modified to include an external porcine pericardial wrap covering the first 1.5 cells (∼12 mm). The aim is to enhance annular sealing, minimize PVL, and derive benefits of a low-profile, self-expanding

valve with supra-annular function. Like the Evolut R valve, the Evolut PRO valve can be recaptured or repositioned to assist in optimal positioning at the level of the aortic annulus. The self-expanding nitinol frame with supra-annular porcine pericardial leaflets is otherwise unchanged from the Evolut R valve design.

Forrest and colleagues[14] described early outcomes with Evolut PRO in 60 patients with symptomatic severe aortic stenosis at increased surgical risk. At 30 days, it demonstrated excellent hemodynamics and mild PVL with 1.7% mortality and 1.7% nonfatal disabling stroke. Paravalvular regurgitation at 30 days was absent or trace in 72.4%, and no more than mild in the remainder of patients. The mean atrioventricular gradient was 6.4 ± 2.1 mm Hg, and EOA was 2.0 ± 0.5 cm^2 at 30 days.

Following the early clinical outcomes at 30 days from the Evolut PRO US Study, follow-up data in 60 patients, which were presented at ACC.18, continued to demonstrate low rates of PVL with 88% of patients showing no or trace PVL at 6 months. In addition, rates of all-cause

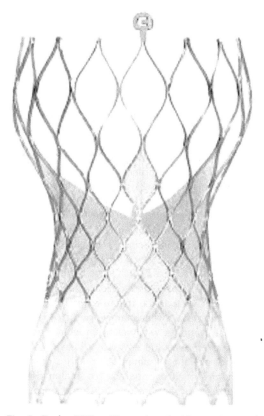

Fig. 3. Evolut PRO+. (*Reproduced with permission of Medtronic, Inc.*)

mortality and disabling stroke were low at 6 months with no instances of coronary obstruction or valve thrombosis. Permanent pacemakers were implanted in 11.7% by 6 months.[15]

At 3-year outcomes, the initial Evolut PRO study patient cohort demonstrated favorable results with no signs of valve deterioration, and very low prevalence of PVL. At 3 years, all-cause mortality was 25.8% (cardiovascular mortality, 16.5%) and the disabling stroke rate was 10.7%. There were no cases of repeat valve intervention, endocarditis, or coronary obstruction. Valve thrombosis was identified in 1 patient 2 years postprocedure and was treated medically. Hemodynamics at 3 years included a mean gradient of 7.2 ± 4.5 mm Hg, an EOA of 2.0 ± 0.5 cm^2, and 88.2% of patients had no or trace PVL. The remaining patients had mild PVL only.[16]

Portico

The Portico (**Fig. 4**) (Abbott, Abbott Park, IL, USA) is a self-expanding valve made of a self-expanding nitinol stent frame, bovine pericardial leaflets, and a porcine pericardial sealing cuff. It can be fully recaptured, repositioned, and retrieved. The valve is deployed at the aortic intra-annular level.[17,18] The transfemoral delivery catheter has an 18F capsule containing the compressed valve and a 12F shaft. The system releases the annular end first. Rapid ventricular pacing is not mandatory during deployment. Loaded onto an 18F delivery system are 23- and 25-mm valves, whereas 27- and 29-mm valves are loaded onto a 19F delivery system.

Initial experience with the transfemoral 23-mm Portico device led to CE mark approval in Europe (November 2012).

Makkar and colleagues[19] 2020 reported results of a randomized, controlled, noninferiority (POR-TICO IDE) trial of the Portico THV system in high- and extreme-risk patients with severe symptomatic AS against other commercially available valves. For the primary safety endpoint at 30 days, the event rate was higher in the Portico valve group than in the commercial valve group. At 1 and 2 years, the rates of the primary efficacy endpoint of nonhierarchical composite of all-cause mortality or disabling stroke were similar between groups.

Fontana and colleagues[20] evaluated the safety profile of the Portico valve with a next-generation low-profile delivery system (FlexNav DS), which includes a hydrophilic-coated sheath (14F and 15F equivalent for 23- or 25-mm and 27- or 29-mm Portico valves, respectively) to facilitate deployment in ≥5-mm-diameter vessels. One hundred eighty high- and extreme-risk patients from a FlexNav DS arm of the PORTICO US IDE trial and the Flex Nav EU CE mark study were assessed for Valve Academic Research Consortium-2 (VARC-2) major complications at 30 days. The rate of major vascular complications was 5.0%, with 4.4% of complications adjudicated as access site-related. Death (0.6%) and disabling stroke (1.1%) were rare. The rate of new permanent pacemaker implantation was 15.4%. Echocardiography revealed a mean gradient of 7.1 ± 3.2 mm Hg, mean valve area of 1.77 ± 0.41 cm^2, no severe paravalvular leak, and a 4.1% rate of moderate paravalvular leak at 30 days.

Myval

The Myval valve (Meril Life Sciences Pvt. Ltd, Chala, Vapi, Gujarat, India) is a balloon-expandable heart valve made of a nickel cobalt alloy frame and bovine pericardium leaflets. The valve has a unique hybrid honeycomb cell design, with open cells on the upper half to ensure the easy access of the coronary ostia and closed cells on the lower half for high radial strength. Upon crimping, this valve design presents a visible "dark and light" band pattern under fluoroscopy. Alternating V-shaped hinges on a hexagonal frame fold, and vertical connectors give Myval THV a unique "Zebra Crossing" appearance under fluoroscopy to help ensure accurate valve positioning and deployment.

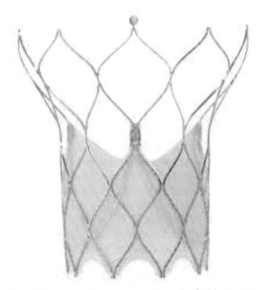

Fig. 4. Portico. (Portico is a trademark of Abbott or its related companies. Reproduced with permission of Abbott, © 2021. All rights reserved.)

The valve comes with an internal PET sealing cuff and an external PET buffing to minimize paravalvular leaks. This CE-approved valve comes in 7 sizes from 20 mm to 29 mm. Currently, Myval THV comes in 9 sizes (20 mm–32 mm diameter). The Myval is directly crimped on a stent balloon delivery system, with a stopper at either end to prevent valve movement and migration during delivery. There is no sheath over the valve; hence, the valve delivery system behaves like a direct stent implantation system without the need for multiple steps and adjustment. The Myval is delivered through a dedicated 14F introducer sheath via a transfemoral approach.

The MyVal-1 study is a first-in-human, prospective, multicenter, single-arm, open-label study of the Myval system for the treatment of severe symptomatic native aortic valve stenosis (n = 30). At 12 months, the study met its primary endpoint for safety and effectiveness with 100% freedom from device-related mortality at 1 year. The investigators reported 100% procedural success, no major adverse events, and marked improvement from baseline to 12 months in quality-of-life scores. There were no new pacemaker implantations, no strokes, and no paravalvular leaks observed in the trial patients.[21] Myval THV was granted CE approval in Europe (May 2019) but is not approved in France and Germany. This device is not approved for sale in the United States.

ACURATE neo2

This self-expanding, supra-annular transcatheter aortic valve design (Boston Scientific, Marlborough, MA, USA) is built on the ACURATE neo platform (Fig. 5) with improved sealing technology that is designed to conform to irregular calcified anatomy and thus further reduce the occurrence of paravalvular leak. Three available sizes (23 mm–27 mm) allow treatment of native annulus diameters from 21 mm to 27 mm. The valve is delivered via a 14F iSLEEVE expandable introducer transfemoral system and is deployed in a "top-down" mechanism that further supports stable placement. In comparison to the previous generation device, the ACURATE neo2 valve system also has an expanded indication in Europe for patients with aortic stenosis, with no specified age or risk level.

Möllmann and colleagues[22] presented a single-arm, prospective, multicenter, non-randomized study at a PCR meeting in London, which was a first investigation of the ACURATE neo2 valve system in patients with severe aortic stenosis (n = 120). Procedural success was achieved in 97.5% of patients with 2 cases of

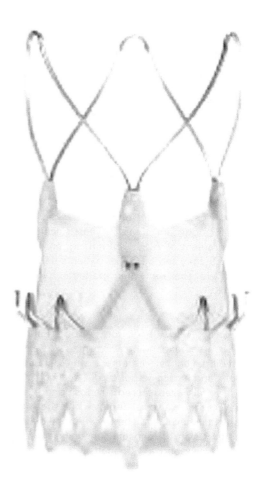

Fig. 5. ACURATE neo2. (©2021 Boston Scientific Corporation or its affiliates. All rights reserved.)

valve-in-valve deployment and 1 conversion to surgery. The rate of all-cause mortality at 30 days was 3.3% (n = 4), and 1.7% (n = 2) experienced a disabling stroke. Major vascular complications occurred in 3.3% (n = 4) and life-threatening/disabling bleeding occurred in 5.0% (n = 6). There were no repeat procedures for valve-related dysfunction. The overall rate of permanent pacemaker implantation was 15.0% (18/120) of patients. Mean aortic valve gradient improved to 9.2 ± 3.7 mm Hg at discharge and was 7.9 ± 3.2 mm Hg at 30 days. No patients were assessed as having severe PVL at 30 days. PVL was described as no/trace (34.0%), mild (60.2%), or moderate (2.9%). The 1-year follow-up to this cohort showed sustained safety and performance of the ACURATE neo2 valve with safety outcomes comparable to those observed in other TAVR studies in similar patient populations.

The ACURATE neo2 Aortic Valve System received CE mark approval in April 2020, and in the United States is undergoing ongoing investigation through the ACURATE IDE clinical trial (NCT03735667).

The SCOPE I trial directly compared TAVR platforms. This study compared TAVR with the self-expanding ACURATE neo valve (n = 372) to the balloon-expandable Sapien 3 valve (n = 367) with the goal of comparing the safety and efficacy among patients with severe aortic stenosis undergoing transfemoral TAVR. The results indicated that TAVR with the self-expanding ACURATE neo valve did not meet criteria for noninferiority compared with the balloon-expandable Sapien 3 valve. TAVR with Sapien 3 was superior for the composite 30-day endpoint, driven primarily by lower rates of acute kidney injury, paravalvular regurgitation, and vascular complications. The ACURATE neo valve had lower transvalvular gradients and a larger EOA.[23]

ALLEGRA

The ALLEGRA valve (Fig. 6) (New Valve Technology, Muri, Switzerland) consists of a self-expanding nitinol stent frame and a sewn-in supra-annular bovine pericardial heart valve for the treatment of severe aortic stenosis. The stent frame has a closed cell, diamond-shaped configuration. The variable cell size distribution allows for better coronary perfusion and easier late coronary guide catheter access. Six radiopaque gold markers are incorporated into the stent frame. These markers indicate the distal part of the semilunar valve to facilitate correct valve positioning. A 12-mm bovine pericardial sealing skirt reduces the risk of significant PVL. The ALLEGRA valve is available in 3 sizes (23, 27, and 31 mm), covering aortic annulus diameter sizes from 19 to 29 mm. The delivery system has an 18F cartridge and a 15F catheter shaft. The prosthesis is released in a 3-step deployment mechanism. Novel implantation technology is designed to facilitate positioning of the ALLEGRA valve and prevent interference with the left ventricular (LV) outflow tract.[24]

First-in-human experience was demonstrated by Wenaweser and colleagues[25] in 2016 in 21 patients with symptomatic severe AS using the ALLEGRA bioprosthesis. Procedural and device success was achieved in 95.2% and 85.7%, respectively. Echocardiographic assessment at discharge showed favorable hemodynamic results with a reduction of the mean transvalvular aortic gradient from 48.0 ± 21 mm Hg to 8.9 ± 3 mm Hg. Trace or less AR was recorded

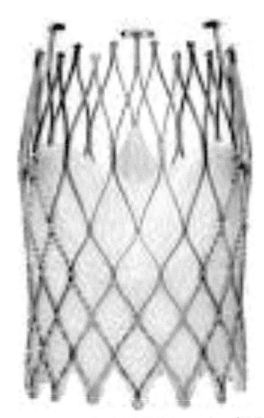

Fig. 6. Allegra valve. (ALLEGRA™ is a product of NVT AG. © 2021 Biosensors Intl. Group. All rights reserved. Used with permission.)

in 90.5% of patients. Permanent pacemaker implantation was required in 23.8% of patients within the first 30 days of follow-up. The ALLEGRA bioprosthesis was able to achieve favorable hemodynamic results and effectively alleviate symptoms at 30-day follow-up. The ALLEGRA THV was CE mark approved in March 2017.

Jagielak and colleagues[24] reported the NAUTILUS study (n = 26) single-arm clinical study designed to assess short-term safety and performance of the ALLEGRA bioprosthesis in high-risk patients with severe AS. The bioprosthesis was successfully implanted in 96% of the cases (n = 25). Echocardiographic assessment confirmed good hemodynamic profile after implantation of the ALLEGRA bioprosthesis. Complications included cardiac tamponade (4%, n = 1) and the need for permanent pacemaker implantation (8%, n = 2). The analysis of procedural aspects showed a short learning effect related to the precise placement of the valve. A significant improvement in clinical symptoms was observed, and no patients died in-hospital or within 30 days of discharge.

Table 1
Innovations in transcatheter heart valve. Above, the latest generation of transcatheter heart valves.

Valve	Intended Use	Deployment Method	Innovation
SAPIEN 3 Ultra	Aortic stenosis	Balloon expandable	Higher sealing "skirt" decreases PVL
Jena Valve	Aortic insufficiency	Self-expanding	First dedicated device for Aortic Insufficiency
Evolut PRO+	Aortic stenosis	Self-expanding	External tissue wrap allows for treatment of larger anatomies
Portico	Aortic stenosis	Self-expanding	Fully recapturable, repositionable, and retrievable
Myval	Aortic stenosis	Balloon expandable	Hybrid honeycomb cell design to allow for easy coronary access
ACURAT neo2	Aortic stenosis	Self-expanding	Improved sealing technology to conform to irregular annular calcium
ALLEGRA	Aortic stenosis	Self-expanding	Variable cell size distribution for enhanced coronary access

Cuevas and colleagues[26] described a European multicenter experience with the ALLEGRA valve in 59 patients with mean Society of Thoracic Surgeons Predicted Risk of Mortality (STS PROM) score of 5.2. The device success was 95%, and 30-day mortality was 1.7%. No stroke or major/life-threatening bleeding occurred. The pacemaker implantation rate was 13.5% at 30 days. Hemodynamic outcomes showed a mean gradient of 7.2 ± 3.5 mm Hg with an EOA of 2.06 ± 0.3 cm^2. Valve performance remained stable at 30 days. More than mild paravalvular leak was present in 5.1% of patients before discharge and 3.4% at 30 days (Table 1).

TRANSCATHETER AORTIC VALVE REPLACEMENT IN BICUSPID VALVES
Introduction
Patients with bicuspid aortic valves account for up to 50% of patients requiring AVR in younger populations but were largely excluded from all pivotal TAVR trials. More recent data, however, suggest that TAVR is safe and feasible in carefully selected bicuspid valves, but the procedure remains challenging from an anatomic and clinical standpoint. The heavily calcified nature of bicuspid stenosis may limit full THV expansion leading to eccentric deployment and PVL. Bicuspid patients are younger on average and may require more than 1 lifetime AVR. Concerns regarding longer-term safety and durability of TAVR thereby impact patient selection decisions. In addition, many of these patients present with concomitant aortopathy that requires surgery.[27–30]

Balloon-Expandable Valves
A retrospective study of 81,822 consecutive patients with AS propensity matched 2691 pairs of patients with bicuspid and tricuspid AS undergoing TAVR with a balloon-expandable valve. Median patient age was 74 years (interquartile range, 66–81), and STS-PROM score was 4.9%. Important findings of the study included the following:

1. At 30 days, all-cause mortality was not significantly different between bicuspid and tricuspid patients undergoing TAVR (2.6% vs 2.5%; hazard ratio: 1.04).
2. At 30 days, the risk of stroke was significantly higher for patients with bicuspid aortic stenosis (2.5% bicuspid AS vs 1.6% tricuspid AS).
3. At 1 year, there was no difference in stroke rate between groups.
4. The risk of procedural complications requiring open heart surgery was higher in patients with bicuspid aortic stenosis (0.9% vs 0.4%).
5. There was no difference in moderate or severe PVL.

These data support the use of TAVR with a balloon-expandable valve in patients with appropriate anatomy.[28] Further randomized data with a surgical comparator arm and long-term durability evaluation are warranted.

Self-Expanding Valves

The Low-Risk Bicuspid Study is the first prospective, single-arm, multicenter study of TAVR using a self-expanding valve (Evolut R/Pro, Medtronic, Gallway, Ireland) in patients with severe bicuspid AS and low surgical risk. One hundred fifty patients met the inclusion criteria for the study and underwent TAVR if anatomy was deemed favorable (mean age, 70.3 years; mean STS-PROM, 1.4%). Of patients, 90.7% had Sievers type 1 valves.

Important exclusion criteria were the following:

1. Patients younger than 60 years old
2. Patients with an ascending aorta diameter greater than 4.5 cm
3. Aortopathy requiring surgery
4. Prohibitive calcification in the LV outflow tract

At 30 days, there was 1 death and 1 disabling stroke. Of note, 15% of patients required a pacemaker following TAVR. Valve hemodynamics were improved in treated patients, and no patients experienced greater than mild aortic insufficiency. These data support the role of TAVR in patients with bicuspid AS. Despite these favorable results, concerns of long-term durability and optimal valve implantation strategies require further study to optimize outcomes.[27]

NEW APPROACHES TO PACING

Minimalist approaches to TAVR have decreased resource utilization and procedure time. Despite this, there has been little innovation in approaches to rapid ventricular pacing. Traditionally, a temporary transcutaneous pacemaker has been placed in the right ventricle. The EASY TAVR[31] trial prospectively assessed pacing using the LV stiff guidewire over which the transcatheter valve is delivered. To facilitate pacing, the cathode of an external pacemaker was attached to the distal end of the guidewire using a crocodile clip, and the anode, a second crocodile clip, was attached to the incised skin site. Important findings from the study are as follows:

1. Mean procedure duration was significantly shorter in patients undergoing LV stimulation (8.4 ± 16.9 minutes vs 55.6 ± 26.9 minutes; $P = .0013$).
2. Effective stimulation was similar between groups (84.9% LV vs 87.1% right ventricular, $P = .60$).
3. 100% of patients in the LV stimulation group underwent successful TAVR.

4. Cost was significantly lower in patients undergoing LV stimulation (€18,807 ± €1318 vs €19,437 ± €2318; $P = .001$).

The Wattson wire is a dedicated guidewire for THV delivery that provides both device delivery support and bipolar pacing, which has received 510k clearance.[32]

UNILATERAL TRANSCATHETER AORTIC VALVE REPLACEMENT ACCESS

Traditionally, transfemoral TAVR has been performed by placing the TAVR delivery system in 1 femoral artery and a second arterial sheath in the contralateral femoral artery (to perform aortic root angiography). Although radial access is an alternate approach to the contralateral femoral artery, it may preclude placement of cerebral embolic protection (CEP). To overcome this, a unilateral access strategy was developed and studied.

Using standard technique, a micropuncture access set (Cook Medical, Bloomington, IN, USA) was used to obtain femoral access. Following placement of an 8F sheath in the femoral artery, a 5F sheath was placed in the inferior aspect of the common femoral artery at least 2 cm below the 8F sheath. The femoral vein is accessed using the modified Seldinger technique for placement of a transvenous pacemaker. In cases of vascular injury, the inferior site was used to perform repair. Hemostasis was achieved using manual pressure at the inferior access site.

This technique was retrospectively compared with bilateral femoral access in 1208 patients (201 unilateral access and 1007 bilateral access). Over a 3-year period, peripheral vascular complications were similar between groups (10.0% bilateral access and 8.6% unilateral access; $P = .543$).[33]

NEW VALVE DEPLOYMENT TECHNIQUES AND FUTURE DIRECTIONS

Cusp-Overlap Technique

Permanent pacemaker implantation following TAVR is an independent risk factor for mortality. Mechanistically, heart block occurs by interaction between the THV and the membranous interventricular septum. Pacemaker implantation rates are historically higher following implantation of a self-expanding valve compared with a balloon-expandable valve.

The cusp-overlap technique is a modified deployment approach for TAVR that attempts to optimize deployment height, minimize interaction with the conduction system, and enable future coronary access.

Fluoroscopically, the right and left coronary cusps are overlapped, isolating the noncoronary cusp (typically in the right anterior oblique imaging plane). This removes parallax and allows clear depth perception and understanding of anatomic relationships to the conduction system. Important principles during valve deployment are to start with a higher valve position, allow the valve to naturally descend during deployment, and use rapid pacing to allow precise deployment of the THV during annular contact and final release.[34] This technique is currently being prospectively studied in the Optimize-PRO registry (NCT04091048).

NEW VASCULAR CLOSURE DEVICES
MANTA Device

Vascular complications owing to large-bore access (14 French to 24 French) are not infrequent and associated with increased morbidity and mortality following TAVR.[35] Contemporary registry data suggest major vascular complication rates of around 2% to 4%.[36] VCD are commonly used to achieve hemostasis following femoral access as an alternative to surgical closure and associated with increased patient comfort, reduced procedure duration, and reduced hospital length of stay.[37] Percutaneous suture-based closure with Perclose ProGlide or Prostar (Abbott Vascular, Abbott Park, IL, USA) is currently most commonly used for large-bore transcatheter access closure.[36,38] The first commercially available, dedicated large-bore percutaneous closure device, the MANTA VCD (Fig. 7) (Teleflex, Wayne, PA, USA), is a collagen-based device designed to close large-bore arteriotomies with outer diameters from 12 French to 25 French.[38] The device is available in 14 French and 18 French. The 14 French is indicated for closure of access sites of 10F to 14F sheaths with maximum diameter of

18 French, and the 18F device is indicated for closure of 15F to 20F sheaths with maximum outer diameter of 25 French.[36] The MANTA device should be avoided with anatomic features such as posterior wall calcification and femoral artery diameter less than 5 mm. The collagen plug is resorbed in several months with a radiopaque marker left in situ. A limitation of the MANTA device is that once deployment is complete, additional devices cannot be deployed in cases of device failure and would then necessitate covered stent or surgical intervention.[36]

The SAFE MANTA IDE study was a prospective, single-arm, multicenter investigation of 263 patients from 20 sites in North America, designed to evaluate the safety and efficacy of the MANTA VCD. Technical success was achieved in 257 (97.7%) patients. In the VARC-2, major vascular complications occurred in 11 (4.2%) cases: 4 (1.5%) received covered stent, 3 (1.1%) had access site bleeding, 2 (0.8%) underwent surgical repair, and 2 (0.8%) underwent balloon inflation. Overall, this study showed safety and efficacy of the MANTA percutaneous VCD in large-bore arteriotomies in patients who underwent TAVR, percutaneous endovascular abdominal aortic aneurysm repair, and thoracic endovascular aortic aneurysm repair.[38] The FDA approved the use of the MANTA device for closure of large-bore arteriotomies in February 2019 following this study. A limitation of this study however was the nonrandomized, single-arm design without comparison to other available VCDs.

Recently, Van Wiechen and colleagues[39] published results of the MASH (MANTA vs Suture-based vascular closure after Transcatheter aortic valve replacement) trial, a pilot RCT of 210 patients comparing MANTA versus 2 ProGlide devices for access site closure following TAVR within 2 European centers. There was no significant difference in access site–related vascular complications between the MANTA versus Pro-Glide groups (10% vs 4%; P = .16) or access

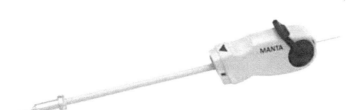

Fig. 7. Manta device. (*Image courtesy of* Teleflex Incorporated. © 2021 Teleflex Incorporated. All rights reserved.)

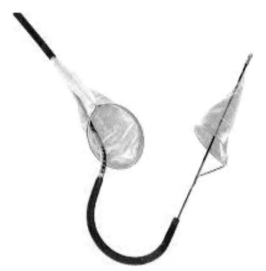

Fig. 8. Sentinel device. (©2021 Boston Scientific Corporation or its affiliates. All rights reserved.)

site bleeding (9% vs 6%; $P = .57$). Bailout in the MANTA group involved covered stents or surgery and additional closure devices in the ProGlide group. This was a small study with a limited number of events, and therefore, further large multicenter RCT with cost-effective analysis are needed to compare collagen-based MANTA VCD versus suture-based ProGlide.

CEREBRAL EMBOLIC PROTECTION

Despite advances in technique, equipment, and operator experience, periprocedural stroke occurs in about 2% of patients after TAVR.[40] The mechanism of stroke is likely embolization of calcified debris from atherosclerotic plaque in the aorta and degenerated aortic valves.[41] To minimize risk of stroke, several CEP devices

have been developed, including filters to capture and remove debris and deflectors to divert debris away from the cerebral circulation.

The Sentinel device (Fig. 8) (Boston Scientific) is the only FDA-approved CEP device in the United States.[41] It is a dual-filter capture device in a 6F delivery catheter that is placed in the brachiocephalic and left common carotid arteries via right radial access over a 0.014-in guidewire.[42] The proximal filter (9–15 mm in diameter) is delivered in the brachiocephalic artery, and a distal filter (6.5–10 mm in diameter) is delivered in the left common carotid artery.[43] A large limitation of the device is that the LV artery remains unprotected.

The SENTINEL trial was a prospective, multicenter, single-blind RCT of 363 patients undergoing TAVR and showed that the device captured embolic debris in 99% of patients; however, reduction in new lesion volume on MRI, stroke, or death was not statistically significant compared with controls.

The TriGuard 3 device (Fig. 9) (Keystone Heart) is a deflection device designed to minimize cerebral embolization by deflecting embolic debris away from the cerebral circulation. It is an over-the-wire system that can be delivered via a 6F femoral sheath with a large filter that covers all 3 cerebral aortic arch vessels. The REFLECT II (Randomized Evaluation of TriGuard 3 Cerebral Embolic Protection After Transcatheter Aortic Valve Implantation) trial evaluated the safety and efficacy of the TriGuard 3 CEP device in patients undergoing TAVR. This prospective, multicenter, single-blind RCT of 220 patients met its primary safety endpoint compared with performance goal, however, did not meet its prespecified superiority efficacy endpoint, as the study was terminated early by the sponsor after the FDA recommended enrollment suspension for unblinded safety data

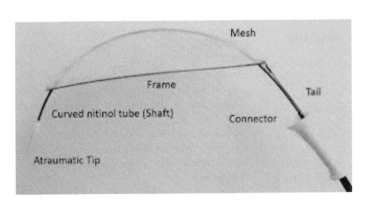

Fig. 9. The TriGuard Device. A dedicated deflection device to minimize cerebral embolization. (Copyright Keystone Heart, A Venus Medtech Company 2021; with permission.)

review.[44] This device is not FDA approved for clinical use at this time, and further large, randomized trials are needed.

There is a paucity of adequately powered RCT showing efficacy of CEP devices and therefore limiting generalized adoption in contemporary practice.[45] The PROTECTED TAVR (Stroke PROTECTion With Sentinel During Transcatheter Aortic Valve Replacement) and BHF PROTECT-TAVR (British Heart Foundation Randomized Trial of Routine Cerebral Embolic Protection in Transcatheter Aortic Valve Implantation) are large studies underway evaluating the efficacy of CEP devices.

CLINICS CARE POINTS

- When evaluating a patient for transcatheter aortic valve replacement, consider new valves with distinct indications.
- When evaluating a patient with a bicuspid aortic valve, perform a computed tomographic scan to assess for transcatheter aortic valve replacement eligibility.
- Consider alternate pacing methods to simplify transcatheter aortic valve replacement implant.

SUMMARY

TAVR has revolutionized the field of AVR. With increasing collaboration from clinicians, researchers, and industry, there has been an explosion in available technology. Continued innovation will not only increase procedural success but also decrease risk. Increased completion will ultimately offer patients the best technology at, it is hoped, a lower price. Despite these advances, long-term durability remains unknown. Further work should be directed to optimizing valve durability, decreasing stroke rates, decreasing pacemaker rates, and facilitating redo TAVR.

DISCLOSURE

C.M. Devireddy: Consultant: Edwards Lifesciences, Medtronic, ReCor Medical, Shockwave Medical.

REFERENCES

1. Carroll JD, Mack MJ, Vemulapalli S, et al. STS-ACC TVT registry of transcatheter aortic valve replacement. J Am Coll Cardiol 2020;76(21):2492–516.

2. Leon MB, Smith CR, Mack M, et al. Transcatheter aortic-valve implantation for aortic stenosis in patients who cannot undergo surgery. N Engl J Med 2010;363(17):1597–607.

3. Mack MJ, Leon MB. Transcatheter aortic-valve replacement in low-risk patients. Reply. N Engl J Med 2019;381(7):684–5.

4. Barbanti M, Costa G. SAPIEN 3 ultra transcatheter aortic valve device: two sides of the moon. JACC Cardiovasc Interv 2020;13(22):2639–41.

5. Francesco S, Caterina G, Tullio P, et al. In-hospital and thirty-day outcomes of the SAPIEN 3 ultra balloon-expandable transcatheter aortic valve: the S3U registry. EuroIntervention 2020;15(14):1240–7.

6. Rheude T, Pellegrini C, Lutz J, et al. Transcatheter aortic valve replacement with balloon-expandable valves: comparison of SAPIEN 3 Ultra versus SAPIEN 3. JACC Cardiovasc Interv 2020;13(22):2631–8.

7. Treede H, Rastan A, Ferrari M, et al. JenaValve. EuroIntervention 2012;8(Suppl Q):Q88–93.

8. Rudolph TK, Baldus S. JenaValve–transfemoral technology. EuroIntervention 2013;9(Suppl):S101–2.

9. Seiffert M, Diemert P, Koschyk D, et al. Transapical implantation of a second-generation transcatheter heart valve in patients with noncalcified aortic regurgitation. JACC Cardiovasc Interv 2013;6(6):590–7.

10. Taramasso M, Pozzoli A, Latib A, et al. New devices for TAVI: technologies and initial clinical experiences. Nat Rev Cardiol 2014;11(3):157–67.

11. Treede H, Mohr FW, Baldus S, et al. Transapical transcatheter aortic valve implantation using the JenaValve system: acute and 30-day results of the multicentre CE-mark study. Eur J Cardiothorac Surg 2012;41(6):e131–8.

12. Silaschi M, Conradi L, Wendler O, et al. The JUPITER registry: one-year outcomes of transapical aortic valve implantation using a second generation transcatheter heart valve for aortic regurgitation. Catheter Cardiovasc Interv 2018;91(7):1345–51.

13. Clawson M. JenaValve Transcatheter Aortic Valve Replacement (TAVR) system designated by FDA as breakthrough device. 2020. Available at: https://www.businesswire.com/news/home/2020 0109005103/en/JenaValve-Transcatheter-Aortic-Valve-Replacement-TAVR-System-Designated-by-FDA-as-Breakthrough-Device. Accessed January 10, 2020.

14. Forrest JK, Mangi AA, Popma JJ, et al. Early outcomes with the evolut PRO repositionable self-expanding transcatheter aortic valve with pericardial wrap. JACC Cardiovasc Interv 2018;11(2):160–8.

15. Williams M. 1-year outcomes with the evolut PRO self-expanding repositionable transcatheter aortic valve with pericardial wrap. JACC 2018;71(11_Supplement).

16. Wyler von Ballmoos MC, Reardon MJ, Williams MR, et al. Three-year outcomes with a contemporary

self-expanding transcatheter valve from the Evolut PRO US Clinical Study. Cardiovasc Revasc Med 2020.

17. Manoharan G, Spence MS, Rodes-Cabau J, et al. St Jude Medical Portico valve. EuroIntervention 2012; 8(Suppl Q):Q97–101.

18. Willson AB, Rodes-Cabau J, Wood DA, et al. Transcatheter aortic valve replacement with the St. Jude Medical Portico valve: first-in-human experience. J Am Coll Cardiol 2012;60(7):581–6.

19. Makkar RR, Cheng W, Waksman R, et al. Self-expanding intra-annular versus commercially available transcatheter heart valves in high and extreme risk patients with severe aortic stenosis (PORTICO IDE): a randomised, controlled, non-inferiority trial. Lancet 2020;396(10252):669–83.

20. Fontana GP, Bedogni F, Groh M, et al. Safety profile of an intra-annular self-expanding transcatheter aortic valve and next-generation low-profile delivery system. JACC Cardiovasc Interv 2020;13(21): 2467–78.

21. Sharma SK, Rao RS, Chandra P, et al. First-in-human evaluation of a novel balloon-expandable transcatheter heart valve in patients with severe symptomatic native aortic stenosis: the MyVal-1 study. EuroIntervention 2020;16(5):421–9.

22. Möllmann H. Transcatheter aortic valve replacement with the ACURATE neo2 valve system:1-year clinical and hemodynamic outcomes. Presented by H. Möllmann at TVT 2019. Chicago (IL), June 13, 2019.

23. Lanz J, Kim W-K, Walther T, et al. Safety and efficacy of a self-expanding versus a balloon-expandable bioprosthesis for transcatheter aortic valve replacement in patients with symptomatic severe aortic stenosis: a randomised non-inferiority trial. The Lancet 2019;394(10209):1619–28.

24. Jagielak D, Stanska A, Klapkowski A, et al. Transfermoral aortic valve implantation using self-expanding New Valve Technology (NVT) Allegra bioprosthesis: a pilot prospective study. Cardiol J 2019.

25. Wenaweser P, Stortecky S, Schutz T, et al. Transcatheter aortic valve implantation with the NVT Allegra transcatheter heart valve system: first-in-human experience with a novel self-expanding transcatheter heart valve. EuroIntervention 2016;12(1):71–7.

26. Cuevas O, Moreno R, Pascual-Tejerina V, et al. The Allegra transcatheter heart valve: European multicentre experience with a novel self-expanding transcatheter aortic valve. EuroIntervention 2019; 15(1):71–3.

27. Forrest JK, Kaple RK, Ramlawi B, et al. Transcatheter aortic valve replacement in bicuspid versus tricuspid aortic valves from the STS/ACC TVT Registry. JACC Cardiovasc Interv 2020;13(15):1749–59.

28. Makkar RR, Yoon SH, Leon MB, et al. Association between transcatheter aortic valve replacement for bicuspid vs tricuspid aortic stenosis and mortality or stroke. Jama 2019;321(22):2193–202.

29. Yoon SH, Bleiziffer S, De Backer O, et al. Outcomes in transcatheter aortic valve replacement for bicuspid versus tricuspid aortic valve stenosis. J Am Coll Cardiol 2017;69(21):2579–89.

30. Yoon SH, Kim WK, Dhoble A, et al. Bicuspid aortic valve morphology and outcomes after transcatheter aortic valve replacement. J Am Coll Cardiol 2020;76(9):1018–30.

31. Faurie B, Souteyrand G, Staat P, et al. Left ventricular rapid pacing via the valve delivery guidewire in transcatheter aortic valve replacement. (1876-7605 (Electronic)).

32. Hensey MA-O, Sathananthan JA-O, Alkhodair A, et al. Single-center prospective study examining use of the Wattson temporary pacing guidewire for transcatheter aortic valve replacement. (1522-726X (Electronic)).

33. Khubber S, Bazarbashi N, Mohananey D, et al. Unilateral Access Is Safe and Facilitates Peripheral Bailout During Transfemoral-Approach Transcatheter Aortic Valve Replacement. (1876-7605 (Electronic)).

34. Ben-Shoshan J, Alosaimi H, Lauzier PT, et al. Double S-Curve Versus Cusp-Overlap Technique: Defining the Optimal Fluoroscopic Projection for TAVR With a Self-Expanding Device. (1876-7605 (Electronic)).

35. Genereux P, Webb JG, Svensson LG, et al. Vascular complications after transcatheter aortic valve replacement: insights from the PARTNER (Placement of AoRTic TraNscathetER Valve) trial. J Am Coll Cardiol 2012;60(12):1043–52.

36. Abbott JD, Bavishi C. In search of an ideal vascular closure device for transcatheter aortic valve replacement. JACC Cardiovasc Interv 2021;14(2):158–60.

37. Tarantini G. MANTA dedicated large-bore vessel closure device. Circ Cardiovasc Interv 2019;12(7): e008203.

38. Wood DA, Krajcer Z, Sathananthan J, et al. Pivotal clinical study to evaluate the safety and effectiveness of the MANTA percutaneous vascular closure device. Circ Cardiovasc Interv 2019;12(7):e007258.

39. van Wiechen MP, Tchetche D, Ooms JF, et al. Suture- or plug-based large-bore arteriotomy closure: a pilot randomized controlled trial. JACC Cardiovasc Interv 2021;14(2):149–57.

40. Butala NM, Makkar R, Secemsky EA, et al. Cerebral embolic protection and outcomes of transcatheter aortic valve replacement: results from the TVT registry. Circulation 2021.

41. Khera R, Girotra S. Cerebral embolic protection devices in transcatheter aortic valve replacement-effective in stroke prevention? JAMA Intern Med 2020;180(5):785–6.

42. Kapadia SR, Kodali S, Makkar R, et al. Protection against cerebral embolism during transcatheter aortic valve replacement. J Am Coll Cardiol 2017; 69(4):367–77.

43. Cubero-Gallego H, Pascual I, Rozado J, et al. Cerebral protection devices for transcatheter aortic valve replacement. Ann Transl Med 2019;7(20):584.

44. Nazif TM, Moses J, Sharma R, et al. Randomized evaluation of TriGuard 3 cerebral embolic protection after transcatheter aortic valve replacement: REFLECT II. JACC Cardiovasc Interv 2021;14(5):515–27.

45. Van Mieghem NM, Daemen J. Reflections on the fate of cerebral embolic protection devices with TAVR: the REFLECT II trial. JACC Cardiovasc Interv 2021;14(5):528–30.

Moving?

Make sure your subscription moves with you!

To notify us of your new address, find your **Clinics Account Number** (located on your mailing label above your name), and contact customer service at:

Email: journalscustomerservice-usa@elsevier.com

800-654-2452 (subscribers in the U.S. & Canada)
314-447-8871 (subscribers outside of the U.S. & Canada)

Fax number: 314-447-8029

Elsevier Health Sciences Division
Subscription Customer Service
3251 Riverport Lane
Maryland Heights, MO 63043

*To ensure uninterrupted delivery of your subscription, please notify us at least 4 weeks in advance of move.